LUMBAR SPINAL STENOSIS

LUMBAR SPINAL STENOSIS

Edited by

Robert Gunzburg, M.D., Ph.D.
Senior Consultant
Department of Orthopedics
Centenary Clinic
Antwerp, Belgium

Marek Szpalski, M.D.
Senior Consultant and Associate Professor
Department of Orthopedics
Centre Hospitalier Molière Longchamp,
Teaching Hospital of the Free University of Brussels
Brussels, Belgium

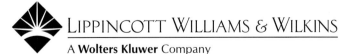 LIPPINCOTT WILLIAMS & WILKINS
A **Wolters Kluwer** Company
Philadelphia • Baltimore • New York • London
Buenos Aires • Hong Kong • Sydney • Tokyo

Acquisitions Editor: Robert Hurley
Associate Developmental Editor: Stephanie Harris
Managing Editor: Susan Rhyner
Production Editor: Deirdre Marino-Vasquez
Manufacturing Manager: Tim Reynolds
Cover Designer: Patricia Gast
Compositor: Maryland Composition
Printer: Maple Press

© **2000 by LIPPINCOTT WILLIAMS & WILKINS**
227 East Washington Square
Philadelphia, PA 19106-3780 USA
LWW.com

Printed in the USA

Library of Congress Cataloging-in-Publication Data

Lumbar spinal stenosis / [edited by] Robert Gunzburg, Marek Szpalski
    p. cm
    Includes index.
    ISBN 0-7817-2380-9
      1. Spinal canal—Stenosis. 2. Spinal canal—Stenosis—Surgery. 3. Lumbar
vertebrae—Surgery. I. Gunzburg, Robert, II. Szpalski, Marek.
    [DNLM: 1. Spinal Stenosis—diagnosis. 2. Lumbar Vertebrae—physiopathology.
3. Spinal Stenosis—therapy. WE 725 L9565 1999]
    RD771.S74.L86 1999   99-044476

Contents

Section VII. Economic and Ethical Considerations in the Management of Spinal Stenosis

Contributing Authors

N. Arafati, Ph.D.   *Service d'Anatomie, Faculte de Medecine Pitie-Salpetriere, 105 Boulevard de L'Hôpital, 75013 Paris, France*

David Attia, M.D.   *Département de Chirurgie du Rachis, Clinique Kennedy, Avenue JF Kennedy, 26200 Montelimar, France*

Christian Bacq, M.D.   *Department of Medical Imaging, Centre Hospitalier Moliére-Longchamp, 142 Rue Marconi, 1190 Brussels, Belgium*

Erik J. Barbaix, M.D.   *Department of Experimental Anatomy, Vrije Universiteit Brussel, Laarbeeklaan 103, 1090 Brussels, Belgium*

Michel Benoist, M.D.   *Consultant Rheumatologist of Paris Hospitals, University of Paris VII, 75116 Paris, France*

Robert S. Biscup, M.D.   *Department of Orthopedic Surgery, Cleveland Clinic Foundation, 9500 Euclid Avenue, Cleveland, Ohio 44195*

Jacques Boulot, M.D.   *Clinique Du Parc, 105 Rue Achille Viadieu, 31400 Toulousse, France*

Jan P. Clarijs, M.D.   *Head, Department of Experimental Anatomy, Vrije Universiteit Brussel, Laarbeeklaan 103, 1090 Brussels, Belgium*

Alvin H. Crawford, M.D., F.A.C.S.   *Director, Pediatric Orthopedics, Children's Hospital, 3333 Burnet Avenue, Cincinnati, Ohio 45229; Professor of Pediatrics, Department of Orthopedics, University of Cincinnati Medical Center, Cincinnati, Ohio 45229*

Henry V. Crock, M.D., F.R.C.S., F.R.A.C.S.   *Consultant Spinal Surgeon, Spinal Disorders Unit, Cromwell Hospital, 2A Pennant Mews, London W8 5JN, United Kingdom*

M. Carmel Crock   *Spinal Disorders Unit, Cromwell Hospital, 2A Pennant Mews, London W8 5JN, United Kingdom*

Phillip de Muelenaere, M.D.   *Orthopedic Surgeon, Muelmed Hospital, Suite 304, Pretorius Str. 577, Arcadia, South Africa 0083*

Patrick J. Depraetere, M.D.   *Heilig-Hartziekenhuis, Gebouw Wilgenstraat (nr.2), 8800 Roeselare, Belgium*

Jean-Pierre Devogelaer, M.D.   *Chief, Department of Rheumatology, Saint-Luc University Hospital, 10 Ave Hippocrate, 1200 Brussels, Belgium; Director, Arthritis Unit UCL5390, Universite Catholique de Louvain in Brussels, Ave Mounier 53, 1200 Brussels, Belgium*

Peter Donceel, M.D., Ph.D. *Department of Occupational and Insurance Medicine, School of Public Health, Katholieke Universiteit Leuven, Kapucinjnenvoer 35/5, 3000 Leuven, Belgium; Chief Medical Advisor, Department of Medical Direction, Christian Sickness Funds, Haachtsesteenweg 579-Postbus 40, 1031 Brussels, Belgium*

Vincent Druez, M.D. *Av. Frans Guillaume 31, Bte 12, 1140 Evere, France*

Marc Du Bois, M.D. *Research Fellow, Department of Occupational and Insurance Medicine, School of Public Health, Katholieke Universiteit Leuven, Kapucinjnenvoer 35/5, 3000 Leuven, Belgium; Medical Advisor, Department of Medical Direction, Christian Sickness Funds, Haachtsesteenweg 579-Postbus 40, 1031 Brussels, Belgium*

Guillaume du Toit, M.D. *Orthopedic Spine Surgeon, 107 Constantiaberg Medi-Clinic, Burnham Road, Plumstead, Cape Town, South Africa 7800*

Jiri Dvorak, M.D. *Abteilung für Neurologie/Spine Unit, Schulthess Clinic, Lengghalde 2, 8008 Zürich, Switzerland*

Jose A. Fernandez de Valderrama, M.D. *Specialist, Orthopedic Surgery and Trauma, General Rodrigo 17, 28003 Madrid, Spain; Former Associate Professor, Surgical Pathology, Universidad Complutense, Madrid, Spain; Former Chief of Orthopedics, Hospital Central Cruz Roja, Madrid, Spain*

Gordon F. G. Findlay, M.D., M.B.ChB., F.R.C.S. *Consultant Neurosurgeon, Walton Centre for Neurology and Neurosurgery, NHS Trust, Lower Lane, Liverpool L9 7LJ, United Kingdom*

Bruce E. Fredrickson, M.D. *Professor of Orthopedic and Neurologic Surgery, Department of Orthopedic Surgery, SUNY Health Science Center—Syracuse, 705 East Adams Street, Syracuse, New York 13202*

J.N.A. Gibson, M.D., F.R.C.S. Orth. *Senior Lecturer, Department of Orthopedic Surgery, The University of Edinburgh, Edinburgh EH10 7ED, United Kingdom; Consultant Spinal Surgeon, Orthopedic Surgery, Princess Margaret Rose Orthopedic Hospital, Edinburgh EH10 7ED, United Kingdom*

M. Gorin, M.D. *Clinique Radiologique, 3 Rue Jules Lefevre, 75009 Paris, France*

Anukul Goswani, M.D. *Surgeon and Clinical Research Fellow, Department of Endoscopic Spinal Surgery, The Spinal Foundation, Arbury Consulting Centre, Manchester Road, Rochdale OL11 4LX, United Kingdom*

Pierre Guigui, M.D. *Department of Orthopedic Surgery, Hôpital Beaujon, 100 Boulevard du General Leclere, 92110 Clichy, France*

Robert Gunzburg, M.D., Ph.D. *Senior Consultant, Department of Orthopedics, Centenary Clinic, Harroniestraat 68, 2018 Antwerp, Belgium*

Philippe Gutwirth, M.D. *Surgeon, Department of Vascular Surgery, Antwerp Blood Vessel Centre, Centenary Clinic, 2018 Antwerp, Belgium*

Olle Hägg, M.D. *Department of Orthopaedics, Sahlgrenska University Hospital, Göteborg University, SE-41345, Göteborg, Sweden*

S. Hansen, M.D. *Service de Chirurgie Orthopédique, Hôpital Pitie-Salpetriere, 83 Boulevard de L'Hôpital, 75013 Paris, France*

Jörg Herdmann, M.D. *Abteilung für Neurochirurgie, Heinrich Heine Universität, D-40001 Düsseldorf, Germany*

William C. Hutton, D.Sc. *Professor, Department of Orthopedics, Emory University, 2165 North Decatur Road, Atlanta, Georgia 30033*

Malcolm I.V. Jayson, M.D. *Professor, Department of Rheumatology, University of Manchester, Oxford Road, Manchester M13 9PT, United Kingdom; Professor of Rheumatology, Rheumatic Diseases Centre, Hope Hospital, Salford M5 8HD, United Kingdom*

Martin T.N. Knight, M.D. *The Spinal Foundation, Arbury Consulting Centre, Manchester Road, Rochdale OL11 4LX, United Kingdom*

H. Knorth, M.D. *Orthopaedic University Clinic, St. Josef Hospital, Gudrunstr. 56, D-44791 Bochum, Germany*

Stephen D. Kuslich, M.D. *Spinology, Inc., 1815 Northwestern Avenue, Stillwater, Minnesota 55082*

C.G. Laudet, M.D. *Service d'Anatomie, Faculté Pitie-Salpetriere, Hôpital Pitie-Salpetriere, 83 Boulevard de L'Hôpital, 75013 Paris, France*

J.-Y. Lazennec, M.D. *Service de Chirurgie Orthopédique, Hôpital Pitie-Salpetriere, 83 Boulevard de L'Hôpital, 75013 Paris, France*

Baudouin Maldague, M.D. *Department of Radiology, Saint-Luc University Hospital, Avenue Hippocrate 10, 1200 Brussels, Belgium*

John A. Malko, Ph.D. *Associate Professor, Department of Radiology, Emory University School of Medicine, Atlanta, Georgia 30322; MRI Physicist, Department of Radiology, Grady Memorial Hospital, 56 Butler Street, Atlanta, Georgia 30335*

L. Maurs, M.D. *Federation de Neurologie, Hôpital Pitie-Salpetriere, 83 Boulevard de L'Hôpital, 75013 Paris, France*

Christian Melot, M.D., Ph.D. *Professor of Biostatistics, Faculty of Medicine, Free University of Brussels, Lennik Road 808, 1070 Brussels, Belgium; Associate Professor of Medicine, Intensive Care Department, Erasme University Hospital, Lennik Road 808, 1070 Brussels, Belgium*

Robert C. Mulholland, M.D. *Special Professor, Department of Orthopedics and Trauma, University Hospital Nottingham, University Park, Nottingham NG7 2RD, United Kingdom; Consultant Surgeon, Spinal Disorders Unit, University Hospital, Queens Medical Center, Nottingham NG7 2RD, United Kingdom*

Everard Munting, M.D., Ph.D. *Professor, Department of Surgery, Universite Catholique de Louvain, 10 Avenue Hippocrate, 1200 Brussels, Belgium; Department of Surgery, Cliniques Universitaires Saint Luc, Avenue Hippocrate 10, 1200 Brussels, Belgium*

Andreas Neekritz *Annastift, Department III, Hannover 30625, Germany*

Margareta Nordin, Dr. Sci. *Director, Occupational and Industrial Orthopedic Center, Hospital for Joint Diseases, Mount Sinai/New York University Medical Center, 63 Downing Street, New York, New York 10014*

Janos T. Patko, M.D., *The Spinal Foundation, Arbury Consulting Centre, Manchester Road, Rochdale OL11 4LX, United Kingdom*

Philippe Peetrons, M.D. *Professor of Radiology, Department of Forensic and Occupational Medicine, University of Brussels, Lennick Road 808, 1070 Brussels, Belgium; Chief, Department of Medical Imaging, Centre Hospitalier, Molière-Longchamps, 142 Rue Marconi, 1190 Brussels, Belgium*

Gilles Perrin, M.D. *Professor, Department of Neurosurgery, Université C. Bernard Lyon I, Domaine Rockfeller, 69373 Lyon, France; Professor of Neurosurgery, Service de Neurochisurgie A, Hôpital Neurologique, 69394 Lyon, France*

Charles E. Pither, M.B.B.S., F.R.C.A. *Consultant, Pain Management Department, and Medical Director, Input Pain Unit, St. Thomas Hospital, Lambeth Palace Road, London SE1 7EH, United Kingdom*

Malcolm H. Pope, Dr.Med.Sc., Ph.D. *Professor, Department of Occupational Medicine, University of Aberdeen, AB25 2ZD, United Kingdom*

Richard Porter, M.D., F.R.C.S., F.R.C.S.E. *Doncaster DN4 7AZ, United Kingdom; Former Professor of Orthopedics, University of Aberdeen, University Medical Building, Aberdeen AB25 2ZD, United Kingdom*

Stephane Ramare, M.D. *Department of Orthopedic Surgery, Pierre et Marie Curie University, 75013 Paris, France; Service d' Chirurgie Orthopédique, Hôpital Pitie-Salpetriere, 83 Boulevard de L'Hôpital, 75013 Paris, France*

B. Roger, M.D. *Service de Radiologie, Hôpital Pitie-Salpetriere, 83 Boulevard de L'Hôpital, 75013 Paris, France; Service de Radiologic, Université Paris 6, 91 Boulevard de L'Hôpital, 75013 Paris, France*

Björn Rydevik, M.D. *Professor and Chairman, Department of Orthopedics, Sahlgrenska University Hospital, Göteborg University, SE-41345 Göteborg, Sweden*

G. Saillant, M.D. *Service de Chirurgie Orthopédique, Hôpital Pitie-Salpetriere, 83 Boulevard de L'Hôpital, 75013 Paris, France*

Abdulrahman Siress, M.D. *Orthopedic Surgeon, American Hospital of Paris, Neuilly, France*

Dan M. Spengler, M.D. *Professor and Chairman, Department of Orthopedics and Rehabilitation, Vanderbilt University Medical Center, D4219 MCN, 1161 21st Avenue South, Nashville, Tennessee 37232*

Reinhard Steffen, M.D. *Associate Professor, Department of Orthopedic Surgery, Ruhr University, St. Josef Hospital, Gudrunstr. 56, Bochkin, Germany 44791; Chief, Department of Orthopedics, Marienkrankenhaus, An St. Swidbert 17, D-40489 Düsseldorf, Germany*

Marek Szpalski, M.D. *Senior Consultant and Associate Professor, Department of Orthopedics, Centre Hospitalier Molière Longchamp, Teaching Hospital of the Free University of Brussels, Rue Marconistraat 142, Brussels 1180, Belgium*

R. Trabelsi, M.D. *Service de Chirurgie Orthopédique, Hôpital Pitie-Salpetriere, 83 Boulevard de L'Hôpital, 75013 Paris, France*

Dimitrios Tsoukas, M.D. *Fellow, Services de Chirurgie et Services Associes, Cliniques Universitaires Saint-Luc Universite Catholique de Louvain, 10 Hippocrate Avenue, 1200 Brussels, Belgium; Surgeon, Department of Orthopedics, Diagnostic and Therapeutic Center of Athens "Hygeia," 4 Erithrov Street and Kifissias Avenue, 15123 Athens, Greece*

Pieter F. van Akkerveeken, M.D., Ph.D. *Director, Rug AdviesCentrum Nederland, Soestdÿkse Weg Zuid 15, 3732 HC De Bilt, The Netherlands*

Jean Pierre Van Buyten, M.D. *Department of Anesthesia and Pain Management, Maria Middelares Hospital, 17 Hospitaal Street, G100 Sint-Niklaas, Belgium*

Peter Van Roy, M.D. *Department of Experimental Anatomy, Vrije Universiteit Brussel, Laarbeeklaan 103, 1090 Brussels, Belgium*

Heiko Visarius, Ph.D. *Director, Medivision, Elmattstr.3, CH-4436 Oberdorf, Switzerland*

Stanislav Vohanka *Neurologicka Klinika FN, Brno Bohunice, Zihlavska 100, CZ-63900 Brno, Czech Republic*

Archibald von Strempel, M.D., D. Eng. *Associate Professor and Medical Director, Annastift, Department III, Heimchenstrasse 1–7, 30625 Hannover, Germany*

Gordon Waddell, M.D., D.Sc., F.R.C.S. *Surgeon, Department of Orthopaedic Surgery, Gladsgow Nuffield Hospital, Beaconsfield Road, Gladsgow G12 OPJ, United Kingdom*

James N. Weinstein, D.O., M.S. *Professor, Department of Community and Family Medicine, Center for Evaluative Clinical Sciences, Dartmouth Medical School, HB 7251, 309 Strasenburgh Hall, Hanover, New Hampshire 03755; Director, Spine Center and Center for Shared Decision Making, The Dartmouth-Hitchcock Medical Center, One Medical Center Drive, Lebanon, New Hampshire 03756*

Paul Wessberg, M.D. *Specialist, Department of Orthopedic Surgery, Sahlgrenska University Hospital, Göteborg University, SE 413 45 Göteborg, Sweden*

Jacques Widelec, M.D. *Department of Medical Imaging, Centre Hospitalier Molière-Longchamp, 142 Rue Marconi, 1190 Brussels, Belgium*

Roland E. Willburger, M.D. *Surgeon, Orthopaedic University Clinic, St. Josef Hospital, and Department of Orthopaedic Surgery, Ruhr University Bochum, Gudrunstr 56, D-44791 Bochum, Germany*

Jan T. Wilmink, M.D., Ph.D. *Professor, Department of Radiology, University Hospital, P. Debyelaan 25, 6202 AZ Maastricht, The Netherlands*

Ralf H. Wittenberg, M.D. *Professor, Department of Orthopedic Surgery, Ruhr University Bochum, Gudrunstr. 56, D-44791 Bochum, Germany; Consultant Senior Surgeon, Orthopaedic University Clinic, St. Josef Hospital, Gudrunstr. 56, D-44791 Bochum, Germany*

Preface

Lumbar spinal stenosis (LSS), whether it is congenital or acquired, is a unique entity in the array of spinal disorders. In this book, a comprehensive review of LSS is presented that takes the reader from basic sciences, clinical presentation, physiopathology, and diagnosis, to conservative and surgical treatment modalities. In addition, economic and ethical considerations surrounding LSS and its management are discussed.

Section I, basics, covers the embryology and development of the spinal canal, as well as the anatomy of the spinal canal, the foramen, and the surrounding ligamentous structures. The biomechanics of the neural arch and of LSS are discussed and lead the reader to the understanding of both physiopathology and clinical presentation.

Neurological symptoms are explained and neurologic claudication is compared to vascular claudication. The *physiopathology* section compares different etiopathological theories: the neurological compression theory and the vascular compression theory.

In the next section, different imaging techniques for diagnosis are described and discussed, from conventional radiology and the computed tomography revolution to the controversy surrounding the use of magnetic resonance instead of myelography. The appreciation of electrophysiological examinations and motion analysis completes the picture.

The reader must understand these theories and the biomechanics of LSS before he or she can understand the *clinical presentation* and physiopathology of LSS. The different classifications and the natural history of LSS are completed with a study of iatrogenic stenosis.

The *conservative treatment modalities* cover rheumatological treatments, physical medicine, and exercise, as well as pure pain management. The *surgical treatment modalities* are comprehensively presented, including the newest techniques proposed to this date. The widely abandoned total laminectomy has been replaced by conservative laminarthrectomy, with its respect of the anatomical structures and, therefore, their biomechanical functions. The need to fuse remains controversial, giving this topic its particularly importance in this book.

Finally, LSS is a very common condition and thus generates high management and disability-related costs, giving rise to both ethical and economic questions. Problems surrounding cost-effectiveness and cost to society are analyzed in the last section and seen in the perspective of the epidemiology of LSS.

Throughout this book the reader is confronted with controversial issues. The comprehensive coverage of all aspects of lumbar spinal stenosis makes this book useful not only for clinicians and researchers, but also for manipulation therapists and those involved with medico-legal issues.

Robert Gunzburg
Marek Szpalski

SECTION I

Basics

Lumbar Spinal Stenosis
edited by Robert Gunzburg and Marek Szpalski
Lippincott Williams & Wilkins, Philadelphia, © 2000.

1

Embryology and Development of the Spinal Canal

Richard Porter

*Department of Orthopaedic Surgery, University of Aberdeen,
Aberdeen AB25 2ZD, United Kingdom*

Understanding the growth of the spinal canal has clinical importance because spinal stenosis is a major factor in certain back pain syndromes. Embryologic studies have shown that the spinal canal is relatively large very early in life. The neural content of the spinal canal probably has a powerful influence on growth of the canal.

EMBRYOLOGIC GROWTH

The conus is located in the lower sacral canal in the first few weeks of intrauterine life. At 10 weeks it begins to rise relative to the vertebral segments, and by 22 weeks it reaches L2.

Up to 10 weeks of intrauterine life, when the spinal cord is within the sacral canal, the cross-sectional area of the spinal canal is the same throughout the whole spine. However, as the conus begins to rise, the distal expansion of the growing canal rises with the ascending conus, until at 22 weeks the distal part of the canal below L2 is proportionally smaller (4). This disproportionate growth between upper and lower lumbar levels continues up to 40 weeks, with the distal extent of the wider proximal canal remaining at L2.

Up to 10 weeks there is very little extradural space throughout the spine. The canal size closely matches the size of the dural sac. After 22 weeks, when the conus has reached L2, the extradural space above L2 remains very small, whereas distal to L2 the extradural space steadily increases in capacity.

The relationship between the size of the canal and the ascending conus, and the increasing extradural space below L2 after 22 weeks, suggests that the spinal cord within the dural sac has a powerful influence on the size and development of the spinal canal.

There is a very close correlation between the sagittal diameter of the fetal brain and the cross-sectional area of the spinal canal before 22 weeks. After 22 weeks, the correlation with brain size is better above L2 than below L2.

The most rapid period of canal growth is between 18 and 36 weeks of intrauterine life. Growth deficiency during this period is likely to have the most significant effect on neural and canal development.

Comparisons between the adult and the fetal spinal canal show that, in cross-sectional area, the adult size is reached very early in life. At L3 and L4 the canal is 80% mature by birth and is fully mature by 1 year of age. At L5, the canal is 50% mature at birth and reaches adult dimensions by 5 years of age. Thus, the proximal lumbar spine matures before the lower levels.

SIGNIFICANT ANTENATAL FACTORS IN THE DEVELOPMENT OF SPINAL STENOSIS

The degree of retardation of canal growth depends on the severity and timing of any adverse effects. We have been able to show that a number of antenatal factors, independently and in combination, are related to a small spinal canal in adult life. These factors include gestational age, small placental weight, greater maternal age, low socioeconomic class, low birth weight, and primiparity (2).

CLINICAL RELEVANCE

Spinal stenosis is an important factor in many back pain syndromes. Although developmental spinal stenosis may remain symptomless throughout life, when other pathologies such as disc protrusion, degenerative change, and segmental displacement supervene, a small canal can become seriously compromised and symptomatic. Developmental stenosis is often the underlying problem.

Growth impairment early in life will permanently stunt growth of the spinal canal because there is no potential for catch-up growth after infancy. Thus, good fetal nutrition and child health care are important if developmental spinal stenosis is to be prevented.

Some patients with spinal stenosis have generalized stenosis throughout the cervical, thoracic, and lumbar spines. Impaired growth could have occurred at any time in fetal life or in the first year of infancy, but the greatest risk for this generalized stenosis would be impairment of fetal growth before 22 weeks. After that time, there is still potential for catch-up growth in the canal below L2.

Others have stenosis only at L3 and L4, with an adequate canal throughout the rest of the spine. It is reasonable to suspect that these patients had growth deficiency at some time between 22 weeks and 1 year of age, because L5 still has catch-up growth up to 5 years of age. An isolated stenosis at L5 would be compatible with growth impairment between 1 and 5 years of age.

Trefoilness occurs at L5 in 15% to 25% of spines. The sagittal diameter in these spines is generally small, and the canal is trefoil in shape (Fig. 1). This suggests that the cause of

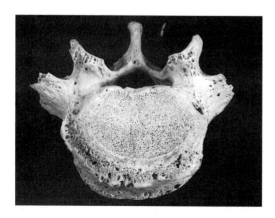

FIG. 1. Fifth lumbar vertebra showing a stenotic trefoil-shaped spinal canal.

trefoilness is linked with a small midsagittal diameter and, therefore, is similarly developmental in origin (1). The midsagittal diameter is affected by early growth, whereas the interpedicular diameter continues to increase up to puberty, which allows a shallow canal to widen into a trefoil shape.

The period of maximum growth of the spinal canal corresponds to the growth curves of the immune and neurologic systems; therefore, it is not surprising that subjects with developmental spinal stenosis sometimes are disadvantaged in health and neurologic status. When compared with subjects who have wider canals, those with spinal stenosis have been found to have more cardiovascular and gastrointestinal symptoms, less postschool qualifications, and poorer performance on vocabulary tests (3). There is more to spinal stenosis than a small spinal canal.

REFERENCES

1. Papp T, Porter RW, Aspden RM. Trefoil configuration and developmental stenosis of the lumbar vertebral canal. *J Bone Joint Surg* 1995;77-B:469–472.
2. Papp T, Porter RW, Craig CE, Aspden RM. Significant antenatal factors in the development of lumbar spinal stenosis. *Spine* 1997;22:1805–1810.
3. Porter RW, Oakshott G. Spinal stenosis and health status. *Spine* 1994;19:901–903
4. Ursu TS, Porter RW, Navaratnam V. Development of the lumbar vertebral canal in utero. *Spine* 1996;21: 2705–2708.

Lumbar Spinal Stenosis
edited by Robert Gunzburg and Marek Szpalski
Lippincott Williams & Wilkins, Philadelphia, © 2000.

2

Anatomy of the Lumbar Canal, Foramen, and Ligaments, with References to Recent Insights

Peter Van Roy, Erik Barbaix, and Jan P. Clarijs

Department of Experimental Anatomy, Vrije Universiteit Brussel, 1090 Brussels, Belgium

The lumbar spinal canal and the intervertebral foramina constitute complex osteofibrous neurovascular tunnels that allow movement and deformation of the spine without loss of their main configuration. They are continuously trimmed by muscular action on symphyses, syndesmoses, and synovial joints, and they are arranged in parallel within one single motion segment while acting in a serial arrangement throughout the entire spinal region (Fig. 1). Along their course, the configuration of these canals is conditioned by several morphologic and biomechanical characteristics of adjacent bony elements and soft tissues, which in turn may reflect constitutional and developmental effects as well as actual physiologic conditions. The lordotic course of the lumbar canal is induced by the forward tilting of the sacrum and by wedge-shaped vertebral bodies and intervertebral discs in the lower lumbar spine. Contemporary research reveals a renewed interest in several morphologic details of the spinal canal and intervertebral foramina and the topographic relationships between bony and soft tissue particularities of surrounding components on the one side and the neural or vascular contents on the other. Aspects of anatomic variability are taken in consideration. Awareness about morphometric variability of the boundaries and the content of the neural canal may be helpful in clinical decision making and in avoiding pitfalls in medical imaging.

A number of recent insights came from contemporary dissection methods, such as cryomicrotomy, and improved methodologic strategy for *in vitro* vascular injections (9,18,36). Cryomicrotomy responds well to the need for correlative topographic anatomic studies, which evolved from the invention of thin-slice medical imaging in computed tomography (CT) and magnetic resonance imaging (36,37). Some anatomic investigations were supported by histologic procedures (14,31,35,55,56). Detailed information about the nerve plexuses within and around the spinal canal in human fetuses was provided by specific coloring techniques based on acetylcholinesterase (14).

BONY ASPECTS

Shape and Morphometric Aspects of the Central Lumbar Spinal Canal

Cross section of the bony lumbar spinal canal shows the canal to be dome shaped in childhood. In adults, the lumbar spinal canal may show an elliptic, rounded triangular, or

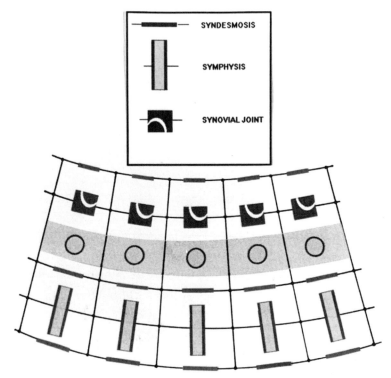

FIG. 1. Model of the central and lateral lumbar spinal canals representing the combined parallel and serial arrangement of symphyses, syndesmoses, and synovial joints that trim the complex osteofibrous neurovascular tunnels.

trefoil configuration (Fig. 2). Commonly, the transition from the thoracic to the sacral spine is characterized by a gradual change from a more circular to a more triangular shape. The trefoil shape of the spinal canal mostly occurs at the fifth lumbar level, to a lesser degree at the fourth lumbar level, and rarely is seen at the third lumbar level.

The trefoil configuration should be considered a developmental feature. The reported absence of trefoil-shaped lumbar canals in newborns (2) is in accordance with findings that a real trefoil shape could not be detected before adulthood (30). Trefoilness results from ventral midpoint thickening of the laminae over their full height, leading to indentation of the basic triangular shape of the central canal and narrowing of the anteroposterior dimensions of the lateral recess (10,39). As a consequence, the pars interarticularis appears as a thickened, sometimes unequally rounded column between the superior and inferior articular processes.

Whereas most of the vertebral bodies of the lumbar spine present slightly concave posterior borders, the posterior borders of the L-4 body are rather straight and those of the L-5 body are straight or slightly convex. When present, this feature may accentuate trefoilness at the L-4 and L-5 levels.

Morphometric data are reported from *in vitro* osteometric studies and *in vivo* measurements using medical imaging. Mean transverse diameters steadily increase from L-1 to L-5 (Fig. 3A–B) (1,22,27,34). An incidence of 78.1% was reported for a spinal canal configuration that presented slightly increasing transverse diameters (A type) (34). A B-type configuration, which was quoted when a single transverse diameter at L-2, L-3, L-4, or L-5 was found to be smaller than that of the vertebra immediately above, was detected in 19.5%. Two levels

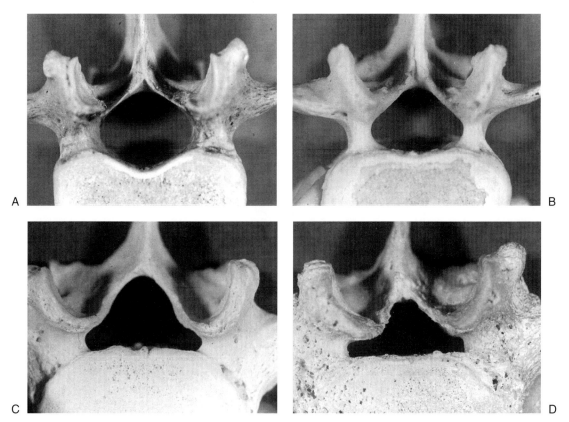

FIG. 2. Variable shapes of the central lumbar canal. **A:** Round; **B:** triangular; **C:** trefoiled; **D:** trefoiled and asymmetric.

of narrower interpedicular distances (type C) or a progressive narrowing of the transverse diameter in the caudal direction (type D) were found in only a few cases. Proximal to spina bifida occulta, the spinal canal tends to be larger than in unaffected spines (29).

The mean transverse diameter was found to be proportional to the vertebral body size (1). Thus, the canal to body ratio can be used to indicate whether measurements of the transverse diameter of the canal may be considered within normal limits for a particular vertebral body size.

Anteroposterior diameters of the lumber spinal canal usually decrease from L-1 to L-3, mostly followed by an increase from L-3 to L-5 (Fig. 3C) (21,22,27,46).

From L-1 to L-3, a small increase of the transverse diameter contrasts with a substantial decrease of anteroposterior diameters. Below L-3, marked increases in the transverse and anteroposterior diameters commonly are observed (27).

Results of a number of morphometric studies are indicative of racial differences in transverse and sagittal diameters of the lumbar spinal canal (Fig. 3A–B) (1,22,34,52).

Cross-sectional areas tend to decrease from L-1 to L-2 and remain rather constant between L-2 and L-4, followed by a marked increase at L-5 (27).

Statistical evidence was presented of correlations between the height of subjects and the interpedicular distances at L-4 and L-5 ($p \leq 0.001$) cross-sectional areas of the central spinal canal at L-4 ($p \leq 0.001$) and L-5 ($p \leq 0.01$), and cross-sectional areas of the dural sac at

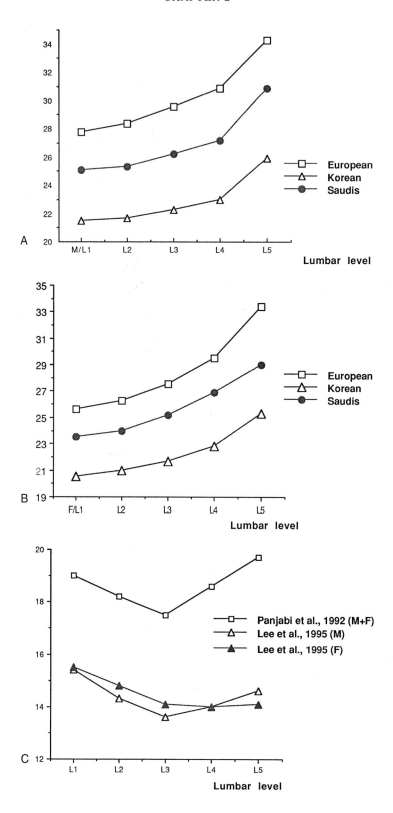

L-3 and L-4 ($p \leq 0.01$). No comparable conclusion was obtained regarding the anteroposterior diameter at these levels (13).

When comparing cross-sectional areas of osseous and nonosseous parts of the spinal canal (15,21), relatively more space for nerve tissue was found in the osseous parts. It is evident that relatively more space around the nerve tissue becomes available toward the caudal end of the lumbar spine. In females, relatively smaller nerve tissue to spinal canal ratios suggest more available space around the nerve tissue than in males, excepted for the L-5 level, where comparable ratios for both sexes were reported. It is clear that the cross-sectional area of the osseous canal always overestimates the available space.

A reduction of the cross-sectional area and anteroposterior diameter of the spinal canal was observed *in vitro* at L-3 to L-4, when moving from flexion to extension and from distraction to compression. This indicates the impact of nonosseous structures on canal dimensions. A reduction of 16% or 40 mm^2 of the cross-sectional area corresponded with a 2-mm reduction of the anteroposterior diameter (45).

With aging, transverse diameters may increase significantly ($p \leq 0.05$) in males but decrease in females (50). The latter probably is related to frequently occurring osteoporotic loss of transverse trabeculae in older females, leading to a more transverse expansion of the vertebral bodies and pedicles. Aging may significantly ($p \leq 0.01$) reduce the anteroposterior diameters at the three lowest lumbar levels in males, whereas in females usually only a restraint reduction is noted.

Left–Right Asymmetries

Systematic observation of listed morphologic features of dried vertebrae revealed a large number of left–right asymmetries (23,51). These findings suggest that spinal motion, especially in the elderly, often is performed in the presence of a combination of facet tropism and asymmetric lever arms for muscles. Facet tropism not only deals with asymmetric shape and inclination, but also with asymmetric size, surface area, implantation, or degenerative enlargement. Perfect symmetry of the spine should not be a basic assumption. Not only tropism of the joint facets but also asymmetries of the pedicles, laminae, and vertebral bodies may influence the shape and size of the neural canals (Fig. 4). Degenerative or pathologic asymmetries may affect the optimal trimming of shape and size of the canals. In the concept of spinal instability proposed by Panjabi (28), degenerative enlargement of zygapophyseal joints causing secondary facet tropism was described as an adaptation of the passive subsystem for a better equilibrium among the passive, the active, and the control subsystems for spinal posture and movement. The clinical appearance of compensatory hypermobility in the neighborhood of a hypomobile motion segment represents a typical example of the longitudinal adaptability between adjacent juncturae of the spine.

EPIDURAL ANATOMY

Posterior Longitudinal Ligament

The posterior longitudinal ligament (PLL) is a typical denticulated flat ligament showing a broad attachment at the level of the intervertebral discs and a narrower course across the

FIG. 3. Transverse and midsagittal diameters of the central spinal canal at lumbar levels. **A:** Transverse diameters in males; **B:** transverse diameters in females; **C:** midsagittal diameters in males and females.

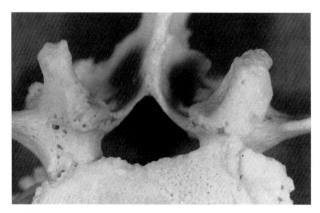

FIG. 4. Example of articular tropism combined with left–right asymmetries of the pedicles and the spinous process.

midportion of the concave posterior wall of the vertebral bodies. Whereas the collagen fibers of the deep layer only span one motion segment, long collagen fibers of the superficial layer cover more than one vertebral segmental level, merging with the annulus fibrosis at the dorsal aspect of the intervertebral discs and showing connections to the endplates (Fig. 5A). The deep part is connected to the margins of the bodies, resulting in a bowstring configuration.

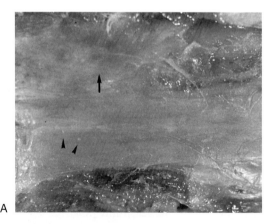

A

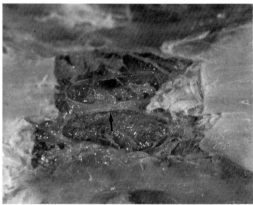

B

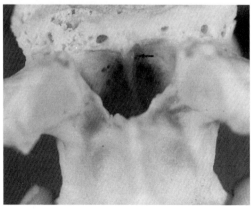

C

FIG. 5. Posterior aspect of the posterior longitudinal ligament (PLL). **A:** Small dots of connective tissue represent the cut lines of filaments of the anterior meningovertebral ligament *(arrowheads)*. The lateral expansion of the PLL *(arrow)* divides the anterior epidural space into anterior and posterior compartments. **B:** Deep sagittal membrane at the midline of the posterior aspect of a lumbar vertebral body *(arrow)*. The compartmental structure contains the medial part of the internal ventral venous plexus in relationship with the basivertebral veins. **C:** Bony septum at the posterior wall of a lumbar vertebral body.

A sagittally oriented membrane (Fig. 5B) connecting the periosteum at the midline of the posterior wall of the vertebral bodies to the deep layer of the ligament was described as a third part of the PLL (35,44). However, interruption of this membrane at the midvertebral level must be considered (18). The sagittal membrane results in a typical T- or Y-shaped aspect of the PLL complex in transverse magnetic resonance images. The vertical part of the T figure in transverse images, which represents the sagittal part of the ligament, disappears at the level of the disc. In contrast, at this level the transverse part of the T figure, which results from the frontally oriented layers of the PLL (horizontal part in the images), becomes wider and thicker. Thus, at the level of the vertebral body only, the sagittal membrane may divide the dorsal concavity into two separate spaces. Not seldomly ossification occurs in this part of the ligament, giving onset to a bony septum at the midline of the dorsal aspect of the vertebral body, separating the nutrient foramina (Fig. 5C). The sagittal membrane is considered clinically significant in the prevention of migration of disc material from one side to another at the level of the vertebral bodies (44). The narrow parts of the PLL behind the vertebral bodies indicate a reduced biomechanical importance. However, it is a suspensory ligament for the dural sac, and the presence of a nerve plexus emanating from the sinuvertebral nerve (6,14) suggests a proprioceptive function of the ligament (31,40).

Due to the dual aspect of the PLL, bowstring over the concavity of the vertebral bodies but firmly attached to the endplates and to the annulus fibrosus of the discs, the part of the anterior epidural space between the PLL and vertebral bodies becomes segmented, whereas the compartment between the PLL and the dural sac normally is uninterrupted.

Anterior Internal Vertebral Venous Plexus

Especially at the level of the vertebral bodies, the epidural space in front of the PLL is filled by the anterior internal vertebral venous plexus (AIVVP) and adipose tissue. Batson's plexus[1] of the spinal canal lies ventrally and laterally from the deep layers of the PLL, closing a distinct paraosseous compartment of the anterior epidural space (44,54). Two parts can be recognized in the AIVVP: a medial venous plexus situated in the dorsal compartment directly behind each vertebral body, and a more individualized lateral vein with longitudinal orientation. The medial part of the AIVVP adheres to the spinal canal by dense connective tissue, whereas the lateral longitudinal vein is attached by loose fibrous tissue (12). The medial part receives the basivertebral veins and is divided into two parts by the sagittal septum in the midline. This medial venous plexus is not continuously present; it is lacking at the level of the intervertebral disc and thus is segmented in the same way as the paraosseous compartment of the ventral epidural space.

The longitudinal vein of the anterior compartment extends laterally along the PLL and receives blood from the more medial situated plexus; this vein has anastomoses with veins from the posterior epidural space and in the intervertebral foramen.

Epidural Membranes

Membranes surrounding the epidural space recently received renewed attention (15,18,35,54). When the dura mater is tilted away from the PLL, a translucent expansion of the superficial layer of the PLL separates a compartment behind the posterior concavity of

---

[1]Batson's plexus is a plexus of valveless veins extending longitudinally in the anterior epidural space, especially behind the dorsal surface of the vertebral bodies, where they receive connections from the basivertebral system inside the bodies (54).

the vertebral body from the compartment between the dural sac and the PLL. Whereas an epidural membrane has been reported in continuity with the superficial layer of the PLL (15), a peridural membrane also was described as a two-layered extradural fibrovascular sheath lining the spinal canal and attaching to the deep layer and sagittal septum of the PLL (54). This peridural membrane was considered a homologue of periosteum in this region, having an important part of the AIVVP extending along its posterior surface.

At the center of the dorsal wall of the vertebral bodies, a pair of basivertebral veins pierce the membrane, coming out of the large nutrient foramina adjacent to the bony septum at the midline. But the expression "fibrous fatty cellular complex" also was suggested to refer to the connective tissue encompassing the medial part of the AIVVP at the level of the vertebral bodies (35). Although it has been hypothesized that the terms epidural membrane and peridural membrane probably have been used to indicate the same tissue (18,35), the medial aspect of the anterior internal venous plexus is situated anteriorly to the translucent lateral extension of the superficial layer of the PLL (Fig. 5A–B).

Laterally, epidural connective tissue presents a loose attachment to the medial aspect of the pedicles; posteriorly, it separates the laminae and ligamentum flavum from the epidural space (54).

Meningovertebral Ligaments

The meningovertebral ligaments represent a heterogeneous group of membranous formations that connect the dura with the PLL and other elements of the spinal canal and prevent the dura from moving far from the vertebral bodies. Since the early descriptions of anterior meningovertebral attachments by Trolard (1888) and Hofmann (1898), little attention has been given to these structures in most anatomy textbooks. However, these structures were revisited recently (4,5,32,35,43,47,54). The way in which the meningovertebral ligaments are referred to as medial and lateral Hofmann's ligaments (5,32,35,47,54), Hofmann–Trolard's ligaments (43), or Trolard's ligaments (4) may lead to confusion.

In his often referred to publication dating from 1898, Hofmann presented a classification of four types of dural attachments. The largest group, termed "ligamenta anteriora durae matris," includes Trolard's median septum as well as a number of paramedian ligaments and filaments in the anterior epidural space between the dural sac and the PLL. The second group, termed "ligamenta dorsolateralia (durae matris)," attaches the posterior aspect of the dural sac to the laminae of the arcus posterior. Hofmann pointed out that these ligaments are common at sacral levels but are rare at lumbar levels. It appears that, later on, the term posterolateral became misunderstood as posterior to the vertebral bodies but within the anterior epidural space. From the original German text and from its illustrations, it is evident that Hofmann described ligaments within the posterior epidural space. He further mentioned the ligamentum interspinale cervicale, which is seen at the cervical level only. Finally, he drew attention to the numerous ligaments that attach the nerve sleeves to the wall of the intervertebral canals (17).

Thus, it is clear that midline ligaments correspond with the "ligamentum sacrale anterius durae matris" originally described by Trolard (49). The name of the ligament is somewhat misleading, as it tends to limit the existence of these ligaments to the sacral levels, but they recently were observed to exist at lumbar and even lower thoracic levels (4). The anterior ligaments may show vault structures extending beyond the midline. Although often present, these meningovertebral ligaments show a large interindividual difference (4,32,47). They vary from loose areolar tissue to clearly individualized ligaments and from pure midsagittal septa to more laterally oriented attachments. Moreover, variation exists at the thoracic, lumbar, and/or sacral levels, where distinct ligaments or septa can be found. A study in our laboratory revealed that in 25 of the 30 spinal canals investigated, the anterior meningovertebral ligament showed a network of filaments, resulting in a double cross vault structure between the PLL and the dura mater (Fig. 6A–C) (4). These meningovertebral ligaments extended from L-3 to the end of the dural envelope. A number of filaments originated from the PLL, reached the dura in an oblique fashion, and returned to the PLL on the contralateral side. A second cross vault consisted of the fibers originating from the dura, reaching the PLL and returning to the dura. Combinations of the double cross vault with other types of central meningovertebral filaments were found: sagittally oriented filaments, a strong ligament at the L5–S1 level, and a strong septum over the entire length. In two cases only loose areolar tissue was observed. At lumbar levels, midsagittal filaments were detected in 44% of the specimens investigated.

Preliminary results of a retrospective study of medial and paramedial attachments in 110 CT scans (16) indicate the presence of a mediosagittal structure below the L-3 level in 43% (Fig. 7 and Table 1). Less numerous medial attachments were seen at disc levels than at surrounding body levels. Due to segmentation of the median part of the AIVVP and of the paraosseous compartment of the ventral epidural space, these structures cannot be central veins at the disc level. Among the numerous median structures at corporal levels, some are black, probably venous structures, and others clearly display a ligamentous aspect. It was hypothesized that these meningovertebral ligaments may play a role as a barrier to transverse displacement of extruded disc material (43).

In addition to pure midline meningovertebral ligaments and lateral ligaments, the lateral root ligaments are of particular value, tethering the nerve root sleeves to the inferior pedicles (Fig. 6D). Reports of posterolateral Hofmann's ligaments are rare (5,17).

Arterial Blood Supply

Anterior branches of segmental arteries provide a longitudinal arterial system on each side of the anterior epidural space. In addition to a number of small vessels to different anatomic components in this area (including the bony cylinder), a larger vessel enters the posterior wall of the vertebral body via the nutrient foramen and reaches the central zone of the endplates to exchange fluid with the intervertebral disc. Anterior and posterior distal radicular branches follow the course of the ventral and dorsal nerve roots. A posterior branch gives connection to the posterior longitudinal arterial system and supplies tissues in the posterior epidural space, neural arch, and intraspinal aspect of the zygapophyseal joints (7,9).

Posterior Epidural Space

The posterior epidural space is a highly variable space between the thecal sac and the neural arches of lumbar vertebrae. At each particular level, its segmented configuration is strongly dependent on the relationship between the laminae and the zygapophyseal joints with the ligamentum flavum (18). Distinction can be made between the lateral parts in front of the oblique course of the laminae that contain the posterior internal vertebral venous plexus (PIVVP) and a central part in front of the spinous process that mainly is filled with adipose tissue.

Ligamentum Flavum

The ligamentum flavum lines an important part of the nonosseous and osseous sections of the posterior epidural region and covers the PIVVP and adipose tissue of the posterior

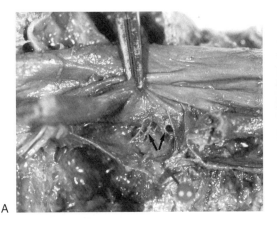

A

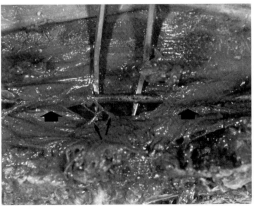

B

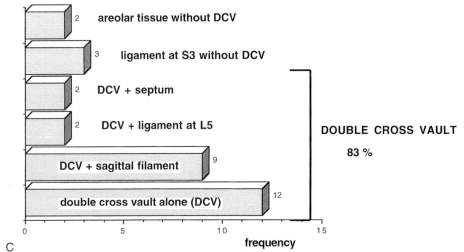

C

areolar tissue without DCV

ligament at S3 without DCV

DCV + septum

DCV + ligament at L5

DCV + sagittal filament

double cross vault alone (DCV)

DOUBLE CROSS VAULT

83 %

frequency

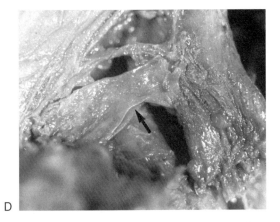

D

FIG. 6. Meningovertebral ligaments. **A:** Cross vault structures of anterior meningovertebral ligament between the posterior longitudinal ligament (PLL) **(bottom)** and the anterior aspect of the dural sac **(top)**. **B:** Combination of cross vault *(small arrows)* and paramedian "ligamenta anteriora durae matris" *(large arrows)*. **C:** Frequency of sacrodural attachments in 30 lumbar spines (4). **D:** Nerve root ligament.

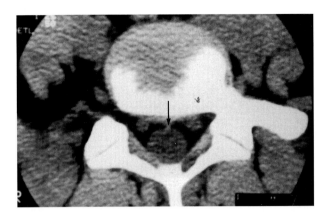

FIG. 7. Typical medial medio-sagittal dural attachment as seen on computed tomography at the endplate of S1 (16).

epidural space. Laterally, it represents the anterior capsule of the zygapophyseal joints and borders the lateral recess and the neural foramen posteriorly.

The large amount of elastin fibers (approximately 80%) explains its typical yellowish aspect and its characteristic thickening when one of its insertions is divided or when adjacent laminae are approximated (55). The ligament spans between the imbricately arranged adjacent laminae and fills the interlaminar space. The capsular portion of the ligament is thinner than the interlaminar portion. The capsular portion may be especially susceptible to different types of hypertrophy (56).

In a recent description, attention was given to a two-layered aspect (26). Both layers are firmly attached to each other. Whereas a more light yellow superficial part fills the interlaminar space with a thickness of about 2.5 to 3.5 mm, a darker yellow deep component of nearly 1-mm thickness borders the spinal canal. The superficial part has a superior attachment that expands from a large insertion at the superior edge and the anteroinferior slope of the upper lamina to a smaller insertion at the superior edge and the anterior part of the posterosuperior slope of the lamina below. The deep component attaches superiorly to a ridge that differentiates the smooth anterosuperior aspect and rough anteroinferior surface of the upper lamina. Its distal insertion reaches the small anterosuperior border of the lamina below. Thus, both layers of the ligament diverge caudally at the level of the upper rim of the lamina. At the lumbosacral transition, a much thinner ligamentum flavum may be found (40).

Due to differences in the morphology and spatial orientation of the laminae in the upper

TABLE 1. *Medial and paramedial dural attachments seen on computed tomographic images*

Lumbar level	No. of images (n = 655)	Medial attachments		Paramedian attachments	
		No.	%	No.	%
L3	71	12	17	12	17
L3–L4	85	4	5	4	5
L4	102	30	29	26	25
L4–L5	102	12	12	11	11
L5	102	71	70	41	40
L5–S1	98	35	36	25	26
S1	95	66	69	41	43

From Heytens et al. (in preparation).

and lower lumbar spine, the coverage of the anterosuperior surface of the lamina increases from the upper lumbar spine to the lower lumbar segments.

The observation of a variable degree of fusion between the left and right leaflets of the ligamentum flavum at the midline (18) indicates that anatomic variability could be an important element to clarify the discussion (18,26,33) as to whether the left and right ligamentum flavum should be considered separate entities (7,18,33,57) or a continuous structure (26). In addition, the interspinous ligament may fill the partial gap between the left and right parts of the ligamentum flavum (33). Both parts of the ligamentum flavum show a transverse angle of less than 90 degrees (18,26,57).

A typical tented recess, which is filled with homogeneous epidural adipose tissue and is rather poorly vascularized, is present in front of the apex of the ligament, to which it is particularly adherent at the midline, where often a vessel enters the posterior epidural space (18).

No significant change in thickness of the ligamentum flavum is expected from change in posture (45).

Posterior Internal Vertebral Venous Plexus

In front of the ligamentum flavum and laminae the posterior epidural space is filled by the PIVVP. In the central recess, the left and right parts of the plexus are separated by a triangular pad of adipose tissue.

Longitudinally oriented vessels of the plexus reach adjacent levels in the spinal canal. Others follow a more transverse course, giving onset to anastomoses with the anterior internal venous plexus or running toward the intervertebral foramen. The PIVVP drains bone and soft tissue of the posterolateral walls of the lumbar canal and gives several anastomoses with its anterior counterpart and with the posterior external vertebral venous plexus. It occupies less space than the AIVVP.

LATERAL RECESS AND INTERVERTEBRAL FORAMEN

Boundaries of the Lateral Neural Canal

The description of the intervertebral foramen as a door at the end of a corridor indicated the presence of a real depth of a neural canal (Fig. 8A–B) connecting the intervertebral

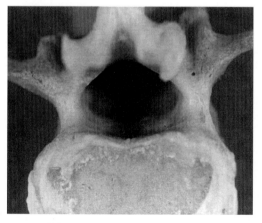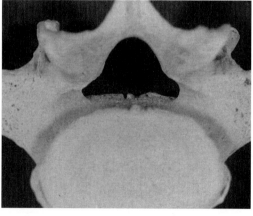

A   B

FIG. 8. Variation of depth of the bony lateral lumbar canal (also note asymmetries).

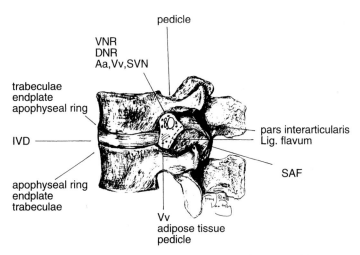

FIG. 9. Boundaries of the lateral recess and intervertebral foramen. DNR, dorsal nerve root; IVD, intervertebral disc; SAF, superior articular facet; VNR, ventral nerve root.

foramen strictu sensu with the lateral aspect of the central spinal canal (8). Every root canal is trimmed by the local symphysis, synovial joints, and syndesmoses.

The nerve root canal has an inverted teardrop- or ear-shaped section and is more oval at the exit (39,41). Its widest part is situated in the subpedicular notch of the upper vertebra where the neural foramen strictu sensu is located (Fig. 9). The anterior wall of the foraminal canal is composed of the posterolateral aspect of the articulating vertebrae and the interposed intervertebral disc. Due to the presence of a real incisura vertebralis superior situated below the level of superior endplate, the morphology of the anteroinferior aspect of the intervertebral foramen strongly depends on the condition of the apophyseal rings and the interposed intervertebral disc. At lower lumbar levels, the intervertebral disc may show a slight physiologic bulging posteriorly, which is accentuated in extension of the lumbar spine. In addition, in the lumbar spine, the outer annulus fibers insert on the body beyond the apophyseal ring. The posterior wall of the neural canal is represented by the ligamentum flavum, the pars interarticularis of the upper vertebra, and the superior articular facet of the vertebra below. The ligamentum flavum in front of the articular facets of the vertebra contributes to reduction of the width in the inferior part of the intervertebral foramen.

Dependent on the level and interindividual variability, the nerve root canal (syn.: radicular canal, neural canal, root canal) starts in its retrodiscal or retrocorporal part, has a shorter or longer parapedicular part in the lateral recess (syn.: lateral canal, lateral nerve canal, subarticular gutter), and finally reaches its foraminal part (7). Whereas nerve roots at higher lumbar levels mostly emerge from the dural sac in the parapedicular zone, L-5 and S-1 nerve roots show a suprapedicular onset. Starting at the upper endplate of the L-5 vertebra and continuing under a broad pedicle, the L-5 neural canal is particularly long and deserves a separate description (38–40).

At the L5–S1 level, the intervertebral canal can differ from those of the higher levels due to the frequent occurrence of variable degrees of unilateral or bilateral sacralization of L-5 that eventually results in fixed bony canals.

A more level-independent classification of the neural canal results from its subdivision into entrance, oblique pedicular, and exit zones (39). In medical imaging, the use of ''zones'' was suggested to locate a lesion in a mediolateral direction within the spinal anatomy. Accordingly, the use of "levels" was proposed for differentiation in a craniocaudal direction (53).

Three clinically important parts of the pedicular zone can be considered: medial, central, and lateral (41). The medial part is continuous with the lateral recess and has a close relationship with the superior articular facet of the vertebra below. The central third lies between the considered pair of pedicles. Horizontal lengths ranging from 8.2 to 10.2 mm and from 8.2 to 12.2 mm were measured at L-4 and L-5 intervertebral foramina, respectively (11). The lateral third is situated near the outer edge of the pedicle in the neighborhood of the posterolateral rim of the upper and lower vertebral bodies. A sharp ridge may be present at the cranial bony aspect of the exit zone. The pedicular zone may be enlarged by trabecular reorganization and lateral spreading of vertebrae in ageing. This predominantly results from osteoporotic changes in older females (50).

Measurements on lateral radiographs revealed mean heights of 14 to 22 mm for the intervertebral foramina at L1–2 and L2–3, and 13 to 20 mm for the intervertebral foramina at L3–4, L4–5, and L5–S1. The mean distance between the ligamentum flavum and vertebral body was 7 mm (41).

Content of the Lateral Neural Canal

Nerve root sleeves display a level-dependent, variable oblique course from their emanation of the thecal sac toward the outer third of the neural canal (7,38,40). In the neighborhood of their origin from the dural sac, short separate meningeal sleeves may be found around the initial course of the ventral and dorsal nerve roots, creating an interradicular foramen. These short sleeves soon merge to create the common dural sleeve that is steeply directed toward the inferior aspect of the pedicle and covers ventral and dorsal nerve roots, the dorsal nerve root ganglion, and the spinal nerve. The mean angle of emerging nerve roots with respect to the central canal in the lumbar spine diminishes from values of 80 degrees at the L1–2 level to 60 degrees at the L3–4 and L4–5 levels, and 45 degrees at the L5–S1 level (7). Nerve root sleeves are shorter in the upper than in the lower lumbar spine (39).

The L-5 nerve roots are relatively thick, and the L5–S1 level usually is characterized by a more reduced foraminal height compared to the other lumbar levels (3,7). Hence, 25% to 30% of the foramen is used for neural tissue at this level, whereas at most lumbar levels 7% to 22% of the foramen is used by neural tissue. Some general statements about the available space in the intervertebral neural canal may be misleading. Observation of the lateral third of the intervertebral foramen alone can give a misleading impression of the real neural content of the foraminal canal (11).

The course inside the neural canal may be altered considerably in the presence of anomalous lumbosacral nerve roots. Deviating configurations may result from an abnormally high or an abnormally low level of emanation (Fig. 10A), conjoined nerve roots that are tented over a pedicle, a double set of nerve roots occupying more space than expected, or a more complex configuration, such as an anastomosis between nerve roots of adjacent levels (24). An incidence of 14% of lumbosacral nerve root anomalies, mostly conjoined nerve roots, encountered at dissection of 100 spinal canals led to the suggestion to use the term variants rather than anomalies (19). Some variation also exists in the position of the dorsal root ganglia relative to the intervertebral foramen. An intraforaminal position seems to be more common at the L-4 and L-5 levels, and an intraspinal localization has to be expected for the S-1 dorsal nerve root ganglion. An intraspinal position of L-4 and L-5 dorsal nerve root ganglia renders them more susceptible to compression from a superior articular facet or a bulging disc. Cases of extraforaminal positions of dorsal root ganglia have been reported at L-4 and L-5 levels (20).

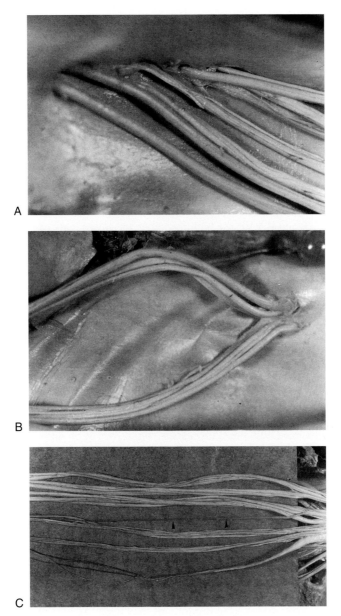

FIG. 10. Devoid of their arachnoidal coverings, multiple nerve roots of the cauda equina reach the dural sleeves. **A:** Unusual number of exiting dural sleeves at sacral levels. **B:** Detail showing anterior and posterior nerve roots leaving the dural sac, initially via separate meningeal sleeves. **C:** Intradural anastomosis between adjacent nerve roots *(arrowheads)*.

The same authors also drew attention to the variable nerve filament contents of ventral and dorsal roots (Fig. 10A–C).

The sinuvertebral nerve(s) and a number of spinal branches of the segmental lumbar artery and radicular veins run through the neural canal at this level. Containing both sympathetic and somatic nerve fibers, the sinuvertebral nerve serves the laterodorsal outer annulus of the intervertebral disc, the PLL, the anterior two thirds of the dural sac, and the anterior vascular plexus (6,14). An overview of patterns of distribution of sinuvertebral nerve within the spinal canal and the according levels of innervation was given by Groen (14).

With an improved strategy for studying vascular details *in vitro*, using injection techniques in strictly controlled and refined dissection conditions, Crock (9) clearly illustrated the typical segmental arrangement of radicular arterial blood supply. Radicular branches were followed from their origin at the lumbar artery along their course through the intervertebral foramen, within the dural sleeves up to their junction with the anterior longitudinal spinal artery on the midline of the cord and conus medullaris or with the posterolateral longitudinal spinal artery at each side. Although these radicular arteries show variance in their diameter, previous reports about a restricted number of segmental radicular arteries have to be revisited. Multiple fine anastomosing arteries exist in human nerve root ganglia, presumably in response to intensive metabolic demand (42). Numerous fine blood vessels, often with a convoluted course, accompany the nerve filaments along their course in the neural canal.

Veins of the AIVVP and PIVVP use both the upper and lower parts of the neural foramen to exit the spinal canal. Crock (9) pointed out that blood flows centrifugally in the radicular veins of the cauda equina. At their connection with the internal venous plexus at the onset of the nerve root sheaths, valvelike structures prevent reflux from the plexus toward the radicular veins.

The remaining space in the foraminal tunnel is filled by adipose tissue and connective tissue. The adipose tissue is assumed to provide a biomechanical supportive function for the structures passing through the intervertebral exit zone (31). Beside additional or missing nerve roots, the degree of lordosis and the effects of ageing on the shape and dimensions of vertebral bodies and intervertebral discs may influence the available exit area.

If the opercula of Forestier and Tinel (48) are considered the medial and lateral parts of the pedicular zone, this course of the canal can be compared to a drum with variable diameter, obtruded by two perforated membranes giving passage to nerve roots, the spinal nerve, and blood vessels entering or exiting the spinal canal. Along its course, an important part of the lateral canal is remarkably filled with connective tissue strands attaching the dural sleeves to the walls of the neural foramen (cf. Hofmann's type 4 attachments), some of them representing a network around the nerve roots and exiting rami.

At the end of the lateral neural canals, one or more transforaminal and corporotransverse ligaments may influence the exit zone of intervertebral foramina. Transforaminal ligaments originate from the inferior or superior articular process or from the capsule of the zygapophyseal joint, run ventrally, and insert either above (superior type) on the posterolateral edge of the intervertebral disc (intermedium type) or distally from it (inferior type). Corporotransverse ligaments originate from the posterolateral aspect of the intervertebral disc and run in a dorsal direction to insert on the transverse process of either the cranial or the caudal vertebra. Regarding their high incidences, these ligaments are no longer considered anomalies. On CT and magnetic resonance images they may be recognized as a single band, a group of bands, or a fan-shaped fibrous structure (25). They may reduce by about 31% the superoinferior distances of the outlets of neuroforamina (3). Further study is needed to clarify their clinical importance with respect to entrapment of neural structures (25).

Considering the complexity of these numerous ligaments, we agree with the report of Hogan (18), who pointed out that the opercula probably represent artifacts that result from preservation techniques, although parts of this network may show membranelike aspects, both in the dissection room and on medical images.

CONCLUDING REMARKS

The question as to whether the epidural space represents a potential or a real space becomes less controversial if a number of typical anatomic features are considered in combination.

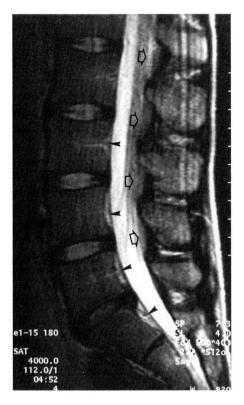

FIG. 11. Level- and intralevel-dependent variable appearance of the anterior *(arrowheads)* and posterior epidural space *(open arrows)* with repetitive compartments.

Along successive vertebral segments, the anterior epidural space, the posterior epidural space, and the lateral neural canal show a variable appearance with repetitive compartments (18). Whereas the anterior epidural space is particularly well developed behind the vertebral bodies, the posterior epidural space and the lateral recess develop their compartmental structure at the transition between two segmental levels (Fig. 11). Thus, the dimensions of the epidural space are not only level dependent, but within one level they also depend on fluctuating bony and/or soft tissue boundaries. Possible anatomic variations of the canals and their content must be added to the typical local morphology, as they appear when passing through different levels of the central spinal canal and through different zones of the lateral neural canals and thus determine the available epidural space. Soft tissues, in turn, may show different fluid contents as a function of time (blood vessels, subarachnoid space). Moreover, through changing postures, spinal shrinkage, and movement, the epidural space is constantly modified at any particular level as a result of the trimming action on the spinal syndesmoses, symphyses, and synovial joints.

REFERENCES

1. Amonoo-Kuofi HS, Patel PJ, Fatani JA. Transverse diameter of the lumbar spinal canal in normal adult Saudis. *Acta Anat* 1990;137:124–128.
2. Atila B, Yazici M, Kopuz C, Baris S, Balçik C. The shape of the lumbar vertebral canal in newborns. *Spine* 1997;22:2469–2472.
3. Bakkum BW, Mestan M. The effects of transforaminal ligaments on the sizes of T11 to L5 human intervertebral foramina. *J Manipulative Physiol Ther* 1994;17:517–522.
4. Barbaix E, Girardin MD, Hoppner JP, Van Roy P, Clarijs JP. Anterior sacrodural attachments: Trolard's ligaments revisited. *Manual Ther* 1996;2:88–91.

5. Bashline SD, Bilott JR, Ellis JP. Meningovertebral ligaments and their putative significance in low back pain. *J Manipulative Physiol Ther* 1996;19:593–596.
6. Bogduk N, Tynan W, Wilson AS. The nerve supply to the human intervertebral disc. *J Anat* 1981;132:39–56.
7. Bogduk N, Twomey LT. *Clinical anatomy of the lumbar spine*. Melbourne: Churchill Livingstone, 1991.
8. Crock HV. Normal and pathological anatomy of the lumbar spinal nerve root canals. *J Bone Joint Surg* 1981; 63-B:487–490.
9. Crock HV. *An atlas of vascular anatomy of the skeleton and spinal cord*. London: Martin Dunitz, 1996.
10. Eisenstein S. The trefoil configuration of the lumbar vertebral canal: a study of South African skeletal material. *J Bone Joint Surg* 1980;62-B:73–77.
11. Giles LGF. A histological investigation of human lower lumbar intervertebral canal (foramen) dimensions. *J Manipulative Physiol Ther* 1994;17:4–14.
12. Gillot C. Radio-anatomie du système azygos inférieur des veines ovariennes et spermatiques. *Phlébologie* 1993; 46:355–388.
13. Gouzien P, Cazalbou C, Boyer B, Darodes de Tailly P, Guenec Y, Sénécail B. Measurements of the normal lumbar spinal canal by computed tomography. *Surg Radiol Anat* 1990;12:143–148.
14. Groen GJ. De innervatie van de wervelkolom bij de mens. *Ned Tijdschr Manuele Ther* 1991;10:48–60.
15. Hasue M, Kikuchi S, Sakuyama Y, Ito T. Anatomic study of the interrelation between lumbosacral nerve roots and their surrounding tissues. *Spine* 1983;8:50–58.
16. Heytens S, Barbaix E, Van Roy P, Clarijs JP. A retrospective study of medial and paramedial attachments in CT-scans: preliminary results. Thesis. September 1999.
17. Hofmann M. Die Befestigung der Dura mater im Wirbelcanal. *Arch Anat Physiol* 1898;403:403–410.
18. Hogan QH. Lumbar epidural anatomy: a new look by cryomicrotome section. *Anesthesiology* 1991;75:767–775.
19. Kadish LJ, Simmons EH. Anomalies of the lumbosacral nerve roots: an anatomical investigation and myelographic study. *J Bone Joint Surg* 1984;66-B:411–416.
20. Kikuchi S, Sato K, Konno S, Hasue M. Anatomic and radiographic study of dorsal root ganglia. *Spine* 1994; 19:6–11.
21. Larsen JL, Smith D. Size of the subarachnoid space in stenosis of the lumbar canal. *Acta Radiol Diagn* 1980; 21:627–632.
22. Lee HM, Kim NH, Kim HJ, Chung IH. Morphometric study of the lumbar spinal canal in the Korean population. *Spine* 1995;20:1679–1684.
23. Lissens J. *Left-right asymmetries of lumbar vertebrae*. Licentiate thesis (in Dutch). Brussels: Vrije Universiteit Brussel, 1996.
24. Neidre A, MacNab I. Anomalies of the lumbosacral nerve roots, Review of 16 cases and classification. *Spine* 1983;8:294–299.
25. Nowicki BH, Haughton VM. Neural foraminal ligaments of the lumbar spine: appearance at CT and MR imaging. *Radiology* 1992;182:257–264.
26. Olszewski AD, Yaszemski MJ, White AA III. The anatomy of the human lumbar ligamentum flavum. *Spine* 1996;21:2307–2312.
27. Panjabi M, Goel V, Oxland T, et al. Human lumbar vertebrae, quantitative three-dimensional anatomy. *Spine* 1992;17:299–306.
28. Panjabi M. The stabilizing system of the spine, Part I. Function, dysfunction, adaptation, and enhancement. *J Spinal Disord* 1992;5:383–389.
29. Papp T, Porter RW. Changes of the lumbar spinal canal proximal to spina bifida occulta. *Spine* 1994;19: 1508–1511.
30. Papp T, Porter RW, Aspden RM. The growth of the lumbar vertebral canal. *Spine* 1994;19:2770–2773.
31. Parke WW. Clinical anatomy of the lower lumbar spine. In: Kambin P, ed. *Arthroscopic microdiscectomy: minimal intervention in spinal surgery*. Baltimore: Urban & Schwarzenberg, 1991.
32. Parke WW, Watanabe R. Adhesions of the ventral lumbar dura: an adjunct source of discogenic pain? *Spine* 1990;15:300–303.
33. Parkin IG, Harrison GR. The topographical anatomy of the lumbar epidural space. *J Anat* 1985;144:211–217.
34. Piera V, Rodriguez A, Cobos A, Hernández R, Cobos P. Morphology of the lumbar vertebral canal. *Acta Anat* 1988;131:35–40.
35. Plaisant O, Sarrazin JL, Cosnard G, Schill H, Gillot C. The lumbar anterior epidural cavity: the posterior longitudinal ligament, the anterior ligaments of the dura mater and the anterior internal vertebral venous plexus. *Acta Anat* 1996;155:274–281.
36. Rauschning W. Computed tomography and cryomicrotomy of lumbar spine specimens: a new technique for multiplanar anatomic correlation. *Spine* 1983;8:170–180.
37. Rauschning W, Bergström K, Pech P. Correlative craniospinal anatomy studies by computed tomography and cryomicrotomy. *J Comput Assist Tomogr* 1983;7:9–13.
38. Rauschning W. Detailed sectional anatomy of the spine. In: Rothman SLG, Glenn WV, eds. *Multiplanar CT of the spine*. Baltimore: University Park Press, 1985:33–85.
39. Rauschning W. Normal and pathologic anatomy of the lumbar root canals. *Spine* 1987;12:1008–1019.
40. Rauschning W. Anatomy and pathology of the lumbar spine. In: Frymoyer JW, ed. *The adult spine: principles and practice*. New York: Raven Press, 1991;1465–1486.
41. Rothman SLG, Glenn WV. *Multiplanar CT of the spine*. Baltimore: University Park Press, 1985.

42. Rydevik BL. The effects of compression on the physiology of nerve roots. *J Manipulative Physiol Ther* 15, 1992;15:62–66.

43. Scapinelli R. The meningovertebral ligaments as a barrier to the side-to-side migration of extruded lumbar disc herniations. *Acta Orthopaed Belg* 1992;58:436–441.

44. Schellinger D, Manz H, Vidic B, et al. Disk fragment migration. *Radiology* 1990;175:831–836.

45. Schönström N, Lindahl S, Willén J, Hansson T. Dynamic changes in the dimensions of the lumbar spinal canal: an experimental study in vitro. *J Orthopaed Res* 1989;7:115–121.

46. Semaan I, Skalli W, Veron S, Templier A, Lavaste F. Anatomie quantitative tridimensionelle du rachis lombaire. *Arch Physiol Biochem* 1998;106:73.

47. Spencer DL, Irwin GS, Miller JAA. Anatomy and significance of fixation of the lumbosacral nerve roots in sciatica. *Spine* 1983;8:672–679.

48. Testut L, Latarjet A. *Traité d'anatomie humaine, Tome III.* Paris: Doin & Cie, 1949.

49. Trolard D. Recherches sur l'anatomie des meninges spinales des nerfs sacrés et du filum terminale dans le canal sacré. *Arch Physiol* 1888;2:191–199.

50. Twomey L, Taylor J. Age changes in the lumbar spinal canal and intervertebral canals. *Paraplegia* 1988;26: 238–249.

51. Van Roy P, Caboor D, De Boelpaep S, Barbaix E, Clarijs JP. Left-right asymmetries and other common anatomical variants of the first cervical vertebra, Part I: left-right asymmetries in C1 vertebrae. *Manual Ther* 1997;2:24–36.

52. Wang TM, Shih C. Morphometric variations of the lumbar vertebrae between Chinese and Indian Adults. *Acta Anat* 1992;144:23–29.

53. Wiltse LL, Berger P, McCullough J. A system for reporting the size and location of a lesion in the spine. Lecture held at the Congress of the International Society for the Study of the Lumbar Spine, Chicago, Illinois, May 20–24, 1992.

54. Wiltse LL, Fonseca AS, Amster J, Dimartino P, Ravessoud FA. Relationship of the dura, Hofmann's ligaments, Batson's plexus, and a fibrovascular membrane lying on the posterior surface of the vertebral bodies and attaching to the deep layer of the posterior longitudinal ligament: an anatomical, radiologic and clinical study. *Spine* 1993;18:1030–1043.

55. Yong-Hing K, Reilly J, Kirkaldy-Willis WH. The ligamentum flavum. *Spine* 1976;1:226–234.

56. Yoshida M, Shima K, Taniguchi Y, Tamaki T, Tanaka T. Hypertrophied ligamentum flavum in lumbar spinal canal stenosis. *Spine* 1992;17:1353–1360.

57. Zarzur E. Anatomic studies of the human lumbar ligamentum flavum. *Anesth Analg* 1984;63:499–502.

Lumbar Spinal Stenosis
edited by Robert Gunzburg and Marek Szpalski
Lippincott Williams & Wilkins, Philadelphia, © 2000.

3

Mechanics of the Neural Arch

William C. Hutton and *John A. Malko

*Department of Orthopedics, Emory University School of Medicine, Atlanta,
Georgia 30033; and *Department of Radiology, Emory University School of Medicine,
Atlanta, Georgia 30322*

The relative motion between the vertebrae can be defined in terms of rotation and translation. As shown in Fig. 1, the rotations consist of torsion (i.e., rotation about the line c-c'), flexion and extension (i.e., rotation about the line b-b'), and lateral bending (i.e., rotation about the line a-a'). One or more of these rotations will generate forces that cause the spine to be compressed or stretched (i.e., displacements in the c-c' direction) or sheared (i.e., displacements in the x-y plane). These forces, in turn, are resisted by the various structures of the lumbar spine (e.g., the apophyseal joints, the ligaments), and can cause failure of one or the other of the structures if the ultimate stress is exceeded (e.g., spondylolysis). Other factors that influence the mechanics are diurnal changes in the disc (i.e., the disc gets bigger during the night when a person lies down to rest). Let us deal with each of these factors in turn.

TORSION

Axial rotation of the lumbar spine is limited to about 1 to 2 degrees of clockwise or counterclockwise rotation, although this may be slightly more if the cartilage on the facet surfaces is thinned (Fig. 2A). Axial rotation of the lumbar spine takes place about a center of rotation in the posterior disc or neural canal (2,6). The center of rotation is determined by mechanical compromise between the different structures resisting rotation. If axial rotation of the lumbar spine were to occur about some axis posterior to the apophyseal joints, it would be resisted most strongly by the fibers of the anterior annulus fibrosus because the posterior annulus would be nearer to the center of the rotation. The apophyseal joints are oriented to resist axial rotation and protect the posterior annulus from the effects of torsion.

FLEXION

The capsular ligaments of the apophyseal joints play the dominant role in resisting flexion of an intervertebral joint (Fig. 2B). In full flexion, as determined by the elastic limit of the supraspinous and interspinous ligaments, they provide ~40% of the joint's resistance. The balance is made up by the disc (~30%), the supraspinous and interspinous ligaments (~20%), and the ligamentum flavum (~10%) (3).

The supraspinous and interspinous ligaments are damaged first in hyperflexion, followed

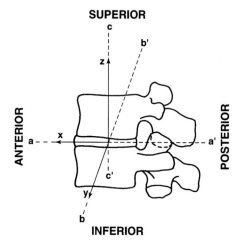

FIG. 1. The three axes of rotation (a-a′, b-b′, and c-c′) and the three directions of translation (x, y, and z) for an intervertebral joint.

by the capsular ligaments and then the disc. However, bending forward and to one side could damage the capsular ligaments first because the component of lateral flexion will produce extra stretching of the capsule away from the side of bending while not affecting the supraspinous and interspinous ligaments, which lie on the axis of lateral bending.

In flexion, as in torsion, the apophyseal joints protect the intervertebral disc. Once the posterior ligaments have been sprained in hyperflexion, the wedged disc is liable to prolapse if subjected to a high compressive force.

COMPRESSION

Experiments using cadaveric lumbar motion segments have shown that, provided the lumbar spine is slightly flattened (as occurs in erect sitting or heavy lifting), all the intervertebral compressive force is resisted by the disc. However, when lordotic postures, such as erect

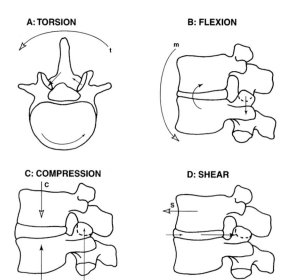

FIG. 2. The apophyseal joints and the intervertebral disc share in resisting torsion, flexion, compression, and shear. The proportional resistance of each structure is represented by the size of the *solid arrowheads*.

standing, are held for long periods, the facet tips do make contact with the laminae of the subjacent vertebra and bear about one sixth of the compressive force (Fig. 2C) (4). This contact may well be of clinical significance because it will result in high stresses on the tips of the facets and possible nipping of the joint capsules, which are well innervated. Disc narrowing results in as much as 70% of the intervertebral compressive force being transmitted across the apophyseal joints. With increasing extension of an intervertebral joint, the compressive force transmitted across the apophyseal joints increases, and it is likely that extension movements are limited by this bony contact. Thus, it is possible that the hyperextension movements could cause backward bending of the neural arch, eventually resulting in spondylolysis, but only as a fatigue fracture.

SHEAR

When an intervertebral joint is loaded in shear (Fig. 2D), the apophyseal joint surfaces resist about one half of the shear force, whereas the disc resists the remaining half (7). However, this passive resistance to shear is complicated by muscle action. The muscle tips attached to the posterior part of the neural arch brace it by pulling downward. This prevents any backward bending of the neural arch and brings the facets together more firmly (12). This means that, in the intact joint, the intervertebral disc is not subjected to shear force (only to pure compression) and that the intervertebral shear force is resisted by the apophyseal joints. This produces a high interfacet force.

This interfacet force is unlikely to produce damage in erect postures because it is resisted across the broad parallel articular cartilage joint surfaces. However, in full flexion, when the shear force is at its highest and the facets are inclined toward one another, there will be high-stress concentrations in the cartilage in the upper margins of the joint, and these could possibly initiate degenerative changes. Also, when an individual marches with a heavy pack, the interfacet force can be high enough to cause spondylolysis as a mechanical fatigue fracture (8).

ARTICULAR TROPISM

If the articular facets of the apophyseal joints are symmetrically oriented (Fig. 3A), they will resist forward shear forces (i.e., forces in the plane of the disc) equally. However, if they are asymmetrically oriented (articular tropism) they will resist forward shear forces unequally (Fig. 3B), and sustained or cyclic shear forces can produce joint rotation toward the side of the more oblique facet. This tendency to rotate might place additional stress on the annulus fibrosus of the intervertebral disc and could be a contributing factor to fatigue damage of these fibers (10).

DIURNAL CHANGES AFFECTING THE NEURAL CANAL

When we sleep, the loading on the intervertebral discs is reduced, and the relatively unopposed disc swelling pressure results in the discs absorbing fluid and increasing in volume (19). The absorbed fluid is expelled during the day when the loading of the spine is increased. Thus, there is diurnal variation in the fluid content and height of the discs as well as the extent of disc bulge (Fig. 4).

The average diurnal variation in human stature is about 19 mm (18), which is mostly attributable to changes in disc height (11). A 19-mm change in structure corresponds to a change of about 1.5 mm in the height of each lumbar disc (1). Changes in disc height are

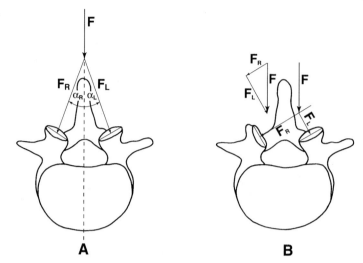

FIG. 3. A: The forces acting on the symmetric facets are shared equally between the facets. **B:** When the facets are asymmetrically oriented (articular tropism), the force on the facets is shared unequally, which can produce rotation (or torsion) of the intervertebral joint in the transverse plane.

caused by fluid exchange and creep deformation of the annulus fibrosus (13). The relative importance of each mechanism probably depends on the severity and duration of loading (1) and factors such as the age and degree of disc degeneration. The diurnal disc height change of 1.5 mm is of a similar magnitude to the normal, age-related narrowing of the lumbar discs (14).

Radial bulging of the disc has been observed to increase after creep loading (13). The size of this increase has not been measured directly, but it may be inferred from the results of Brinckmann and Horst (5). They altered the volume of the disc by either injecting fluid into it or fracturing the vertebral body endplate. They found that the change in radial bulging was

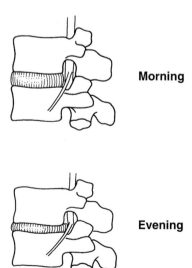

Morning

Evening

FIG. 4. Compared to morning, the disc in the evening is thinner and bulges more.

about one third of the change in disc height. This suggests that the diurnal reduction in disc height of 1.5 mm is accompanied by an increased radial bulge of about 0.5 mm. For comparison, the increased radial bulge caused by increasing the compressive force on the spine from 300 N (lying in bed) to 1,000 N (light manual work) is only about 0.2 mm (5). Diurnal bulging will have clinical implications when the central or root canal is stenotic. The width of the intervertebral foramen is normally about 8 to 10 mm (16), but it can be much less in the root canal and the lateral recess.

The experimental evidence can be summarized as follows: with creep, as occurs in walking during the day, the intervertebral discs lose height and bulge more (Fig. 4). In life, these changes will depend on the severity of loading on the spine: heavy labor will have a greater effect and in less time than sedentary activity.

An magnetic resonance image (MRI)-based protocol has been used to measure disc volume over time in subjects as their disc adjusted to various load changes (15). The most interesting of these load changes were those brought about by having the subjects carry a 20-kg backpack for 3 hours. Disc volumes were measures by taking MRI scans at strategic times during a protocol that involved walking with a 20-kg backpack for 3 hours and resting for 3 additional hours while lying in the MRI scanner. These studies allowed the measurement of disc volume as it recovered after removal of the backpack. These measurements showed that there is a substantial volume decrease caused by carrying the backpack and then a gradual increase in volume after removal of the backpack. These data showed that after removal of the backpack, the normal disc undergoes volume changes in the 3% to 7% range (mean 5%). By assuming an initial 75% fluid content, the mean of 5% volume change translates into a corresponding mean of 7% fluid change.

SPONDYLOLYSIS

In spondylolysis, a break occurs in one or both sides of the narrowed region of the neural arch, the pars interarticulars (17,20). Although spondylolysis occurs most commonly in the neural arch of the fifth lumbar vertebra, upper lumbar vertebrae may be affected. Associated with spondylolysis is the tendency to spondylolisthesis, which can take place (without a break occurring in the neural arch) either as a result of erosive changes in the apophyseal joints or in association with elongation of the neural arch.

To produce a spondylolytic fracture, sufficient stress must be generated across the pars interarticulars. This stress is caused by forces acting on that part of the neural arch behind the pars interarticulars. Using free body analysis, it can be shown that there are two forces acting on a lumbar intervertebral joint: (i) a compressive force and (ii) a shear force (12). It is the shear force that is relevant to the neural arch (and spondylolysis).

If we assume that the soft tissues outside the spine make no significant contribution to resisting the shear force in the plane of the lumbar joint, there are two structures within the spine that oppose this shear force: (i) the intervertebral disc and (ii) the neural arch of the lumbar vertebra through its inferior articular processes. Experiments showed that the intervertebral shear is resisted about equally between the intervertebral disc and the neural arch (12), although this proportion changes as the disc (a viscoelastic structure) creeps with time. Using free body analysis and knowing that the intervertebral shear force is shared about equally between the disc and the neural arch, the force on the apophyseal joints can be calculated, as can the force exerted by the muscle slips attached to the neural arch. However, as noted previously, this passive resistance to shear is complicated by muscle action. The muscle tips attached to the posterior part of the neural arch brace it by pulling downward. This prevents any backward bending of the neural arch and brings the facets more firmly together (12).

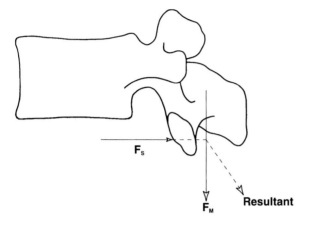

FIG. 5. In the normal joint, there is little shear force on the disc (see text), but a high interfacet force. This interfacet force combines with the force exerted by the muscle slips attached to the neural arch to give a resultant force that acts down the plane of the laminae. When there is a spondylolytic fracture, the mechanics are disturbed and all the shear force acts on the disc, which tends to produce spondylolisthesis.

This means that, in the intact joint, the intervertebral disc is not subjected to shear force (only to pure compression) and that the intervertebral shear force is resisted by the apophyseal joints; this produces a high interfacet force. Experiments using cadaveric vertebrae showed that the neural arch is a relatively strong structure that is well able to resist the combination of these two forces (9), one from the apophyseal facets and the other from the muscle slips on the neural arch (Fig. 5) that are applied to it in life. Further experiments using cadaveric vertebrae showed that the pars interarticulars of the neural arch is vulnerable to mechanical fatigue (8).

Thus, the neural arch, at the pars interarticulars, has something to spare in terms of strength, and spondylolytic fractures seems most commonly due to fatigue. A spondylolytic fatigue fracture can occur in the fully flexed or partially flexed postures, provided a cyclic loading situation is set up: walking for long periods with a heavy pack and bending forward continually lifting weights are such situations.

REFERENCES

1. Adams MA, Dolan P, Hutton WC. Diurnal variations in the stresses in the lumbar spine. *Spine* 1987;12:130–137.
2. Adams MA, Hutton WC. The relevance of torsion to the mechanical derangement of the lumbar spine. *Spine* 1981;6:241–248.
3. Adams MA, Hutton WC, Stott JRR. The resistance to flexion of the lumbar intervertebral joint. *Spine* 1980;5: 245–253.
4. Adams MA, Hutton WC. The effect of posture on the role of the apophyseal joints in resisting intervertebral compressive force. *J Bone Joint Surg* 1980;62B:358–362.
5. Brinkman P, Horst M. The influence of vertebral fracture, intradiscal injection and partial discectomy on the radial bulge and height of human lumbar discs. *Spine* 1985;10:138–145.
6. Cossette JW, Farfan HF, Robertson GH, Wells RV. The instantaneous centre of rotation of the third lumbar intervertebral joint. *J Biomech* 1971;4:149–53.
7. Cyron BM, Hutton WC, Stott JRR. Spondylolysis—the shearing stiffness of the lumbar intervertebral joint. *Acta Orthop Belg* 1980;45:459–469.
8. Cyron BM, Hutton WC. The fatigue strength of the lumbar neural arch in spondylolysis. *J Bone Joint Surg* 1978;60B:234–238.
9. Cyron BM, Hutton WC. Variations in the amount and distribution of cortical bone across the partes interarticulars of L5: a predisposing factor in spondylolysis. *Spine* 1979;4:163–167.
10. Cyron BM, Hutton WC. Articular tropism and stability of the lumbar spine. *Spine* 1980;5:168–172.
11. De Pukey P. The physiological oscillation of the length of the body. *Acta Orthop Scand* 1935;6:338.
12. Hutton WC, Stott JRR, Cyron BM. Is spondylolysis a fatigue fracture? *Spine* 1977;2:202–229.
13. Koeller W, Finke F, Hartmann F. Biomechanical behaviour of human intervertebral discs subjected to long-lasting axial loading. *Biorheology* 1984;21:675–686.
14. Koeller W, Muehlhaus S, Meir W, Hartmann F. Biomechanical properties of human intervertebral discus subjected to axial dynamic compression influence of age degeneration. *J Biomech* 1986;19:807–816.

15. Malko JA, Hutton WC, Fajman WA. An *in vivo* magnetic imaging study of changes in volume (and fluid content) of the lumbar intervertebral discs during a simulated diurnal load cycle. *Spine* 1999;24:1015–1022.
16. Panjabi MM, Takata K, Goel VK. Kinematics of lumbar intervertebral foramen. *Spine* 1983;8:348–357.
17. Stewart TD. The age incidence of neural arch defects in Alaskan natives, considered from the standpoint of etiology. *J Bone Joint Surg* 1953;35A:937–950.
18. Tyrrell AR, Reilly T, Troup JDG. Circadian variation in stature and the effects of spinal loading. *Spine* 1985; 10:161–164.
19. Urban JP, McMullin JF. The water content of post-mortem intervertebral discs. *Spine* 1988;13:179–187.
20. Wiltse LL, Widell EH, Jackson DW. Fatigue fracture: the basis lesion in isthmic spondylolisthesis. *J Bone Joint Surg* 1975;57A:17–22.

Lumbar Spinal Stenosis
edited by Robert Gunzburg and Marek Szpalski
Lippincott Williams & Wilkins, Philadelphia, © 2000.

4

Biomechanics of Spinal Stenosis

Malcolm H. Pope

*Department of Occupational Medicine, University of Aberdeen,
Aberdeen AB25 2ZD, United Kingdom*

Low back pain and sciatica continue to occur at epidemic proportions, and our populations are getting older. An important etiology of low back pain and sciatica in older people is degenerative lumbar spine stenosis (often secondary to degenerative spondylolisthesis) caused by compression of exiting nerve roots by bone or soft tissue elements. Degenerative stenosis may be the most common cause of sciatica in those 50 years of age or older. In the older patient with degenerative changes of the lumbar spine, one of the most frequent causes of compression of the neural elements within the thecal sac is spinal stenosis. This is important because the spinal canal contains the conus terminalis and the cauda equina. Pressure on these structures may represent an emergency for the patient.

Lumbar spinal stenosis often is classified using four anatomic sites for neural compression: central, lateral recess, foraminal, and far out. Lateral stenosis is defined as an entity in which a nerve root, dorsal root, ganglion, or spinal nerve is entrapped in its pathway. Spinal stenosis often is classified into either congenital or acquired. The most common etiology of the latter kind of degenerative spinal stenosis is due to osteophyte formation, disc bulging, facet joint hypertrophy, lamella subluxation, or ligamentous thickening (9). Ultimately, these are all due to altered mechanical forces.

FUNCTIONAL ANATOMY AND STENOSIS

Measurements of the size and shape of the lumbar canal have resulted from interest in the etiology of spinal stenosis. Ultrasonic studies have shown that patients with lumbar disc herniation have narrower diameters than patients with less severe back symptoms whose diameters, in turn, are less than those in symptom-free subjects (14). Hurme et al. (4) found little correlation among radiographic measures of canal size, stature, or age. Only the interpedicular distances and the anteroposterior diameter of the intervertebral foramen at L3 were greater in males than in females. In all patients, the size of the canal was smaller for those with a pathologic myelogram than in either patients with low back pain or cadavers.

Iatrogenic changes can occur. Spondylolisthesis can occur after surgical reduction of the facet joints during decompression for spinal stenosis of the lumbar spinal canal or nerve roots. It is most common at the L4–5 level and probably results from the high compression and shear forces found at this level. This is probably due to lumbar lordosis and the lack of ligamentous support of the pelvis compared to the L5–S1 level (1,2). Grobler et al. (3) used midpedicle and superior endplate computed tomographic cuts to show that the coronal

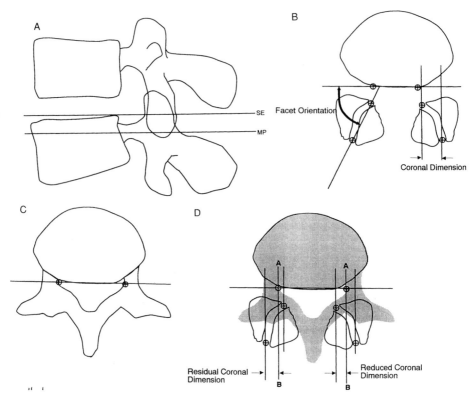

FIG. 1. A: Computed tomographic cuts were taken through the level of the superior endplate of L5 (SE) and the midpedicle (MP) of L5. The SE cut is used to characterize the facet joint morphology, whereas the MP cut is used to define the coronal extent of the spinal canal and the lateral extent of an ideal pedicle-to-pedicle decompression. **B:** Diagrammatic representation of a computed tomographic cut at the superior endplate of L5. Facet joint orientation and facet joint coronal dimension are measured from this cut. These measurements are based on the coronal plane, which is identified from points marked on the back of the vertebral body. **C:** Diagrammatic representation of computed tomographic cut through the MP of L5. The medial border of each pedicle defines the lateral extent of a pedicle-to-pedicle decompression, which restores the coronal dimension of the spinal canal at L4-5. **D:** Superimposition of the SE and MP cuts allows accurate representation of facet joint and pedicle spatial relationships. Using this technique both the amount of joint to be resected (the reduced coronal dimension medial to the line AB) and the amount remaining (the residual coronal dimension lateral to line of AB) can be calculated.

dimension of the facet joint in degenerative spondylolisthesis is less than that of the normal population. This probably increases the stresses on the facet joint and compromises its antero-posterior stability. Furthermore, surgical decompression to restore the coronal dimensions of the canal reduces the coronal dimension of the facet joint (Fig. 1).

DEGENERATIVE CHANGES

Of increasing importance are the degenerative changes in the aging population. Schmorl and Junghanns (17) found an increasing incidence of vertebral osteophytes from the third decade onward. Osteophytes were found in 90% of all males older than 50 years and all females older than 60 years. Osteophytes also are associated with disruption of the intervertebral disc (8). Kirkaldy-Willis and Farfan (6) showed the importance of degenerative instability in the etiology of spinal stenosis. Knutson (8) and Junghanns (5) reported the instability that can be associated with disc degeneration. The altered dimensions of the motion segment leads to altered kinematics. However, the term instability is poorly defined, although Pope and Panjabi (13) suggested that instability is a mechanical entity and should be related to a loss of stiffness rather than to a clinical presentation. Kirkaldy-Willis et al. (7) pointed out that the degenerative process initially is dysfunction followed by instability and then by restabilization. The unstable phase alters both the kinetics and the kinematics of the motion segment. This phase is associated with disc height reduction, ligamentous laxity, and facet joint degeneration, which in turn leads to an even more abnormal range of motion. Remodeling (osteophyte formation) eventually will restabilize the motion segment, but stenosis may ensue. Kirkaldy-Willis contrasted lateral nerve root entrapment in which the superior facet impinges on the spinal nerve in the lateral canal to a fixed mode of nerve root entrapment with little segmental motion. Thus, the whole of the degenerative process described by Kirkaldy-Willis can result in spinal stenosis.

NEUROPHYSIOLOGY

The altered motion segment biomechanics due to degeneration or other causes of stenosis can lead to abnormal loads on the neurologic structures. These loads alter the conduction of action potentials in the nerves. Olmarker and Rydevik (11) found that double-level nerve root compression, which is the most common, had a large effect on reduction of nerve impulse conduction as compared to one vertebral segment. Takahashi et al. (19) found that double-level compression of the cauda equina can cause impairment of blood flow, not only at the compression sites but also in the intermediate nerve segments located between the two compression sites. This phenomenon occurs even at very low contact pressures. Porter and Ward (16) pointed out that the kinematics of an individual unstable motion segment will determine the pattern of symptoms.

OCCUPATIONAL FACTORS

Porter and Bewley (15) showed that a factor in the degenerative change associated with stenosis is heavy manual work. Clinical practice shows that very few of such patients are sedentary workers. There is a higher incidence in males, which could be related to heavier manual work in this group. Heavy manual work (lifting, twisting, carrying, bending) loads the motion segment abnormally and causes remodeling (Wolff's law). Thickening of the ligamentum flavum or ossification can be responsible for the stenosis, and diffuse idiopathic spinal hyperostosis can precipitate stenosis when it is associated with a congenitally small canal. However, a 10-year prospective study of the canal size by Porter and Bewley (15) showed that canal size is not a predictor for back pain in general but is a predictor for severe back pain in early working life.

BIOMECHANICS

The spine is a slender column that must be supported by the muscles for it to have adequate stability. With the muscles absent, a ligamentous spine will buckle at loads of 14 N. Thus, it is self-apparent that the muscles are extremely important, particularly in preventing adverse motion that can lead to spinal stenosis. Likewise, physical therapy may be indicated so as to improve muscular stabilization.

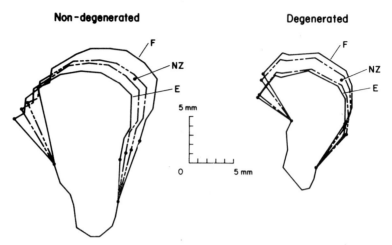

FIG. 2. Changes in the right intervertebral foramen in flexion-extension for normal and degener-ated specimens. F and E, flexion and extension under applied moments of 7.5 Nm; NZ, neutral zone.

Axial loading of the spine, particularly if associated with some bending due to lifting a burden, can displace an unstable segment and lead to symptoms. Pure axial compression of cadavaric spines decreases the cross-sectional area of the canal by an average of 50 mm (14,18). The spinal canal is markedly affected by flexion and extension. Knutson (8) used myelography in a stenotic patient and demonstrated a loss of impingement and restoration of a patent canal in the flexed position. Likewise, anatomic studies confirmed that between flexion and extension there is an average change of 40 mm in the cross section of the canal. Panjabi et al. (12) showed in cadaveric studies that the size of the foramina increased in flexion whereas the size decreased in extension. In addition, they found that nondegenerated specimens had a relatively large intervertebral foramina as compared to the degenerated specimens (Fig. 2) The foramina opened during flexion by 24% and closed during extension by 20%. The changes due to lateral bending and axial rotation were less significant.

Thus, extension seems to affect both the lateral and central canal. In severe stenosis, even the slightest degree of extension may compress neural elements, especially in degenerated specimens. In such specimens, flexion increases the available space by reducing the disc bulge and by stretching the ligamentum flavum; however, extension reduces the space as the ligamentum flavum buckles. When the spine extends, the L5 nerve root may be compressed between the superior facet and the disc.

Clinical observations show that patients with stenosis have problems with walking. Inter-mittent claudication will be one of the limiting factors in their life. Lordosis could be a factor in the increased symptoms during walking, although this has not really been proven (10). The stenotic canal seems to reduce further while walking, as in vivo measurements show that the epidural pressure increases by approximately 20 mm Hg with each step (20). This is probably due to the complex rotary movement in the spinal segments that occurs during walking that, in turn, reduces the canal cross section.

DISCUSSION

Biomechanical considerations in spinal stenosis in terms of etiology, pathomechanics, and treatment are of vital importance. The facet joints are essential for control of normal motion and serve as a control of anteroposterior slippage because of their orientation. The surgeon must consider carefully the orientation of the facet joint during decompression to avoid reduction of the coronal area and the possibility of progressive anterior slip. Occupational factors such as heavy manual work have some relevance to the increase of spinal stenosis, but further work is needed to concentrate on these issues and to weigh the relative importance of these factors against congenital factors. Should screening of canal size be done on those beginning a life of heavy manual work? Biomechanical studies have demonstrated the importance of spinal loading, such as axial loading, on reduction of canal size, particularly in a forward flexed position. Studies also have demonstrated the pathomechanics of canal reduction during extension. This is exacerbated during walking, leading to shutting of the canal and symptoms of intermittent claudication.

REFERENCES

1. Adams MA, Hutton WC. The effect of posture on the role of the apophysial joints in resisting intervertebral compressive forces. *J Bone Joint Surg* 1980;62B:358–362.
2. Adams MA, Hutton WC. The mechanical function of the lumbar apophyseal joints. *Spine* 1983;8:327–329.
3. Grobler LJ, Robertson PA, Novotny JE, Ahern JW. Decompression for degenerative spondylolisthesis and spinal stenosis at L4-5. The effects on facet joint morphology. *Spine* 1993;18:1475–1480.
4. Hurme M, Alaranta H, Aalto T, Knuts L-R, Vanharanta H, Troup D. Lumbar spinal canal size of sciatica patients. *Acta Radiol* 1989;30:353–358.
5. Junghanns H. Spondylolisthesen ohne Spalt im Zwischengelenkstuck. *Arch Orthop Unfall Chir* 1930;29: 118–127.
6. Kirkaldy-Willis WH, Farfan HF. Instability of the lumbar spine. *Clin Orthop* 1982;165:110–113.
7. Kirkaldy-Willis WH, Wedge JH, Yong-Hing K, Tchang S, de Korompay V, Shannon R. Lumbar spinal nerve lateral entrapment. *Clin Orthop* 1982;169:171–178.
8. Knutson F. The instability associated with disc degeneration in the lumbar spine. *Acta Radiol* 1944;25:593–609.
9. Naylor A. Factors in the development of the spinal stenosis syndrome. *J Bone Joint Surg* 1979;61B:306–309.
10. Negrini S, Frigo C, Sibilla P. Variations of lordosis of the adolescent spine during gait. *Proc Int Soc Study Lumbar Spine* 1997;24:16.
11. Olmarker K, Rydevik B. Single- versus double-level nerve root compression. An experimental study on the porcine cauda equina with nerve impulse conduction properties. *Clin Orthop* 1992;279:35–39.
12. Panjabi M, Takata K, Goel V. Kinematics of lumbar intervertebral foramen. *Spine* 1983;4:348–354.
13. Pope MH, Panjabi M. Biomechanical definitions of spinal instability. *Spine* 1984;21:2046–2052.
14. Porter RW. Spinal stenosis and neurogenic claudication. *Spine* 1996;21:2046–2052.
15. Porter RW, Bewley B. A ten year prospective study of vertebral canal size as a predictor of back pain. *Spine* 1994;19:173–175.
16. Porter RW, Ward D. Cauda equina dysfunction: the significance of multiple level pathology. *Spine* 1992;17: 9–15.
17. Schmorl G, Junghanns H. Die gesunde und kranke Wirbelsaule im Rontgenbild. *Fortschr Geb Rontgenstr* 1932; 46:361–362.
18. Schönström N, Bolender NF, Spengler DM. The pathomorphology of spinal stenosis as seen on CT scan of the lumbar spine. *Spine* 1985;10:806–811.
19. Takahashi K, Olmarker K, Holm S, Porter RW, Rydevik B. Double-level cauda equina compression: an experimental study with continuous monitoring of intraneural blood flow in the porcine cauda equina. *J Orthop Res* 1993;11:104–109.
20. Takahashi K, Kagechika K, Takino T. Changes in epidural pressure during walking in patients with lumbar spinal stenosis. *Spine* 1995;20:2746–2749.

SECTION II

Classification and Etiology

Lumbar Spinal Stenosis
edited by Robert Gunzburg and Marek Szpalski
Lippincott Williams & Wilkins, Philadelphia, © 2000.

5

Congenital versus Acquired Lumbar Canal Stenosis

Henry V. Crock and M. Carmel Crock

Spinal Disorders Unit, Cromwell Hospital, London W8 5JN, United Kingdom

Until the middle of the 20th century, little attention was paid to clinical problems arising from spinal stenosis. In 1945, Sarpenyer (7) described congenital strictures of the lumbar canal with spastic diplegia in nine young children and one adult. In 1954, Verbeist (11), a neurosurgeon from the University of Utrecht in Holland, published his article, ''A radicular syndrome from developmental narrowing of the lumbar vertebral canal,'' which dealt with seven cases. The interpedicular distances in each case were normal compared with measurements from x-rays of 100 asymptomatic Dutch patients. Although the title of the article included the phrase ''developmental narrowing of the lumbar vertebral canal,'' Verbeist concluded that the stenosis was due to encroachment on the spinal canal by the articular processes. He actually was describing degenerative lumbar canal stenosis, which by far is more common than so-called congenital stenosis. Verbeist (12) went on to publish a seminal monograph on ''Neurogenic Intermittent Claudication,'' in which he described an instrument called a stenosimeter for measuring the dimensions of the spinal canal at operation. Epstein and Malis (3) published an article on ''Compression of spinal cord and cauda equina in achondroplastic dwarfs.'' The first American article dealing with nerve root compression associated with narrowing of the lumbar spinal canal was not published until 1962 (2). It was an extremely important article in which attention was drawn to thickening of the laminae as a contributing cause of the stenosis. The importance of this observation still is overlooked frequently, as evidenced by the fact that radiologic reports rarely mention laminal dimensions. An important contribution from Schatzker and Pennal (8) in Canada followed in 1968 in their article ''Spinal stenosis: a cause of cauda equina compression.'' They made the statement that ''a midline laminectomy never completely relieves the compression in spinal stenosis. This is the most important and fundamental fact to appreciate in the treatment'' (Fig. 1). However, the greater part of the credit for drawing attention to spinal stenosis as a crippling form of spinal disease was accorded to Verbeist during his long life.

Congenital lumbar stenoses are rare. They usually are identified in infancy and childhood and often are associated with generalized disorders such as achondroplasia. Stenoses may develop in several areas of the vertebral column and often lead to serious neurologic deficits, such as quadriplegia or paraplegia. Congenital hemivertebrae often occur at the thoracolumbar and cervicothoracic junctions, where progressive kyphotic deformities may develop during growth and can lead to compression of the spinal cord. The kyphosis may be controlled, in some cases by posterior spinal fusion alone, performed in early childhood.

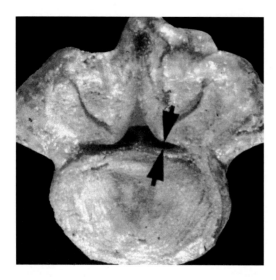

FIG. 1. Specimen from the lumbar spine showing features of central canal and bilateral nerve root canal and foraminal stenosis. Note the laminal hypertrophy and osteoarthritic changes in the facet joints and the thickened ligamentum flavum. (Courtesy of Professor W. Kirkaldy Willis, University of Saskatoon.)

Patients with these deformities are best treated by specialists in the management of spinal deformities, because complex procedures involving combined anterior and posterior spinal operations with the use of internal fixation sometimes are required to correct the deformities and prevent spinal cord injury with paraplegia. Congenital stenoses at the cervicocranial junction are rare but associated with severe cord compression that leads, if untreated, to quadriparesis and death.

Diastematomyelia is another important cause of spinal canal stenosis. Until the advent of computed tomographic examination it often went undiagnosed.

In recent years, awareness of the importance of spinal stenosis has increased, as witnessed by the growing numbers of monographs published on the condition as it affects different segments of the vertebral column (1,5,6,13).

The main focus of attention in this chapter is directed at the increasingly common problem of acquired lumbar canal stenosis. The condition occurs essentially in two forms: lateral canal stenosis and central canal stenosis. It is extremely rare for central canal stenosis to occur in isolation. Lateral canal stenosis is best described using the terms foraminal and nerve root canal stenoses, which usually are bilateral.

In assessing the degree of lumbar canal stenosis over the years, there have been many efforts made to measure various diameters of the spinal canal from plain radiographs. Jones and Thompson (4) constructed ratios based on the products of measurements of four diameters: two related to the spinal canal and two related to the vertebral bodies. From these measurements they constructed tables on the basis of which they identified large normal canals or small normal canals. Verbeist had attempted to measure the anteroposterior diameter of the lumbar canal at surgery. Others drew attention to the importance of narrowing of the interlaminar spaces and of the distances between the medial margins of the inferior facets at an affected level. With the development of modern imaging techniques, the usefulness of these different methods of mensuration has decreased. In 1985, Schönström et al. (10) concluded from their study on the pathomorphology of spinal stenosis that bony measurements alone did not reliably identify patients with spinal stenosis. They claimed that the size of the dural sac is a more reliable measure of stenosis. Although it is conceded that there are developmental differences in the size of the lumbar canal, ranging from small to large, it seems reasonable to conclude that it is necessary for some added pathologic change related to a narrow canal to develop before symptoms of spinal stenosis are produced (9).

Review of the normal anatomy of the roof of the spinal canal, the spinal canal itself, and its contents is essential if the pathologic bases of spinal stenosis are to be understood. The essential features of the roof of the lumbar canal are depicted in Figs. 1 and 2. The interlaminar space is wide. The capsular fibers of the facet joints are shown with capsular extensions running along the inferior margins of the superior lamina at the interspace. Below the facet joints, on both sides, extrasynovial fat pads can be seen. The ligamentum flavum is depicted in the interlaminar space, and its relation to the undersurface of the superior lamina is drawn in with dotted lines. There is a wide gap between the spinous processes, with that space occupied by the supraspinous and interspinous ligaments. The inferior laminal margin is partly covered by the inferior attachment of the ligamentum flavum. The depth between the laminal cortices is normally approximately 3 to 4 mm, whereas the depth of the inferior margin of the superior lamina at the interspace is likewise on the order of 4 to 5 mm.

In cases of spinal stenosis, dramatic pathologic changes in the roof of the canal occur, depending on changes in the height of the intervertebral disc itself. When the height is significantly decreased as a result of disc resorption, the interlaminar space is reduced. Laminal hypertrophy occurs, and the medial margins of both facet joints approach the midline, obstructing the view of the ligamentum flavum, which becomes thickened and buckles anteriorly into the spinal canal. This buckling contributes to the hourglass deformity of the dural sac, which can be seen on magnetic resonance images in the coronal, sagittal, and transverse planes. Hypertrophy of the laminal margins often reaches proportions between 15 and 20 mm. In addition, gangliform extrusions from the facet joints and from the region of the interspinous ligament contribute to obstruction of the spinal canal. In many cases, crescentic osteophytic outgrowths from the posterior surface of the inferior lamina related to the inferior aspects of the facet joints will develop. Radiologic reports rarely mention the laminal dimensions, which is essential information for the practicing surgeon.

In cases where the interlaminar space has been greatly reduced, shingling of the inferior

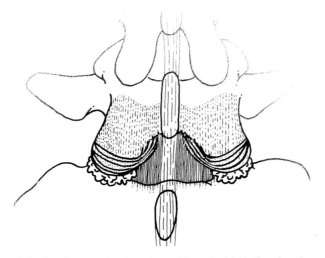

FIG. 2. Drawing of the lumbosacral spine viewed from behind showing the normal anatomic features of the interspinous ligaments and ligamentum flavum. Note the capsular fibers of the facet joints and their extensions along the inferior margin of the L5 lamina. The extrasynovial fat pads are shown below the lower margins of the facet joints.

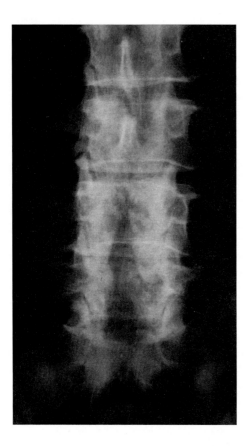

FIG. 3. Anteroposterior radiograph of the lumbar spine of a 63-year-old man presenting with severe symptoms of cauda equina claudication following two previous laminectomies. The first laminectomy was performed 20 years ago and the second 10 years before this x-ray radiograph was taken. Note regrowth of bone covering the dural sac. The laminal margins measured 27 mm at reoperation.

lamina beneath the upper lamina often will occur, and ossification of the deeper layers of the ligamentum flavum frequently is associated with it. Within the spinal canal, distortions of the nerve root canals and intervertebral foramina will result from changes in the orientation of the facet joints, particularly if there is an associated loss of intervertebral disc height. In this case, the superior facet will sublux upward toward the inferior margin of the pedicle of the superior vertebra, thereby contributing to the foraminal and nerve root canal stenoses, which usually are bilateral.

The surgeon should have a clear view in mind of the concept of the nerve root canal, which will vary in length depending on the point of takeoff from the dural sac of the nerve root sheath and on the length of its course to the intervertebral foramen just below the inferior margin of the pedicle to which it is related. In many cases, the floor of the nerve root canal will be distorted by the bulging remnants of annular fibers that intrude into the canal in cases of disc resorption.

Throughout their courses, the lumbar nerve roots are surrounded by the perineural veins of the internal vertebral venous plexus. Obstruction to theses venous pathways always occurs in cases of spinal stenosis. One of the principal aims in surgery is to relieve the perineural venous obstructions. In the presence of kissing spines, pathologic changes occur in the interspinous ligament system, with buckling and thickening of the ligament that are aggravated by gangliform changes and ectopic calcification and ossification. In such cases, the component of central canal stenosis is severe. This must be dealt with surgically, as described in Chapter 24.

In cases of spondylolysis, acquired foraminal and root canal stenoses also exist. Although the laminal pseudoarthroses usually are asymmetric, quite often the patient's symptoms are bilateral.

In patients whose symptoms have not been adequately relieved by appropriate decompressions in the lower lumbar canal, radiculography still finds a place in investigation, as an associated thoracic canal stenosis is easily overlooked.

In recent years, one of the most common causes of acquired lumbar canal stenosis results from complications of multiple spinal operations, particularly those that involved the use of internal fixation devices in association with decompressive procedures and spinal fusion, with subsequent surgery to remove the internal fixation devices. In these cases, damage to the paraspinal muscles often is extreme, and they are replaced with dense white scar tissue of fibrocartilaginous consistency, in which ectopic bone formation occurs, which further obstructs the canal. Hypertrophy of the laminal margins in such cases often will exceed 25 mm (Fig. 3). Until there is widespread awareness that this condition is produced by the inappropriate use of internal fixation devices in degenerative diseases of the spine, particularly when used in cases in which there have been several previous failed surgical procedures, repeated operations will continue to fail.

REFERENCES

1. Andersson BJ, McNeill W. *Lumbar spinal stenosis.* St. Louis: Mosby-Year Book, 1992.
2. Epstein JA, Epstein BS, Lavine L. Nerve root compression associated with narrowing of the lumbar spinal canal. *J Neurol Neurosurg Psychiatry* 1962;25:165–176.
3. Epstein JA, Malis LI. Compression of spinal cord and cauda equina in achondroplastic dwarfs. *Neurology* 1955; 5:875–881.
4. Jones RAC, Thompson JLG. The narrow lumbar canal: a clinical and radiological review. *J Bone Joint Surg Br* 1968;50:595–605.
5. Nixon JE. *Spinal stenosis.* London: Edward Arnold/Hodder & Stoughton, 1991.
6. Postacchini F. *Lumbar spinal stenosis.* New York: Springer-Verlag, 1989.
7. Sarpenyer MA. Congenital stricture of the spinal canal. *J Bone Joint Surg* 1945;27:70–79.
8. Schatzker J, Pennal GF. Spinal stenosis: a cause of cauda equina compression. *J Bone Joint Surg Br* 1968;50: 606–618.
9. Schlesinger EB, Taveras JH. Factors in the production of cauda equina syndromes in lumbar discs. *Trans Am Neurol Assoc* 1953;78:263.
10. Schönström NSR, Bolender NF, Spengler DM. The pathomorphology of spinal stenosis as seen on CT scans of the lumbar spine. *Spine* 1985;10:806–811.
11. Verbeist H. A radicular syndrome from developmental narrowing of the lumbar vertebral canal. *J Bone Joint Surg Br* 1954;36:230–237.
12. Verbeist H. *Neurogenic intermittent claudication.* Amsterdam: Elsevier Science, 1976.
13. Yonenobu K, Sakou T, Ono K. *OPLL: ossification of the posterior longitudinal ligament.* Tokyo: Springer-Verlag, 1997.

Lumbar Spinal Stenosis
edited by Robert Gunzburg and Marek Szpalski
Lippincott Williams & Wilkins, Philadelphia, © 2000.

6

Classification of Canal and Lateral Stenosis of the Lumbar Spine

Pieter F. van Akkerveeken

Rug AdviesCentrum Nederland, 3732 HC De Bilt, The Netherlands

To avoid comparing apples and oranges, terms in research must have the same meaning to everyone and, therefore, must be clearly defined. Similarly, a classification of pathologic entities is needed to enable researchers to compare studies properly and to support clinicians in deciding on a rational treatment. This chapter describes a taxonomy of lumbar stenosis, providing a comprehensive system with clearly defined terms, pathologic entities, and clinical syndromes. It is primarily aimed at the clinician who will find its use helpful to understanding the problem of stenosis in daily practice.

The use of certain terms seems to be subject to fashion. This is sometimes the consequence of a rediscovery: as early as 1891 Gowers (13) described that ''narrowing of the foramina may damage the nerve roots'' and ''radiating pains are produced, sometimes even a descending neuritis.'' Indeed, in the 1920s this concept was applied in clinical practice by Putti (27). He described extensively the pathology, clinical presentation, and treatment of what nowadays is called ''lateral degenerative stenosis'' without using the word ''stenosis.'' His experience and knowledge became obscured by the publication of Mixter and Barr (25); the era of the disc had begun.

In the 1960s the old knowledge was rediscovered: Epstein (9) described clinical entities related to entrapment of the nerve roots in what he called the lateral recess. Meanwhile, the use of the term stenosis had become widespread after the publications of Verbiest (33) in the early 1950s. Thus, the term ''lateral recess stenosis'' was created and became ''en vogue.'' In fact, what Putti had reported in the 1920s was redescribed in new terms.

In order to make an appealing classification, one sometimes has to bow to common use and include a popular term that may be linguistically incorrect. For example, Verbiest (35) originally used the term ''narrowness'' instead of ''stenosis,'' which is linguistically incorrect in the context of a narrow lumbar vertebral canal. However, the term narrowness never became commonly used.

A good system of classifications has to fulfill the following criteria:

- Terms must be well defined and appeal to common use.
- Classifications have to be easy to use and provide the clinician with information related

Reprinted with permission from van Akkerveeken PF. A taxonomy of lumbar stenosis with emphasis on clinical applicability. *Eur Spine J* 1994;3:130–136.

to the indication for treatment. In other words, the clinician should gain by the use of a classification.

• A classification should be based on one criterion, and the various classifications needed for a given problem have to form a coherent system.

TERMINOLOGY

A number of common terms are frequently used in daily practice, but often incorrectly. Therefore, key terms such as stenosis, neurogenic intermittent claudication, nerve root compression, and radiculopathy are discussed and defined.

Stenosis

According to Verbiest (34,35), stenosis is an abnormal narrowing of cavities, tubular organs, orifices, or valves capable of producing disease through its influence on the contents. Stenosis may be divided into two subclasses: transport stenosis and compressive stenosis. Transport stenosis is related to fluids and gases and manifests itself at a distance. Compressive stenosis involves compression of fixed living tissue and damage of the contents in a narrowed area, which in itself may cause effects at a distance. Lumbar stenosis is clearly a form of compressive stenosis.

Compression of nervous tissue may take place at two opposite sides of that tissue or may be circumferential. Kirkaldy Willis and Yong Hing (18) agree with this definition, although they mention only the opposite parts of the canal as the cause of compression and thus do not consider circumferential compression.

When the dura and cauda equina in the vertebral canal are compressed, central or preferably canal stenosis is present (1). In the case of entrapment of a nerve root in its pathway, one speaks of lateral stenosis (30). According to this definition the term lateral stenosis has to also be used when a nerve root is entrapped in the vertebral canal, as in lateral recess stenosis. The term nerve root pathway is therefore preferable in a classification to the term nerve root canal, which anatomically cannot cover lateral recess stenosis.

Neurogenic Intermittent Claudication

This entity is defined by Verbiest (34) as the onset of pain, tension, and weakness upon walking in one or both legs, which progressively increase until walking becomes impossible, then subsequently disappear after a period of rest. This definition implies that the causative symptoms are not present at the start of walking and that they occur after walking a small distance. Also, the symptoms should disappear after a short rest. Reading this definition carefully, one notes that the combination of pain, tension, and weakness has to be present for the diagnosis of neurogenic intermittent claudication. Therefore, the term atypical leg pain was introduced (30) for patients with only pain, for those with motor or sensory disturbances, for those in whom the leg pain decreases during sitting or squatting but does not completely disappear, and for other patients who are able to walk long distances without having to stop, although the pain in the leg increases in the first minutes of walking.

Nerve Root Compression

Patients with nerve root compression demonstrate a radicular syndrome. The clinical presentation is characterized by pain in one or both legs, often in a segmental pattern. The patient has positive signs of nerve root compression and may have a neural deficit of one nerve root. The following signs of nerve root compression (also called irritation) may be found at physical examination:

- Lasègue's test was first described by Forst (12). The affected leg is raised passively in an extended position, and at the moment of pain in the leg, the knee flexes, and subsequently hip flexion is noted. If pain persists during the second part of the maneuver, the leg pain is probably not radicular but caused by other spinal disorders or by hip joint disease. If, however, leg pain occurs only during the straight leg raising, it is assumed that the pain is radicular.
- The straight leg raising test has been described by Lazarevic (19). The affected leg is raised passively with the knee extended. When pain occurs, the angle between the extended leg and the table is noted. Often the buttock of the affected side will come up from the table at the moment of maximum straight leg raising. The same test is applied to the other leg: when raising the nonaffected leg produces pain in the affected leg, the so-called crossed leg sign is positive. This test is also called the well leg raising test of Fajerszajn (39). A positive test is considered pathognomonic for nerve root compression.
- Kemp test: In a standing position the patient bends slightly backward, tilting the trunk to one side while the examiner stands behind the patient. While holding the patient in this unstable position with his or her arms around the shoulders of the patient, he or she suddenly exerts pressure in a downward direction. Subsequently, the test is done toward the other side. The test is positive if the patient experiences leg pain during the maneuver to the homolateral side (16).
- In the bowstring test, also known as the Cram test (4), the patient may be supine or seated. The painful leg is raised while the knee is nearly fully extended. During this maneuver the sciatic nerve is pressed in the popliteal space. The test is positive if the leg pain increases during the latter part of the maneuver (8).
- For the Bragard test, the patient lies supine. The leg is raised until just below the point at which the leg pain is reproduced or increased. At that point the foot is passively dorsiflexed. If this maneuver increases the leg pain, the test is positive.
- In the Naffziger test, manual compression of the jugular veins provokes the leg pain (26).
- Patrick's test has to be negative in patients with radicular pain. The hip of the patient is passively brought into flexion, abduction, and exorotation, then subsequently extended. If pain increases during this maneuver, the hip is probably the cause of the leg pain (9).

Radiculopathy

A patient with neurologic signs of decreased function of one nerve root, a so-called nerve root deficit, has radiculopathy. Whether signs of nerve root compression are present or absent is not relevant for this diagnosis. In contrast, a patient with positive signs of nerve root compression does not necessarily have a nerve root deficit. Also, radiculopathy may occur without pain. In some patients a minor degree of radiculopathy may only be detected by neurophysiologic testing such as electromyography or evoked potentials.

PATHOLOGIC ANATOMY

The Vertebral Canal

The anterior wall consists of the posterior aspect of the vertebral body and the intervertebral disc covered by the posterior longitudinal ligament. This ligament is present mainly in the median part.

The posterior wall consists of the lamina and ligamentum flavum. The lamina viewed laterally is obliquely oriented in such a way that its proximal part is directed anteriorly and the distal part posteriorly. The ligamentum flavum is attached to the lamina distally at the anterior aspect and proximally at the posterior aspect. Laterally, the vertebral canal is partly open and partly covered by the pedicle and the medial aspect of the facet joint.

Theoretically, the anteroposterior diameter, the transverse diameter, or both may be too narrow. Indeed, in clinical practice all three possibilities have been described, although in developmental stenosis most frequently a narrowness of the anteroposterior diameter is observed (31). When both diameters are too small, circumferential stenosis is present.

Verbiest (33) was the first to recognize that the vertebral canal may be too narrow without any pathologic process: developmental stenosis. At birth, only a cartilaginous spinal column is present. During growth ossification gradually occurs. This process ends around the time that the adolescent becomes an adult. When the dimensions of the bony vertebral canal are very small, symptoms may occur at the age of about 18 years. When, however, only a mild narrowness is present, the stenosis may be asymptomatic for many years and become symptomatic when the available space has been decreased by pathologic processes such as degeneration. Therefore, Verbiest (34) differentiated between what he called ''absolute'' and ''relative'' stenosis. Absolute stenosis is present when the anteroposterior diameter of the vertebral canal in the midline (''midsagittal diameter'') is 10 mm or less. Patients with absolute stenosis have symptoms by definition: only very rarely has absolute stenosis been observed by Verbiest in asymptomatic people. The onset of symptoms is usually in late adolescence. Relative stenosis is characterized by a midsagittal diameter of 10 to 12 mm. This occurs frequently in asymptomatic people. When contributing factors are present, such as osteophyte formation at the articular processes or disc margins, a circular disc bulge due to loss of disc height and thickening of the ligamentum flavum, symptoms may arise. Diameters between 12 and 14 mm form an area of controversy, as a diameter of more than 14 mm is definitely normal. Also, the size of the neural contents should be taken into consideration, because in the case of a very small cauda equina even 10 mm may be sufficient. However, it has been demonstrated that the size of the dural sac with the neural contents does not correlate with the osseous dimensions of the lumbar canal (29).

Schönström and co-workers (29) found experimentally during gradual constriction of the dural sac that the intrathecal pressure started to increase at a cross-sectional area of 75 ± 30 mm^2. While examining patients with canal stenosis an average cross-sectional area of 90 ± 35 mm^2 was clinically observed. Furthermore, this area decreased under axial load to 50 ± 30 mm^2 and varied from extension to flexion to 40 ± 20 mm^2. This may explain why patients have symptoms during standing and walking, which disappear during sitting.

The Pathway of the Nerve Root

Although the term nerve root is often used in a broad sense, strictly speaking it is only the part proximal to the dorsal root ganglion, consisting of a dorsal and a ventral rootlet. Beyond the dorsal root ganglion it is called the spinal nerve, which ends in the lumbosacral plexus. The pathway of the nerve root, including the dorsol root ganglion and the spinal nerve, begins at the point where the nerve root sheath leaves the dural sac and ends at the point where the spinal nerve leaves the intervertebral foramen.

Burton (2) recognized two zones: central and foraminal. Zindrick et al. (40) divided this pathway into three zones, which they called subarticular, pedicle, and exit. The exit zone is equal to the foraminal zone of Burton. Furthermore, they described a zone located outside

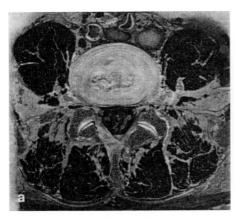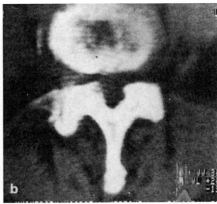

FIG. 1. A: Anatomy of the entrance zone, also called the lateral recess. The nerve root with its sheath has just left the dural sac and is located in the entrance to the nerve root canal. Anteriorly it may be trapped by a disc protrusion, and posteriorly by changes of the articular facets. **B:** Computed tomographic section partly through the upper endplate of L5 and partly through the disc L4–5. The *right side* shows osteophytes at the articular facet impinging on the L5 nerve root in the entrance zone. (Reprinted with permission from *Der Orthopäde* 1993; 22:202–210.)

the foramen: entrapment of the spinal nerve at that location is called by Wiltse et al. (38) "the far-out syndrome."

Crock (5) has defined the lateral distal end of the pathway as "the doorway of a passage to the intervertebral foramen." The pathway itself is defined by him as the nerve root canal. Lee and co-workers (20) used the term "lateral lumbar spinal canal." However, if one wishes to include the lateral recess in a classification of entrapment of the nerve root, the term nerve root pathway is preferable to the term lateral spinal canal. This pathway is divided into three parts: the entrance zone, the mid zone, and the exit zone.

The entrance zone (Fig. 1) is the area of the vertebral canal, medial and/or anterior to the superior articular process. This zone has no medial or lateral walls. Entrapment of a nerve root in this zone may be caused by disc protrusion and/or by degenerative changes of the facet joint leading to osteophytes and synovial swelling: lateral recess stenosis.

The mid zone (Fig. 2) is the area anterior to the pars interarticularis medial and caudal to the pedicle. The anterior wall of this zone is the posterior aspect of the vertebral body. The lateral wall is the pedicle. The posterior wall is the pars interarticularis. The mid zone has no medial wall. The dorsal root ganglion is situated in this zone.

The exit zone (Fig. 3) is the area located at the lateral aspect of the pedicle. The anterior wall is the posterior aspect of the vertebral body and the intervertebral disc. The posterior wall is the lateral margin of the inferior articular process of the vertebra above and the superior articular process of the vertebra below. The superior wall is the caudal margin of the pedicle above, and the inferior wall is the cephalad margin of the pedicle below. The dorsal root ganglion and/or the beginning of the spinal nerve are located in this zone.

To solve the semantic confusion I propose using in clinical classifications the term nerve root pathway instead of the term intervertebral canal. This pathway has a beginning, the entrance zone or osteum internum, followed by the mid zone or pedicle zone, the exit zone or osteum externum, and the far lateral zone. Furthermore, I propose abandoning the term intervertebral foramen, in particular in descriptions of radiographs, because it is a two-dimensional concept. Although etymologically the word "foramen" could also be used for a canal,

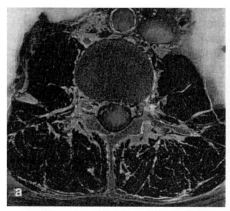
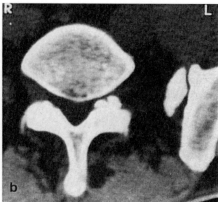

FIG. 2. The mid zone. **A:** Anatomic transverse section through a lumbar segment in the proximal one third of the vertebral body. The dorsal root ganglion is located in the mid part of the nerve root canal, anteriorly bordering the posterior aspect of the vertebral body and posteriorly the upper part of the facet joint. **B:** Computed tomographic section through a comparable level. Osteophytes on the *left side* are clearly impinging on the dorsal root ganglion. (Reprinted with permission from *Der Orthopäde* 1993;22:202–210.)

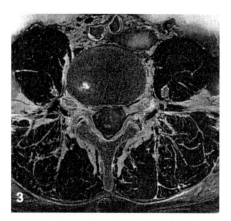
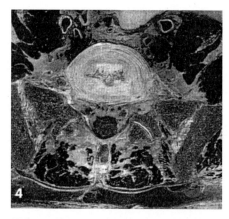

FIG. 3. The exit zone. The spinal nerve is just located at the exit of the nerve root canal. It is posterior to the psoas muscle and the disc, and anterior to the facet joint. At this position the spinal nerve may be trapped by a lateral disc protrusion or osteophytes at the vertebral body. (Reprinted with permission from *Der Orthopäde* 1993;22:202–210.)

FIG. 4. The far lateral zone. This anatomic transverse section demonstrates at the L5–S1 level a ligament between the sacrum and the disc on the *right side,* producing a triangular space in which the nerve root is located. The nerve root is not able to escape when this space is filled by a lateral disc protrusion. This is located well outside the intervertebral foramen. Osteophytes at this level may cause a similar problem. (Reprinted with permission from *Der Orthopäde* 1993;22: 202–210.)

most authors define the word foramen in a two-dimensional sense: a window without thickness. As such, it is identical to the exit zone or the osteum externum.

CLASSIFICATIONS INVOLVING ANATOMIC VARIABLES

A classification based on the localization of the abnormal narrowing:

- Ostium internum or entrance zone (lateral recess)
- Pedicle zone or mid zone
- Ostium externum or exit zone
- "Far lateral" zone (strictly speaking no narrowing) (Fig. 4).

A classification based on the pathologic anatomy of the narrowness: one factor only or a combination of factors may cause the stenoses:

- Ligaments
  Ligamentum flavum: hypertrophy, calcification, ossification
  Ligamentum longitudinale posterius: calcification
- Disc
  "Bulging" annulus in the case of severe degeneration
  Severe loss of disc height
  Protrusion
- Facet joint
  Synovitis with synovial hypertrophy and effusion
- Bone
  Articular process: osteophyte formation, uncommon shape or orientation
  Vertebral body: osteophyte formation posteriorly or laterally
  Lamina: hypertrophy, spondylolysis with granulation tissue.

Pathobiomechanics

The biomechanics of a lumbar motion segment as a whole may be of relevance to entrapment, as in the case of fixed rotational deformity, described by Farfan (11), and of segmental hypermobility, described by Kirkaldy Willis (17) as dynamic stenosis. These are controversial issues and need further study.

SYMPTOMS AND SIGNS

Entrapment of a lumbar nerve root in its pathway may be caused by any space-occupying lesion, such as metastasis in the pedicle or osteophytes. Furthermore, it may be the result of a deformity, congenital or acquired, for example, as in burst fractures of the vertebral body. Also, variation in shape, size, and orientation of articular processes, as in developmental stenosis, may cause stenosis.

Pathology may be present without causing symptoms or signs: asymptomatic pathology. People without any symptoms or signs may have diminished space for the nerve root somewhere along its pathway. This has been demonstrated on caudography (10,15,24), computed tomography (CT) (37), and magnetic resonance imaging (MRI). MacNab (22) concluded that "the patient may have a lateral recess stenosis that involves both sides at several levels, yet his complaint may be unilateral and monoradicular." Differentiating between symptomatic and asymptomatic lateral stenosis may be very difficult, and this dilemma can only be solved by nerve root sheath infiltration applied as a diagnostic test (6,21,30,31).

Entrapment of a nerve root by degenerative changes may cause pain, a neural deficit of that nerve root, or a combination of symptoms and signs.

Pain is usually located in one leg, although back pain, present during standing and walking and absent in a sitting posture, may be the only feature of stenosis (34). The leg pain may be present at rest, without signs of nerve root compression or neural deficit, so-called atypical leg pain (30). The leg pain may be present at rest, in combination with a positive Lasègue's test: such a patient has nerve root compression. Finally, leg pain may be present on walking only, as in patients with neurogenic intermittent claudication.

Neural deficit may be permanent in the sense of motor weakness, sensory changes, or absent reflexes of one specific nerve root: radiculopathy (36). Neural deficit may be present on walking only: neurogenic intermittent claudication (34). However, patients with lateral stenosis can demonstrate neurogenic intermittent claudication while also demonstrating signs of radiculopathy.

Patients with degenerative lateral stenosis may thus present with one or a combination of four clinical syndromes: neurogenic intermittent claudication, radiculopathy, nerve root compression, and atypical leg pain. These four clinical syndromes are characterized by the presence or absence of typical findings in the history and at physical examination. They may occur in combination or not. For example, entrapment of one nerve root in the mid zone may cause a history of intermittent claudication, while at physical examination signs of radiculopathy are observed. The emphasis is on diagnosing these syndromes clinically without using imaging techniques.

Atypical Leg Pain

Patients may present with back pain and radiating pain in the buttock, greater trochanter, and posterolateral or posterior aspect of the thigh. Sometimes the pain may radiate below the knee, along the lateral aspect or the posterolateral aspect of the calf, into the ankle. Incidentally, a patient feels pain in the foot, resembling a segmental pattern. Leg pain may be constantly present and in some patients is aggravated by walking and standing. Nevertheless, patients may be able to walk without interruption. The leg pain may decrease by sitting or bending forward, and for these patients bike riding is comfortable. In others, at rest or even in a bending position the leg pain may persist. Signs of nerve root compression are negative, and signs of a neurologic deficit are absent.

A classification based on clinical presentation:

Pain
  Present at rest
    • Nerve root compression
    • Atypical leg pain
  Only on walking
    • Neurogenic intermittent
      claudication
Lasègue's test
  Negative
    • Atypical leg pain

  Positive
    • Nerve root compression
Nerve root function
  Impaired at rest
    • Radiculopathy
  Only on walking
    • Neurogenic intermittent
      claudication
A combination of these factors.

CLINICAL RELEVANCE

After conservative treatment of radicular syndromes, patients are completely free of their symptoms, while still demonstrating, on CT, images of the disc protrusion unchanged from the pretreatment examination. Also, people without any symptoms and no history of nerve root entrapment may demonstrate radiographic signs of narrowness of the nerve root pathway. In other words, lateral lumbar stenosis may occur without causing symptoms: the pathomorphologic changes may not correlate with the clinical symptoms. This phenomenon seems to be related to age. These observations pose a problem for the clinician managing a patient with pain in a leg but without localizing neurologic signs and, indeed, the majority of patients with nerve root entrapment due to lateral stenosis presents clinically with only pain, not located segmentally. This diagnostic problem can be solved by selective nerve root sheath infiltration. This method has been described by MacNab (21), and its diagnostic value was later defined (30). In experienced hands a high reliability and very high sensitivity, in combination with sufficient specificity, are observed. The positive predictive value in degenerative lateral stenosis proved to be around 90% (30).

Neurophysiologic examination, including motor and sensory evoked potentials, can in a number of patients define the nerve root responsible for the neural deficit. Dvorak and co-workers (7) and Herdmann and co-workers (14) demonstrated in 65% of patients with stenosis a significant delay (> 2 SD) in motor conduction time to the leg muscles, and in 80% of patients in whom F-waves were recorded. However, in many patients pain is the only feature, and at neurophysiologic examination no signs of neural dysfunction are observed. Even in the case of a dysfunction, the affected nerve root may not be the one that is causing the symptoms! Therefore, the clinical symptoms and signs have to be correlated meticulously with morphologic and neurophysiologic data to answer the question of whether the neurologic deficit is a sign of a manifest entrapment or a ''scar'' of an earlier healed lesion.

Surgical decompression of every radiographically demonstrated level with stenosis is not indicated. In many patients a two- or three-level laminectomy is necessary. MacNab (23) demonstrated in 97% of patients 10 years after laminectomy signs of denervation of the erector spinae muscle, and thus these patients are left with an unstable back due to the lack of good muscular control. Therefore, one should keep the decompression to a minimum, preferable only to the symptomatic level. This is possible because in the majority of patients only one level is symptomatic as demonstrated by diagnostic nerve root sheath infiltration (3,22): only a very limited decompression is needed, directed at the symptomatic nerve root, using an interlaminar approach without denervation of the paraspinal muscles.

Some surgeons may decompress all locations of stenosis on the assumption that they may become symptomatic at a later date, in other words, ''preventive surgery.'' This is unjustified. With an average follow-up of more than 5 years only 1 of 15 patients with multilevel degenerative lateral stenosis became symptomatic at a different level after decompression of only the symptomatic nerve root (32). Besides, in those patients back pain is a minor problem compared with patients treated by wide laminectomy (30).

Knowing which nerve root is symptomatic and the exact location of the entrapment is essential when surgical treatment is being considered. In particular, in the case of entrapment in the exit or far lateral zones, decompression is difficult using a medial approach and necessitates a very wide laminectomy and even facetectomy, while a small, effective decompression can be carried out using a lateral approach (28,30).

To make a diagnosis in patients with suspected lateral stenosis, the following use of the presented classifications is suggested:

1. After the clinical analysis on the basis of data from history and physical examination, define the clinical syndrome being presented. When signs of radiculopathy are present,

the neurologic level may be defined at this stage, for example, an L5 radiculopathy on the right side.

2. Choose imaging techniques on the basis of the clinical diagnosis to provide the pathomorphology of the diagnosis:

   • The location of an abnormal narrowing can be defined for each lumbar segment. Also, the question can be answered of whether a combination of canal stenosis and lateral stenosis is present.
   • When surgical decompression is indicated, the anatomical structures causing the stenosis can be described in detail, enabling the surgeon to make a concise plan of approach preoperatively.

3. Assess whether the observed morphology indicates a symptomatic entrapment or not. In particular, this is important with multilevel anatomical changes indicating stenosis. In the majority of cases, only one level is symptomatic. Selective nerve root sheath infiltration, and in some patients neurophysiologic examination, may differentiate between symptomatic and asymptomatic stenosis.

REFERENCES

1. Arnoldi CC, Brodsky AE, Cauchoix J, et al. Lumbar spinal stenosis and nerve root entrapment syndromes. Definition and classification. *Clin Orthop* 1976;115:4–6.
2. Burton CV. On the diagnosis and surgical treatment of lumbar subarticular and farout lateral spine stenosis. In: Watkins RG, Collins JS, eds. *Lumbar discectomy and laminectomy.* Rockville, MD: Aspen, 1987;195–203.
3. Castro WHM, van Akkerveeken PF. Der diagnostische Wert der selektiven lumbalen Nervenwurzelblockade. *Z Orthop* 1991;129:374–379.
4. Cram RH. A sign of nerve root pressure. *J Bone Joint Surg Br* 1953;35:192–195.
5. Crock HV. Normal and pathological anatomy of the lumbar spinal nerve root canals. *J Bone Joint Surg Br* 1981;63:487–494.
6. Dooley JF, McBroom RJ, Taguchi T, MacNab I. Nerve root infiltration in the diagnosis of radicular pain. *Spine* 1988;13:79–83.
7. Dvorak J, Herdmann J, Theiler R, Grob D. Magnetic stimulation of motor cortex and motor roots for painless evaluation of central and proximal peripheral motor pathways. Normal values and clinical application in disorders of the lumbar spine. *Spine* 1991;16:955–960.
8. Dyck P. Sciatic pain. In: Watkins RG, Collis JS, eds. *Lumbar discectomy and laminectomy.* Rockville, MD: Aspen, 1987;5–14.
9. Epstein JA. Diagnosis and treatment of painful neurological disorders caused by spondylosis of the lumbar spine. *J Neurosurg* 1960;17:991–998.
10. Falconer MA, McGeorge M, Begg AC. Observations on the cause and mechanism of symptom production in sciatica and low back pain. *J Neurol Neurosurg Psychiatry* 1948;11:13–26.
11. Farfan HF. *Mechanical disorders of the low back.* Philadelphia: Lea & Febiger, 1973.
12. Forst JJ. *Contribution à l'étude clinique de la sciatique.* Thèse 33, Université de Paris, 1883.
13. Gowers WR. *A manual of diseases of the nervous system,* 2nd ed. Reprinted by Hafner, Darien, CT, 1893.
14. Herdmann J, Dvorak J, Volanka S. Neuro-physiological evaluation of disorders and procedures affecting the spinal cord and cauda equina. *Curr Opin Neurol Neurosurg* 1992;5:544–548.
15. Hitselberger WE, Witter RM. Abnormal myelograms in asymptomatic patients. *J Neurosurg* 1968;28:204–206.
16. Kemp A. Diagnosis and treatment of lumbar hernia nuclei pulposi (in Dutch). *Ned Tijdschr Geneeskd* 1953; 97:3116–3121.
17. Kirkaldy Willis WH. *Managing low back pain.* New York: Churchill Livingstone, 1984.
18. Kirkaldy Willis WH, Yong Hing K. Lateral recess, lateral canal and foraminal stenosis. In: Watkins RG, Collis JS, eds. *Lumbar discectomy and laminectomy.* Rockville, MD: Aspen, 1987;245–253.
19. Lazarevic LJ. Ischias postica Cotumni. Ein Beitrag zu deren Differentialdiagnose. *Allg Wien Med* 1884;29: 425–429.
20. Lee CK, Rauschning W, Glenn W. Lateral lumbar spinal canal stenosis: classification, pathologic anatomy and surgical decompression. *Spine* 1988;13:313–320.
21. MacNab I. Negative disc exploration. *J Bone Joint Surg Am* 1971;53:891–903.
22. MacNab I. The pathogenesis of spinal stenosis. In: Hopp E, ed. *Spinal stenosis.* Philadelphia: Hanley & Belfus, 1987.
23. MacNab I, Cuthbert H, Godfrey CM. The incidence of denervation of the sacrospinalis muscles following spinal surgery. *Spine* 1977;2:294–298.

24. McRae DL. Asymptomatic intervertebral disc protrusion. *Acta Radiol* 1956;6:9–27.
25. Mixter WJ, Barr JS. Rupture of the intervertebral disc with involvement of the spinal canal. *N Engl J Med* 1934;211:210–215.
26. Naffziger HC, Jones OW. Desmoid tumors of the spinal cord: report of four cases with observation: a clinical test for the differentiation of the source of radicular pain. *Arch Neurol Psychiatry* 1935;33:941–944.
27. Putti V. On new conceptions in the pathogenesis of sciatic pain. *Lancet* 1927;2:53–60.
28. Ray CD. Far lateral decompression for stenosis, the paralateral approach to the lumbar spine. In: White AH, Rothman RH, Ray CD, eds. *Lumbar spine surgery.* St. Louis: Mosby, 1987;175–187.
29. Schönström N. *The narrow lumbar spinal canal and the size of the cauda equina in man. A clinical and experimental study.* Thesis, University of Göteborg, 1988.
30. Van Akkerveeken PF. *Lateral stenosis of the lumbar spine.* Thesis, University of Utrecht, 1989.
31. Van Akkerveeken PF. The diagnostic value of nerve root sheath infiltration. *Acta Orthop Scand Suppl* 1992; 251:61–63.
32. Van Akkerveeken PF. Decompression of only the symptomatic nerve root in patients with radiological signs of entrapment at multiple lumbar levels. A long term follow up. 2nd Annual Meeting, European Spine Society, Rome, Italy, October 17–19 1991. *Abstracts Book,* 1994.
33. Verbiest H. Sur certaines formes rares de compression de queue de cheval. In: *Hommage à Clovis Vincent.* Paris: Maline, 1949:161–174.
34. Verbiest H. *Neurogenic intermittent claudication.* New York: Elsevier, 1976.
35. Verbiest H. Lumbar spinal stenosis: morphology, classification, long term results. In: Weinstein J, Wiesel SW, eds. *The lumbar spine.* Philadelphia: WB Saunders, 1990;546–589.
36. Weinstein PR, Ehni G, Wilson CB. *Lumbar spondylosis.* Chicago: Year Book, 1977.
37. Wiesel SW, Tsourmas N, Feffer HI, Citrin CM, Patronas M. The incidence of positive CT-scans in an asymptomatic group of patients. *Spine* 1984;9:549–552.
38. Wiltse LL, Guyer RD, Spencer CW, et al. Alar transverse process impingement of the L5 nerve: the far out syndrome. *Spine* 1984;9:31–41.
39. Woodhall B, Hayes GJ. The well-leg raising test of Fajerszajn in the diagnosis of ruptured intervertebral disc. *J Bone Joint Surg Am* 1950;32:786–792.
40. Zindrick MR, Wiltse LL, Rauschning W. Disc herniations lateral to the intervertebral foramen. In: White AH, Rothman RH, Ray CD, eds. *Lumbar spine surgery.* St. Louis: Mosby, 1987;195–208.

Lumbar Spinal Stenosis
edited by Robert Gunzburg and Marek Szpalski
Lippincott Williams & Wilkins, Philadelphia, © 2000.

7

Lumbar Spinal Stenosis in Metabolic Bone Diseases

Jean-Pierre Devogelaer and *Baudouin Maldague

*Departments of Rheumatology and *Radiology, Saint-Luc University Hospital, 1200 Brussels, Belgium*

Narrowing of the spinal canal may develop as a complication in a large variety of conditions leading to bony outgrowth of the spine. The vast majority of such conditions are degenerative in origin (i.e., osteoarthritis). However, osteoarthritis may not represent the primary event responsible for the bony outgrowth, but it may constitute a secondary event. Several conditions are associated with or cause bony outgrowth of the spine (Table 1). Some of them can be due to metabolic bone diseases, but these conditions are either rare or, if relatively frequent, they are rarely complicated by spinal stenosis.

The clinical manifestations of spinal stenosis in metabolic bone diseases are similar to those occurring in conditions of other etiologies, beyond the specific symptoms linked to the primitive disease: neurogenic claudication, numbness, and muscle weakness in the legs. Radicular pain can occur frequently. In severe cases, spinal stenosis may lead to cauda equina syndrome. Physical examination is not specific; for example, decreased mobility of the lumbar spine is often observed, whereas demonstrable motor and sensory nerve deficits are rather uncommon. In the metabolic bone diseases as in degenerative conditions, spinal stenosis of the lumbar segment can be divided into three groups on the basis of its anatomic location: stenosis of the central canal, stenosis of the subarticular or lateral recesses, and stenosis of the neural foramina, but it has less therapeutic implications, e.g., particularly for Paget's disease of bone, in which medical therapy is of utmost importance. Any of these locations may be affected to different degrees, either isolated or simultaneously (Tables 2 and 3).

Diffuse idiopathic skeletal hyperostosis (DISH), also called Forestier's disease (9,23), is a disorder characterized by bony proliferation of spinal and extraspinal structures. The most characteristic spinal changes are asymptomatic ossification predominantly of the right ligaments on the anterolateral aspect of the vertebral bodies. Calcification and ossification of extraspinal ligaments and tendons may occur, with bone proliferation at the attachment of ligaments and tendons to bone. However, the association of ''spinal'' DISH with spinal stenosis also has been described (3). The spinal stenosis may be due to peculiar hypertrophic changes in the apophyseal joints (chiefly involving the inferior joints) (3) and ossification of the ligamentum flavum (3,4,12), but also to calcification and ossification of the posterior longitudinal ligament of the spine (15,22,23), which has been described in up to 50% of patients (22). Although lumbar involvement occurs in almost all cases of DISH, spinal stenosis at this level seems to be rare (12). The inclusion of DISH in metabolic diseases relies on the

TABLE 1. *Several conditions associated with or causing bony outgrowth of the spine*

Diffuse idiopathic skeletal hyperostosis (DISH)
Paget's disease of bone
Ankylosing spondylitis
Acromegaly
Hypoparathyroidism, pseudohypoparathyroidism
Fluorosis
Ochronosis
Sternocostoclavicular hyperostosis
X-linked hypophosphatemic osteomalacia

association of this condition with obesity, diabetes mellitus (13), increased concentrations of retinoic acid and vitamin A in the plasma (7,19), and prolonged etretinate therapy (20,28). When long-term therapy with such compounds is started, it has been proposed that a lateral x-ray film of the thoracic spine be taken every year (28) because bone scintigraphy has been disappointingly insensitive to the changes of hyperostosis (28). Other authors, however, have not found any influence of prolonged oral retinoid use on the frequency and severity of spinal abnormalities in adults (26).

Endemic fluorosis is a chronic fluorine intoxication found in certain parts of the world (Punjab, Morocco), where there is excessive fluorine in the water (up to 14 parts per million) and soil. In the spine, fluorosis may be complicated by calcification of various ligaments, particularly the ligamenta flava and intertransverse and interspinous ligaments, leading to the production of large numbers of osteophytes (25). The vertebral bodies become slightly larger than normal, with much lipping. The anterior and posterior longitudinal ligaments may be thickened and calcified to a varying degree. The spinal canal may be extremely narrowed in the cervical segment, but less so in the thoracic and lumbar segments (25). This kind of complication is not seen in our western regions, neither sporadically nor after the usually time-limited therapeutic use of sodium fluoride in osteoporosis.

The association of ectopic calcification/ossification and hypoparathyroidism states is well known. Paravertebral ligamentous ossification (PVLO) has been described in idiopathic hypoparathyroidism (1). Severe ossification of the posterior longitudinal ligament (OPLL) has been observed in idiopathic hypoparathyroidism and in pseudohypoparathyroidism (18). OPLL is a type of PVLO first reported by Japanese authors (16). There is some correlation between the incidence of PVLO and the length of time during which the hypoparathyroidism has not been treated, but no significant relationship could be found between the severity of biochemical abnormalities before vitamin D therapy and the incidence of PVLO. Moreover, the incidence of hypoparathyroidism does not seem to be significantly higher among PVLO patients than among normal controls. The vast majority of patients with PVLO have normal parathyroid function, whereas some patients with a long-standing untreated hypoparathyroidism do not have PVLO. It is suggested, therefore, that hypoparathyroidism is an aggravating, rather than a causative, factor in the genesis of PVLO (18). It is possible, however, that OPLL could explain some of the neurologic manifestations consistent with nerve root compression in some patients suffering from idiopathic hypoparathyroidism or pseudohypoparathyroidism. Computerized tomography or magnetic resonance imaging of the spine should be performed in these rare cases.

Spinal stenosis is a rare complication of adult X-linked hypophosphatemia accounting for only 4% of cases of this rare condition, whereas spondylosis similar to that in DISH amounts to 12% (10). It is more prevalent in men (10). Spinal stenosis has been described at the cervical level, where it is due to PVLO (mainly Japanese patients) (29). In white patients,

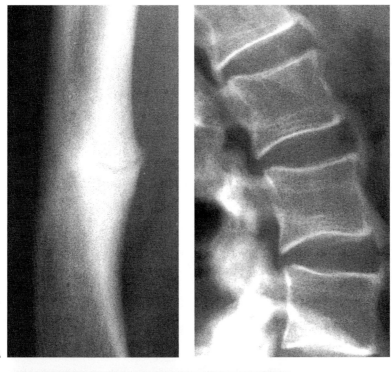

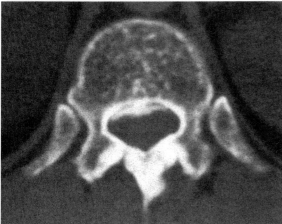

FIG. 1. Male adult suffering from X-linked hypophosphatemic osteo-malacia. **A:** Looser-Milkman zone at the medial part of the femoral shaft. **B:** Ossification of the para-vertebral ligaments similar to dif-fuse idiopathic skeletal hyperosto-sis and ossification of the posterior longitudinal ligament (OPLL) are seen at the *upper part* of the image. **C:** Confirmation of OPLL by com-puted tomographic scan.

new bone formation within the spinal canal at the thoracic level (osseous overgrowth of the facet joints, thickening of the laminae) was deemed responsible for the stenosis and, more rarely, ossification of the ligamentum flavum at the lumbar spine (Fig. 1) (2). Once again, there was no obvious correlation between the severity and extent of the intraspinal new bone observed on computed tomography and that present around the vertebral column or elsewhere on conventional radiographs (2).

The spine is one of the most common skeletal sites to be affected by Paget's disease (14); therefore, it is not surprising that neurologic complications have been frequently reported. Cord or nerve root symptoms are more frequently described when Paget's disease is situated

TABLE 2. *Causes of central lumbar stenosis*

Achondroplasia: developmental narrowing of the interpediculate distance
DISH: hypertrophic changes related to OA in the apophyseal joints
DISH ⎱
Fluorosis ⎰ thickening of the ligamentum flavum

DISH ⎱
Hypoparathyroidism-pseudohypoparathyroidism ⎰ ligamentous calcification or ossification
X-linked hypophosphatemia

Paget's disease ⎱
Fluorosis ⎰ diffuse bone overgrowth

Fluorosis ⎱
X-linked hypophosphatemia ⎰ osteophytes in the vertebral body
DISH

DISH, diffuse idiopathic skeletal hyperostosis; OA, osteoarthritis.

in the thoracic spine than in the cervical spine. This is probably because the width of the vertebral canal is narrowest in this area of the column, and, therefore, more easily deformed by the bony overgrowth and thickening. Characteristically, when spinal cord compression is present, three to five adjacent vertebrae are involved by the pagetic process (5). Patients usually complain of a slowly progressive impairment of the spinal cord function. The symptoms may arise from the disc or the facet distraction, or they may be due directly to Paget's disease of bone itself, root impingement, or vascular compromise by distortion or by stealing (5).

However, the lumbar spine is a more common site of Paget's disease, with this pagetic localization affecting up to 50% of patients (14). An enlargement of the vertebral body is commonly observed. Most frequently, it is symmetric and visible on anteroposterior radiographs and is seen more easily on lateral radiographs. However, as an increase in vertebral height is never seen, probably because of gravity, weight bearing, and other stresses on the spinal column, and because the pagetic bone is ''soft,'' the pagetic vertebra takes the appearance of a flattened vertebral body, which can compromise the integrity of the intervertebral foramens, affect the blood supply to the spinal cord or the nervous roots, or lead to narrowing of the width of the vertebral canal. When the lumbar spine involvement is associated with compression of neural elements, the pagetic disease characteristically involves a single vertebra, whereas several vertebrae are involved in other parts of the spine (24). Neurologic complications are relatively rare when compared to the frequency of the spinal involvement. The vast majority of patients suffering from Paget's disease of the spine have no symptoms. When a patient is symptomatic, this does not mean automatically that the pagetic involvement of the vertebra is immediately responsible for the symptoms. In our experience, the vertebral deformity attributable to the pagetic involvement frequently favors some prolapse of the intervertebral disc, potentially provoking by itself an entrapment of the nervous roots. Osteo-

TABLE 3. *Causes of foraminal or lateral recesses stenosis*

Causes of foraminal narrowing
    Discal herniation (may be due to Paget's disease of the vertebral body)
    DISH: osteophytosis involving the vertebral body or the articular processes
    Synovial cysts, tumors
    Spondylolisthesis
Causes of subarticular or lateral recesses stenosis
    DISH ⎱
    Paget's disease ⎰ bone hypertrophy about the apophyseal joint

DISH, diffuse idiopathic skeletal hyperostosis.

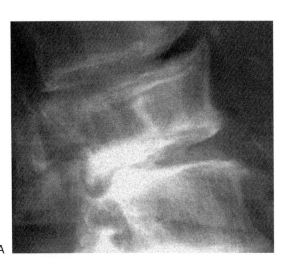
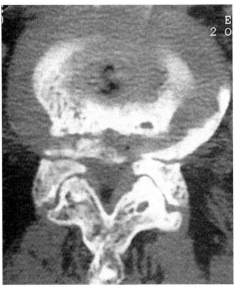

A   B

FIG. 2. A: Posteriorly slipped pagetic vertebra L3 on L4. **B:** Circumferential bulging of the discovertebral junction. No severe spinal stenosis was observed at the level of the pagetic vertebral body.

phytosis, secondary to disc degeneration, also might be responsible for compression of nervous tissue. Of course, a pagetic collapsed vertebra can encroach the spinal canal (Fig. 2). The increased vascularity of the pagetic lesions may deprive the spinal cord or the nervous root of its blood supply (Fig. 3), culminating in a spinal artery steal syndrome (8). The spinal canal can become progressively narrowed because of pagetic vertebral body collapse and

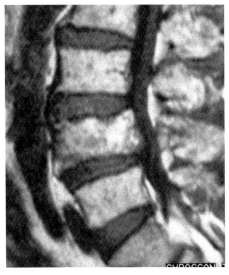
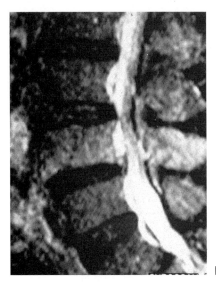

A   B

FIG. 3. Paget's disease of L4. No bony spinal stenosis at the height of the vertebral body is seen on computed tomographic scan. **A,B:** The T1- and T2-weighted sagittal magnetic resonance images show significant thickening of the ventral epidural space with enlarged epidural veins impinging on the thecal sac.

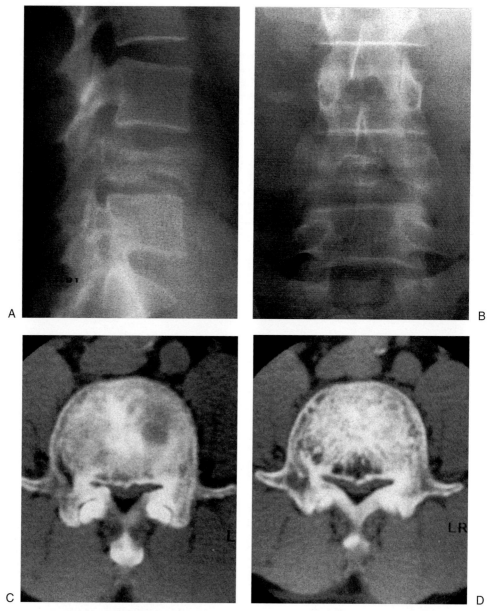

FIG. 4. A,B: Vertebral body collapse of pagetic L4 leading to spinal stenosis from osseous origin, visible on computed tomographic scans **(C,D)**.

formation of new bone backward into the vertebral canal. The pagetic process can involve the neural arches, which can increase in thickness and thus further reduce the aperture of the intervertebral foramina and/or the spinal canal (Fig. 4). Finally, some authors have described a pagetic extension into the ligamentum flavum or epidural fat (26), but this should be a rare event.

From records over the last 20 years, we retrospectively retrieved the case histories of 20 pagetic patients who had complaints of spinal stenosis (Fig. 5). Six of these patients suffered

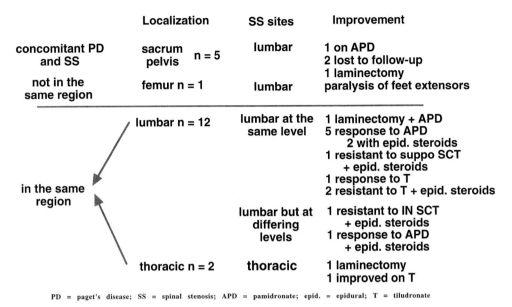

	Localization	SS sites	Improvement
concomitant PD and SS	sacrum pelvis n = 5	lumbar	1 on APD 2 lost to follow-up 1 laminectomy
not in the same region	femur n = 1	lumbar	paralysis of feet extensors
in the same region	lumbar n = 12	lumbar at the same level	1 laminectomy + APD 5 response to APD 2 with epid. steroids 1 resistant to suppo SCT + epid. steroids 1 response to T 2 resistant to T + epid. steroids
		lumbar but at differing levels	1 resistant to IN SCT + epid. steroids 1 response to APD + epid. steroids
	thoracic n = 2	thoracic	1 laminectomy 1 improved on T

PD = paget's disease; SS = spinal stenosis; APD = pamidronate; epid. = epidural; T = tiludronate

FIG. 5. Twenty cases suffering from Paget's disease and spinal stenosis.

from Paget's disease in a skeletal region too distant from the spine (hemipelvis, sacrum, or femur) for the symptoms to be ascribed to Paget's disease itself. The clinical symptoms were attributed to osteoarthritic spinal stenosis. However, one of these patients clearly improved with pamidronate therapy (Fig. 5). Twelve patients suffered from lumbar spinal stenosis corresponding to a lumbar vertebral involvement by Paget's disease (ten at a corresponding level and two at a differing level when comparing symptoms and Paget's disease level). Six patients dramatically improved in the long term (more than 1 year) after pamidronate therapy and could walk without any further intermittent claudication. Two patients received salmon calcitonin for 6 months (one by intranasal spray and the other by suppositories) without any significant long-standing improvement. One patient underwent laminectomy immediately after pamidronate therapy. Another patient became asymptomatic after tiludronate therapy. Two other patients on tiludronate did not respond, and one of these patients required laminectomy. Two patients suffered from thoracic cord symptoms caused by pagetic vertebral involvement. One patient with very severe Paget's disease of the spine required an extensive laminectomy; however, this was before the availability of modern therapies for Paget's disease. Since then, there has been no recurrence of symptoms while on salmon calcitonin and later on tiludronate. The other patient improved dramatically while on long-term (years) intermittent tiludronate therapy. Even if these data pertain to a retrospective study, and even if in some cases a placebo effect cannot be excluded completely, it remains that our data confirm the scant data of the literature implying that in pagetic patients suffering from spinal stenosis, medical therapy (calcitonin or bisphosphonates) should be started promptly and maintained for weeks, before considering any surgical decompressive intervention (5,8,11,17,21,27).

REFERENCES

1. Adams JE, Davies M. Paravertebral and peripheral ligamentous ossification: an unusual association of hypoparathyroidism. *Postgrad Med J* 1977;53:167–172.

2. Adams JE, Davies M. Intra-spinal new bone formation and spinal cord compression in familial hypophosphata-emic vitamin D resistant osteomalacia. *Q J Med* 1986;61:1117–1129.

3. Arlet J, Abiteboul M. Rétrécissement du canal rachidien et hyperostose vertébrale ankylosante. *Rhumatologie* 1981;33:73–80.

4. Arlet J, Abiteboul M, Mazières B, et al. Sténose acquise des canaux lombaires et hyperostose vertébrale. *Rev Rhum* 1983;50:635–641.

5. Chen J-R, Rhee RSC, Wallach S, et al. Neurologic disturbances in Paget disease of bone: response to calcitonin. *Neurology* 1979;29:448–457.

6. Clarke PR, Williams HT. Ossification in extradural fat in Paget's disease of spine. *Br J Surg* 1975;62:571–572.

7. Dougados M, Leporho MA, Esmilaire L, et al. Taux plasmatiques des vitamines A et E au cours de la maladie hyperostosique, la spondylarthrite ankylosante et la polyarthrite rhumatoïde. *Rev Rhum* 1988;55:251–254.

8. Douglas DL, Duckworth T, Kanis JA, et al. Spinal cord dysfunction in Paget's disease of bone. Has medical treatment a vascular basis? *J Bone Joint Surg* 1981;63B:495–503.

9. Forestier J, Rotes-Querol J. Senile ankylosing hyperostosis of the spine. *Ann Rheum Dis* 1950;9:321–330.

10. Hardy DC, Murphy WA, Siegel BA, et al. X-linked hypophosphatemia in adults: prevalence of skeletal radio-graphic and scintigraphic features. *Radiology* 1989;171:403–414.

11. Herzberg L, Bayliss E. Spinal-cord syndrome due to non-compressive Paget's disease of bone: a spinal-artery steal phenomenon reversible with calcitonin. *Lancet* 1980;ii:13–15.

12. Johnsson KE, Petersson H, Wollheim FA, Säveland H. Diffuse idiopathic skeletal hyperostosis (DISH) causing spinal stenosis and sudden paraplegia. *J Rheumatol* 1983;10:784–789.

13. Julkunen H, Heinonen OP, Pyorala K. Hyperostosis of the spine in an adult population. Its relation to hyperglycae-mia and obesity. *Ann Rheum Dis* 1971;30:605–612.

14. Kanis JA. *Pathophysiology and treatment of Paget's disease of bone.* London: Martin Dunitz Ltd., 1991.

15. Malghem J, Nagant de Deuxchaisnes C, Rombouts-Lindemans C, et al. Ossification du ligament longitudinal postérieur cervical. *J Belge Radiol* 1979;62:69–77.

16. Mitsui H, Sonozaki H, Juji T, Kabata K. Ankylosing spinal hyperostosis (ASH) and ossification of the posterior longitudinal ligament (OPLL). *Arch Orthop Trauma Surg* 1979;94:21–23.

17. Nicholas JJ, Helfrich DJ, Cooperstein L, Goodman M. Clinical and radiographic improvement of bone of the second lumbar vertebra in Paget's disease following therapy with etidronate disodium: a case report. *Arthritis Rheum* 1989;32:776–779.

18. Okazaki T, Takuwa Y, Yamamoto M, et al. Ossification of the paravertebral ligaments: a frequent complication of hypoparathyroidism. *Metabolism* 1984;33:710–713.

19. Periquet B, Lambert W, Garcia J, et al. Increased concentrations of endogenous 13-cis-and all-trans-retinoic acids in diffuse idiopathic skeletal hyperostosis, as demonstrated by HPLC. *Clin Chim Acta* 1991;203:57–66.

20. Pittsley RA, Yoder FW. Retinoid hyperostosis: skeletal toxicity associated with long-term administration of 13-cis-retinoic acid for refractory ichthyosis. *N Engl J Med* 1983;308:1012–1014.

21. Porrini AA, Maldonado Cocco JA, Morteo OG. Spinal artery steal syndrome in Paget's disease of bone. *Clin Exp Rheumatol* 1987;5:377–378.

22. Resnick D, Guerra J, Robinson CA, Vint VC. Association of diffuse idiopathic skeletal hyperostosis (DISH) and calcification and ossification of the posterior ligament. *Am J Roentgenol* 1978;131:1049–1053.

23. Resnick D, Shapiro RF, Weisner KB, et al. Diffuse idiopathic skeletal hyperostosis (DISH) (ankylosing hyperos-tosis of Forestier and Rotes-Querol). *Semin Arthritis Rheum* 1978;7:153–187.

24. Schmidek HH. Neurologic and neurosurgical sequelae of Paget's disease of bone. *Clin Orthop* 1977;127:70–77.

25. Singh A, Dass R, Singh Hayreh S, Jolly SS. Skeletal changes in endemic fluorosis. *J Bone Joint Surg* 1962; 44B:806–815.

26. Van Dooren-Greebe RJ, Lemmens JAM, De Boo T, et al. Prolonged treatment with oral retinoids in adults: no influence on the frequency and severity of spinal abnormalities. *Br J Dermatol* 1996;134:71–76.

27. Wallace E, Wong J, Reid IR. Pamidronate treatment of neurologic sequelae of pagetic spinal stenosis. *Arch Intern Med* 1995;155:1813–1815.

28. Wilson DJ, Kay V, Charig M, et al. Skeletal hyperostosis and extraosseous calcification in patients receiving long-term etretinate (Tigason). *Br J Dermatol* 1988;119:597–607.

29. Yoshikawa S, Shiba M, Suzuki A. Spinal-cord compression in untreated adult cases of vitamin D resistant rickets. *J Bone Joint Surg* 1968;50A:743–752.

Lumbar Spinal Stenosis
edited by Robert Gunzburg and Marek Szpalski
Lippincott Williams & Wilkins, Philadelphia, © 2000.

8

The Natural Evolution of Degenerative Lumbar Spinal Stenosis

Michel Benoist, *Pierre Guigui, and †Abdulraham Siress

*Paris Hospitals, University of Paris VII, 75116 Paris, France; Department of Orthopedic Surgery, *Hôpital Beaujon, 92110 Clichy, France; and †American Hospital of Paris, Nevilly, France*

The purpose of this review is to present current information on the natural course of lumbar spinal stenosis (LSS). Numerous studies have been devoted to the clinical presentation and diagnostic value of the various symptoms and signs. Much of the literature has focused on the diagnosis accuracy of the different imaging studies, including myelography, computed tomographic (CT) scan, and magnetic resonance imaging (MRI). Corroboration of clinical findings with results of imaging studies have made the diagnosis of LSS more accurate. As the population becomes older, this condition is encountered more frequently, but the epidemiology of LSS is largely unknown. Surgery rates are increasing internationally. However, the effectiveness of surgical management for lumbar stenosis is still a matter of controversy. According to a recent meta-analysis of the literature, reports of surgical outcome vary greatly across studies (22). Some authors have reported deterioration of initially good results with time (12,21). Complications or worsening of symptoms may follow surgical procedures. At the present time, there is no scientific evidence of the effectiveness of surgical management for LSS.

Because of the relative unpredictability of surgical treatment at the individual level, good knowledge of natural evolution is crucial. It is important to determine the factors that influence the course of the disease, such as age, sex, duration and type of baseline clinical symptoms, and site and severity of the stenosis. Unfortunately, and in contrast with numerous surgical series, few studies have dealt with natural evolution. Moreover, no randomized study has compared short- and long-term results of medical versus surgical treatment. Such studies obviously are difficult to conduct in an older population with a high rate of comorbidity and mortality and with variable lifestyles and socioeconomic conditions. There also are ethical concerns. For example, it is difficult to advise surgery to an old patient with mild symptoms. To evaluate the current information on this topic, it is necessary to research the pertinent data reported in the literature.

ANECDOTAL REPORTS

There are a few reports of successful nonsurgical treatment of LSS. Jones and Thompson (11) studied 13 cases. Three patients were treated conservatively; two of these patients were unchanged or improved. The third patient was lost to follow-up. Blau and Logue (4) reported two nonoperated cases; one patient was unchanged after 10 years, and the other had a slight deterioration after 7 years. In a review of 70 cases, Tile et al. (20) described two patients for whom surgery had been considered and who had a favorable outcome with medical treatment. Rosomoff and Rosomoff (17) reported the case of a 70-year-old man who had a complete block at L3–4 noted on myelography but who fully recovered without surgery. Postacchini (16) observed 12 untreated patients with central stenosis followed for 3 to 12 years. All patients underwent myelography, CT scanning, and MRI. Stenosis was at one level in seven cases and at two or more levels in five cases. Compression was severe in seven cases and moderate in five cases. Radicular symptoms worsened in two cases with severe stenosis, remained unchanged in six, and disappeared in four. Of the latter four cases, three had moderate stenosis. The present author (MB) interviewed by telephone 21 patients treated conservatively in the past 10 years. Seven had been operated on; the others were either unchanged or improved (2).

These anecdotal observations have no scientific value. but they indicate that some patients do not deteriorate with time and are able to tolerate their disability without surgical decompression. Moreover, there are a few nonrandomized long-term patient-based studies that describe the natural evolution of LSS and the efficacy of medical treatment.

STUDIES ON THE NATURAL COURSE OF LUMBAR SPINAL STENOSIS: REVIEW OF THE LITERATURE

We shall now review the few available studies in chronological order. The first attempt to study the natural history of LSS was made by Porter and associates (15) in 1984. The study concerned patients considered to have entrapment of the nerve root in the root canal. Patients were selected according to four criteria: severe constant root pain to the lower leg, pain unrelieved by bed rest, minimal tension signs, and patient age over 40 years. Root entrapment syndrome was recognized in 249 patients. Radiologic signs of degenerative changes were seen in 80% of the patients. No active treatment was given to the majority of the patients with the exception of back school attendance in 22%. Fourteen percent received one or several steroid epidural injections. Ten percent were operated on and underwent decompression of the root canal. The 24 operated patients were assessed after 1 year. There was a complete recovery in only three patients. Fifteen patients were moderately improved and six were unchanged. Ninety percent were not operated on. Their progress was assessed by a mail questionnaire to which 75% replied. After 3 years, 78% still had some leg pain, but most of them were not bothered enough to undergo surgery. The clinical criteria used in this study to identify root entrapment now are recognized as classic clinical signs of lateral stenosis. However, the diagnosis was based solely on clinical symptoms and signs. Myelography was only performed in the operated group. The study was done before the common use of CT scan and MRI. In the majority of patients, the diagnosis of lateral stenosis was not verified by imaging studies and consequently remained uncertain.

Johnsson and associates (9) compared the clinical course of 44 patients treated surgically with that of 19 patients treated conservatively for central LSS. All patients had lumbar myelography with water-soluble contrast. The 19 untreated patients were advised to have surgery,

TABLE 1. *Follow-up estimation by visual analog scale (0–100)*

	No.	Worse %	Unchanged %	Improved %
Not operated	19	10	58	32
Operated with moderate stenosis	30	20	7	57
Operated with severe stenosis	14	36	0	64

From ref. 9.

TABLE 2. *Follow-up estimation by clinical examination*

	Worse %	Unchanged %	Improved %
Not operated	1	37	58
Operated with moderate stenosis	0	36	63
Operated with severe stenosis	1	29	64

From ref. 9.

but some of them declined or were excluded by the anesthesiologist. Patients were divided into three groups according to the severity of the stenosis at myelography: 19 nonoperated patients with a moderate stenosis, 30 operated patients with a moderate stenosis, and 14 operated patients with a complete block. The midsagittal diameter of the contrast column was similar in the nonoperated group and in the operated group with moderate stenosis; thus, these two groups were comparable. The mean follow-up time was approximately 3 years for the untreated patients and 4 years for the surgically treated group. Results judged by a visual analog scale are presented in Table 1. Most of the nonoperated patients were unchanged or improved. Only 10% of the nonoperated patients felt worse versus 20% in the operated group with moderate stenosis. Table 2 shows the results evaluated by a nonindependent surgeon. Interestingly, the rate of improvement (approximately 60%) was similar in the three groups. At follow-up, the level of pain and the use of analgesics did not differ significantly. However, walking capacity improved significantly more for patients after surgery than in the untreated group. The overall results of of the study were as follows. Of the untreated patients, 30% improved and 60% remained unchanged. After surgery, 60% improved and 25% deteriorated. However, as indicated by the authors, the conclusions of this study must be interpreted with a critical mind. First, it is not a randomized study. Second, the starting level of pain is not indicated. Third, the walking capacity at diagnosis was more impaired in the operated group. Finally, the radiographic findings were more pronounced in the surgically treated patients. More precisely, there was significantly more degenerative spondylolisthesis in the operated group with moderate stenosis (n = 12) than in the nontreated group (n = 5). Moreover, the outcome assessment was made by a nonindependent observer and was based on subjective opinion.

In another article, Johnsson et al. (10) reported the natural course of 32 patients studied prospectively. The mean follow-up time after myelography was 4 years, and the mean patient age was 60 years. All patients were advised to have surgical decompression. Thirty declined surgery and two were excluded by the anesthesiologist. About 75% of the patients had neurogenic claudication; the others had radicular pain or mixed symptoms. Outcome measures, completed by the patient, included a visual analog scale to appreciate the overall evolution and a second visual analog scale to evaluate the level of pain. Results also were assessed by clinical examination. Walking capacity was evaluated by visual analog scale and by measuring the walking distance on a level surface from start to onset of symptoms. Five patients were lost to follow-up (three died). The overall estimation of results at final follow-up by visual analog scale is presented in Table 3. Four patients (15%) worsened; the 23 remaining patients

TABLE 3. *Estimation of results by visual analog scale (0–100)*

No. of patients	Worse [% (n)]	Unchanged [% (n)]	Improved [% (n)]
27	15% (4)	70% (19)	15% (4)

From ref. 10.

TABLE 4. *Level of pain at follow-up*

Mild	19%
Moderate	70%
Severe	11%

From ref. 10.

were unchanged or improved. As shown in Table 4, all patients were still complaining of back and/or leg pain, which was severe in three patients. The walking distance of the whole group was unchanged, but was worse in 30% of the patients. The overall results of the study were as follows: 70% were unchanged, 15% improved, and 15% were worse. The authors correlated the midsagittal diameter of the contrast column with the clinical evolution. Interestingly, the four patients who worsened had the narrowest anteroposterior (AP) diameter (Table 5).

The natural course of 91 nonoperated patients was presented at the annual meeting of the International Society for the Study of the Lumbar Spine by Herno and associates (6) in 1996. This was a retrospective study with a mean follow-up time of 8 ± 3 years. Patients were divided into four groups according to the radiologic findings: 11 block stenosis, 40 moderate stenosis (anteroposterior diameter < 10 mm), 18 mild stenosis (AP diameter 10 to 12 mm), and 22 lateral stenosis. The outcome measures were based on the Oswestry questionnaire and on the walking capacity determined by the treadmill test. The level of pain in the back and legs before and after walking on the treadmill was assessed on a visual analog scale. At follow-up the overall patient subjective evaluation was as follows: 27 were unchanged, 41 improved, and 23 were worse. The mean Oswestry score was 31 ± 16. The score did not differ significantly according to the radiologic findings or follow-up time. The level of pain before and after walking on the treadmill did not differ between the radiologic groups. No difference in walking capacity was noted among the four groups. The final conclusion of the study was that, for these 91 patients, the natural course was benign and that the subjective and physical condition was unchanged.

In another study, Herno and associates (5) compared in a matched pair format the outcome of surgically treated and nonsurgically treated patients. They were able to form 54 similarly matched pairs. The matching criteria included sex, age, duration of symptoms, and myelographic findings. The major symptoms were neurogenic claudication, leg pain, and mixed symptoms. The myelographic findings were graded in four categories: total block, subtotal block (AP diameter < 10 mm), moderate stenosis (AP diameter 10 to 12 mm), and lateral stenosis. Assessment of results was based on the Oswestry score, and estimation of the functional status was based on clinical examination. Statistical analysis of the results determined that the mean Oswestry score was similar in the whole population and in women. However, the score was significantly better in operated men. The functional status was good

TABLE 5. *AP diameter and clinical evolution*

VAS result	No. of patients	AP diameter (mm)
Worse	4	4.7
Unchanged	19	6.8
Improved	4	8.2
Total	27	

AP, anteroposterior; VAS, visual analog scale.
From ref. 10.

TABLE 6. *Outcome of the nonsurgical group (n = 58)*

	Better	Same	Worse
Low back pain compared to baseline	41	38	20
Leg pain compared to baseline	44	42	12

From ref. 1.

in both groups. There was no correlation of the outcome with age, central (n = 35) versus lateral (n = 19) stenosis, and presence or absence of coexisting illness. This study has major limitations. As indicated by the authors, it is retrospective, and the starting level of pain and disability is unknown. Moreover, in 37 patients in the conservatively treated group, the pain was not severe enough to require an operation. This observation casts some doubt on the reliability of the matching.

Herno et al. (7) presented a longitudinal analysis of 38 nonoperated patients with LSS at the 1997 annual meeting of the International Society for the Study of the Lumbar Spine. Nineteen women and 19 men were examined for the first time in 1989 and for the second time in 1995. Most of them had one or several coexisting diseases. The radiologic findings were graded according to the severity and site of the stenosis as central (n = 27) or lateral (n = 11). The mean Oswestry score of all 38 patients was 34.3 in 1989 and 33.4 in 1995. The overall alterations in the patients conditions was judged on (i) physical condition, (ii) ability to perform daily activities, (iii) walking capacity on a treadmill, and (iv) pain on a visual analog scale after the treadmill test. Taken together, these parameters show that the overall condition remained almost unchanged. However, the patients with complete block noted on myelography worsened. In the authors' opinion, patients with block stenosis require surgical decompression.

Saal et al. (18) studied 52 patients with a follow-up ranging from 2 to 8 years. All patients had radiculopathy and restriction of walking capacity, with evidence of central stenosis with or without lateral stenosis on imaging studies. Treatment included analgesics, epidural injection, and physiotherapy. Outcome was assessed by an independent observer by questionnaire and telephone interview. Thirty-three of the 52 patients had a pain level controlled with nonnarcotic analgesics with no or minimal walking restriction. The remaining patients received epidural and physical therapy. There was no neurologic deterioration. Four patients were treated surgically. The authors concluded that patients with nonoperative treatment can avoid surgery and that medical and physical treatments are associated with better results than natural history by itself as reported by other authors. Unfortunately, no correlation was made in this study between the outcome and the clinical symptoms at diagnosis and with the site and severity of the stenosis.

The Maine Lumbar Spine study assessed the outcome after 1 year of surgical and nonsurgical management of LSS (1). One hundred forty-eight patients were enrolled in this prospective cohort study and followed at 3.6 and 12 months by questionnaire and telephone interview. Outcome measures were based on patient-reported symptoms of leg and back pain, functional status disability, and satisfaction with care. Eighteen patients (12%) dropped out; of these, nine were surgically treated and nine were medically treated. Tables 6 and 7 summarize the

TABLE 7. *Outcome of the surgical group (n = 72)*

	Better	Same	Worse
Low back pain	77	17	5
Leg pain	78	15	6

From ref. 1.

TABLE 8. *Subjective assessment of the conservative group*
(n = 18)

Worse	Unchanged	Improved
11%	45%	44%

From ref. 8.

outcomes at 1 year of the nonsurgical and the surgical groups. Twenty-eight percent of the nonoperated patients and 55% of the operated patients were improved. However, the surgical group on average had more severe symptoms and imaging findings at baseline. Consequently, the authors identified a group of nonoperated and operated patients with similar moderate symptoms at baseline. In this group of moderately symptomatic patients, surgical treatment resulted in greater improvement. Approximately 20% of the operated patients were not improved and some of them worsened. As indicated by Nachemson (14), the shortcomings of this study include the short follow-up, the absence of data on the imaging studies, the numbers of eligible patients not entered in the study, and the absence of follow-up by an independent examiner. These observations preclude any valuable conclusion.

In contrast to the Maine Lumbar Spine study, Hurri et al. (8) focused on the long-term prognosis of LSS. Seventy-five of 134 patients with LSS diagnosed by myelography between 1978 and 1982 were followed up in 1993. Forty-eight had died and 11 could not be reached. Outcome was assessed by telephone interview using a structured questionnaire. Estimation of the disability was made according to the Oswestry score and by subjective assessment by the patient (improved, unchanged, or worse). Stenosis was severe (< 7.0 mm) in 32 patients (26 operated) and moderate (7 to 10.5 mm) in 43 patients (31 operated). Tables 8 and 9 summarize the subjective assessments of both groups. The authors concluded that therapy, as such, did not correlate with the disability at outcome. In contrast, the severity of the stenosis predicted disability independently of the treatment. The major shortcoming of this study is the loss of a significant number of patients at follow-up.

CONCLUSIONS

Results of these studies suggest that a substantial proportion of patients do not automatically deteriorate and will remain unchanged or even improved if they are helped by medical means. They also suggest that patients with severe baseline symptoms, block stenosis, and degenerative spondylolisthesis tend to deteriorate and require surgical decompression (8–10). However, the studies reviewed in this chapter are retrospective and thus carry with them the problems of missing data and the stability of the population. In the studies comparing medical and surgical treatment, the lack of precise information on baseline clinical symptoms and/or the imaging data preclude any clear-cut conclusions. Therefore, at the present time no scientifically based recommendations can be made to LSS patients at diagnosis. Similarly, predictors of success or failure of medical and surgical treatment still need to be identified.

TABLE 9. *Subjective assessment of the operated group*
(n = 57)

Worse	Unchanged	Improved
18%	19%	63%

From ref. 8.

However, the input given by the retrospective studies provide invaluable information to organize prospective randomized studies with an appropriate methodology. Such studies should be able to determine different variables, clinical or radiologic, that influence the natural evolution. As already mentioned, randomized studies are difficult to conduct in this older population, mainly for ethical reasons. However, as suggested by Berthelot et al. (3), such studies could proceed by stages with cohorts reviewed every 6 to 12 months. Patients with disabling pain and functional status will be proposed randomization to surgery or no surgery.

Relevant variables include age, gender, socioeconomic and occupational conditions, comorbidity, as well as adequate baseline clinical symptoms. Pathoanatomic definition must be clearly documented. This includes the anatomic location of the stenosis (central and/or lateral) and classification according to the etiology (primary or secondary). Myelography traditionally has been used for diagnosis of LSS and still currently is performed before surgery. However, possible adverse reactions and poor visualization of the lateral recess explain why CT scan and/or MRI now are commonly used as first-line imaging studies. The number of stenotic and unstable levels as well as diameter and area measurements must be defined and measurements made by independent examiners demonstrating satisfactory inter- and intraobserver reproducibility.

Lumbar spinal stenosis is a specific subgroup of low back pain, and outcome measures must be adapted to its characteristics to appreciate accurately efficacy of treatment and allow comparison with natural evolution. Evaluation of physical impairments such as neurologic abnormalities or Lasègue's sign do not reflect properly the functional status and disability. The patient's entered outcome measures are essential in evaluating this particular subgroup. In the authors' current practice, outcome measures include five items: (i) the cumulative illness rating scale to detect a potential comorbidity (13), (ii) a psychological evaluation using the self-rating depression scale, (iii) a generic health status index such as SF36 to evaluate both physical and nonphysical impairment (23), (iv) a condition-specific health status index as proposed by Stucki et al. (19), and (v) two visual analog scales, one to evaluate low back pain and the other to evaluate radicular pain. The ability of disease-specific outcome measures such as the Oswestry low back pain questionnaire to document treatment efficacy in LSS has not been demonstrated. Condition-specific health status indexes seem more appropriate and adapted to this unique category of low back pain patients. The authors currently are using a self-administered questionnaire adapted from that of Stucki and colleagues. The combined use of these indexes in clinical trials of patients with LSS is strongly recommended by the authors.

REFERENCES

1. Atlas SJ, Deyo RA, Keller RB, et al. The Maine Lumbar Spine study. Part III: 1 year outcomes of surgical and nonsurgical management of lumbar spinal stenosis. *Spine* 1996;21:1787–1795.
2. Benoist M. Unpublished data.
3. Berthelot JM, Bertrand-Vasseur A, Rodet D, et al. Lumbar spinal stenosis. A review. *Rev Mal Osteoartic* 1997; 64:337–348.
4. Blau JN, Logue V. The natural history of intermittent claudication of the cauda equina. *Brain* 1978;101:211–222.
5. Herno A, Airaksinen O, Saari T, et al. Lumbar spinal stenosis: a matched pair study of operated and nonoperated patients. *Br J Neurosurg* 1996;10:461–465.
6. Herno A, Nevalainen S, Saari T, et al. *The natural course of 91 nonoperated patients with lumbar spinal stenosis*. Presented at the annual meeting of the International Society for the Study of the Lumbar Spine, Burlington, June 25–29, 1996.
7. Herno A, Nevalainen S, Saari T, et al. *The longitudinal analysis of 38 nonoperated patients with lumbar spinal stenosis*. Presented at the annual meeting of the International Society Society for the Study of the Lumbar Spine, Singapore, June 2–6, 1997.
8. Hurri H, Slatis P, Soini J, et al. Lumbar spinal stenosis: assessment of long-term outcome 12 years after operative and conservative treatment. *J Spinal Disord* 1998;11:110–115.

9. Johnsson KE, Uden A, Rosen I. The effect of decompression on the natural course of spinal stenosis. A comparison of surgically treated and untreated patients. *Spine* 1991;16:615–619.

10. Johnsson KE, Rosen I, Uden A. The natural course of lumbar spinal stenosis. *Clin Orthop* 1992;279:82–86.

11. Jones RAC, Thompson JLP. The narrow lumbar canal. A clinical and radiological review. *J Bone Joint Surg* 1968;50B:595–605.

12. Katz JN, Lipson SJ, Chang LC, et al. Seven to 10 year outcome of decompressive surgery for degenerative lumbar spinal stenosis. *Spine* 1996;21:92–98.

13. Linn BS, Linn M, Currel L. Cumulative illness rating scale. *J Am Geriatr Soc* 1968;16:622–626.

14. Nachemson A. Point of view. *Spine* 1996;21:1794–1795.

15. Porter RW, Hibbert C, Evans C. The natural history of root entrapment syndrome. *Spine* 1984;9:418–421.

16. Postacchini F. Lumbar spinal stenosis. Long-term results. In: Wiesel SW, Weinstein JN, Herkowitz H, Dvorak J, Bell G, eds. *The lumbar spine, volume 2.* Philadelphia: WB Saunders, 1990:766–781.

17. Rosomoff H, Rosomoff R. Nonsurgical aggressive treatment of lumbar spinal stenosis. *Spine* 1987;3:383.

18. Saal JS, Saal JA, Parthasarathy R, et al. *The natural history of lumbar spinal stenosis. The results of nonoperative treatment.* Presented at the annual meeting of the International Society for the Study of the Lumbar Spine, Singapore, June 2–6, 1997.

19. Stucki G, Daltroy L, Liand M, et al. Measurement properties of a self-administered outcome measure. *Spine* 1996;21:796–803.

20. Tile M, McNeil SR, Zains RK, et al. Spinal stenosis: results of treatment. *Clin Orthop* 1976;115:104–108.

21. Tuite GF, Stern JD, Doran SE, et al. Outcome after laminectomy for lumbar spinal stenosis. Part 1: Clinical correlations. *J Neurosurg* 1994;81:699–706.

22. Turner JA, Ersek K, Herron L, Deyo R. Surgery for lumbar spinal stenosis. Attempted meta-analysis of the literature. *Spine* 1992;17:1–8.

23. Ware JE, Sherbourne CD. The MOS 36-item short form health survey (SF36). I. Conceptual frame work and item selection. *Med Care* 1992;30:473–483.

Lumbar Spinal Stenosis
edited by Robert Gunzburg and Marek Szpalski
Lippincott Williams & Wilkins, Philadelphia, © 2000.

9

Stenosis and Cauda Equina Syndrome

Olle Hägg and Björn Rydevik

*Department of Orthopaedics, Sahlgrenska University Hospital, Göteborg University,
SE-413 45 Göteborg, Sweden*

Cauda equina syndrome (CES) can be defined as the clinical entity in which mechanical compression of the nerve roots of the cauda equina, including the centrally located sacral nerve roots, results in vesical, rectal, and sexual dysfunction together with dysesthesia of corresponding cutaneous areas. If the compression occurs at levels where lumbar nerve roots are present, motor and sensory deficits in the lower extremities can be part of the clinical syndrome. However, this discussion will mainly focus on the consequences of sacral nerve root compression. Whereas the neurogenic claudication is the main clinical presentation and indication of surgery in spinal stenosis, the urogenital and rectal manifestations seldom are reported in the literature. The true frequency of these symptoms may be underestimated because most patients with spinal stenosis are older, and both patient and surgeon might assign urogenital and rectal dysfunction to other age-related diseases. The clinical presentation can range from acute complete CES to chronic incomplete CES.

EFFECTS OF COMPRESSION ON CAUDA EQUINA NERVE ROOTS

Mechanical compression of the lumbar and sacral nerve roots in spinal stenosis is a slowly developing phenomenon (24). It appears that cauda equina nerve roots can progressively adjust to increasing compression and become more resistant to acute compression (14). Moreover, slow and gradual deformation of nerve roots is better tolerated than rapid deformation (Fig. 1) (22). These facts probably explain why the cauda equina can still function even in cases of spinal stenosis with very severe narrowing of the spinal canal, as evidenced by magnetic resonance imaging, myelography, or computed tomography. A series of investigations using a porcine model demonstrated that in acute graded compression of the cauda equina, there is a pressure threshold between 50 and 75 mm Hg at which changes in both afferent and efferent conduction are induced (27). Investigations of intraneural blood flow in cauda equina nerve roots during graded compression revealed that blood flow in the venules was impaired at low pressure levels of 5 to 10 mm Hg (19). Compression for 2 hours at 50 mm Hg resulted in edema formation in the spinal nerve roots (20) as well as impairment of the nutritional supply to the cauda equina (21). As a general finding in several of these investigations, it was noted that rapid onset of compression had a more profound effect than slow onset (0.05 to 0.1 vs. 20 s). These observations thus provide a biologic correlate to the clinical observations that slowly developing, chronic compression may be fairly well tolerated by cauda equina nerve roots in contrast to acute, rapid deformation.

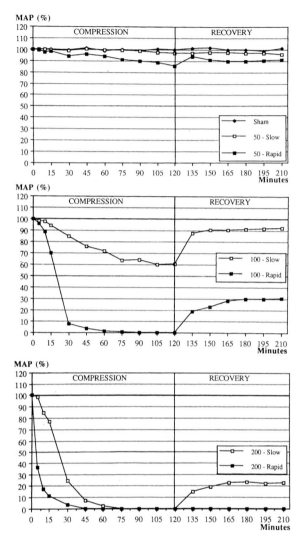

FIG. 1. Data on motor conduction in pig cauda equina nerve roots from *in vivo* experiments. The diagrams show the average amplitude of the fastest conducting nerve fibers expressed as a percentage of the baseline value. Data are presented as monitored during 2 hours of compression and 1.5 hours of recovery for sham compression and for rapid and slow onset of compression at 50, 100, and 200 mm Hg. Note that the functional deterioration is more pronounced following rapid onset than slow onset of compression, especially at 100 mm Hg compression. These data indicate that slow and gradual deformation of nerve roots is better tolerated than rapid deformation. MAP, muscle action potential. (From ref. 22, with permission.)

CHRONIC INCOMPLETE CAUDA EQUINA SYNDROME: BLADDER, GENITAL, AND RECTAL DYSFUNCTION

Whereas acute complete CES has been reported as a consequence of central lumbar disc herniations (7,15,28,30,32), the corresponding complication seems to be a very rare event in spinal stenosis (18).

Bladder dysfunction was studied prospectively in a recent investigation (25). It was found that 80% of 108 male patients with spinal stenosis had micturition problems. In another study, ten male and ten female patients with bladder dysfunction were investigated after surgery (4). At the 6-month follow-up, 12 patients reported subjective improvement of micturition. Bladder dysfunction has been investigated urodynamically (29) and electrophysiologically (9) both before and after decompressive surgery. Genital dysfunction has been described in case reports as walking-induced intermittent priapism in conjunction with bladder incontinence (1,8,10,26). The symptoms had the potential to resolve after surgery. Fecal incontinence was not reported in a Swedish survey of 163 cases (11), but it is described in a case report as exercise-provoked symptomatology (6).

There are no prospective studies addressing either rectal or genital dysfunction. The few case reports concerning genital dysfunction discuss only priapism. Sexual dysfunction, male or female, has not been discussed in the literature. There are reasons to assume that these kinds of symptoms may be more frequent than is known at present (34). Even if the mean age is about 65 years for subjects with central lumbar spinal stenosis (12), this condition is not uncommon in younger individuals. In the study by Jönsson and Strömqvist (12), the youngest patients were 37 years of age. Thus, central spinal stenosis may occur in populations that are sexually active. Well-designed prospective studies in this area are needed to elucidate the true prevalence of vesical, genital, and rectal dysfunction in conjunction with lumbar spinal stenosis.

ACUTE POSTOPERATIVE CAUDA EQUINA SYNDROME

Acute CES is a severe complication after decompressive surgery (2). It has been reported in 1 of 50 patients (13) and 4 of 96 patients (16). The most common cause in these studies is reported to be an epidural hematoma. However, it also has been described as an effect of a free autogenous fat graft (3,17,31), unrecognized incomplete decompression (35), and an unrecognized arachnoid cyst above the level of decompression (33).

In our institution we encountered three cases of acute postoperative CES in 217 cases (1.4%) of operated cases of spinal stenosis during the last 2 years. In these three cases, the CES developed secondary to epidural hematoma formation (Fig. 2) 1 to 3 days after surgery despite the use of an active epidural suction drainage. There were no intraoperative complications, and there was no excessive blood loss to indicate CES. We conclude that the only way to prevent this potentially disastrous complication is by regular postoperative neurologic examinations during the first days after surgery.

TIMING OF DECOMPRESSION FOR ACUTE CAUDA EQUINA SYNDROME

When discussing the clinical evaluation of a patient with a suspected CES and the timing of decompression, the underlying pathophysiologic effects of compression on spinal nerve roots should be considered. It seems well established that the degree of nerve injury is, at least to some extent, dependent on the duration of compression (23,27). Delamarter and co-workers (5) described observations obtained in a canine model for cauda equina compression. They subjected the cauda equina to varying degrees of constriction and followed the recovery after decompression at various time points ranging from immediately after application of the constriction up to 1 week after the onset of compression. They did not find any significant differences in the degree of recovery after early versus late decompression.

In a clinical situation, there are no reasons to delay the decompression any more than necessary. Appropriate preoperative examinations of the patient must be performed, but because an epidural hematoma is the most common cause of postoperative CES, in most cases there is no need to perform computed tomography or magnetic resonance imaging, which

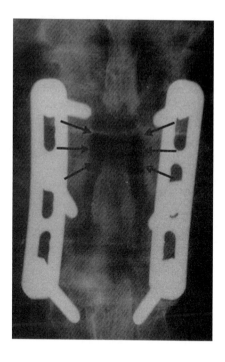

FIG. 2. Myelogram from the anteroposterior view of the lower lumbar spine 2 days after decompression of spinal stenosis at L4–5 and L5–S1 including instrumented fusion in a patient who developed acute postoperative cauda equina syndrome. Note that there is a myelographic defect indicating epidural compression at the L4–5 level. Surgical decompression revealed an epidural hematoma causing pronounced compression of the dural sac at that level.

would only delay a necessary acute decompression further. The issue of reversibility of neural injury as a result of cauda equina compression is very complex, with factors such as magnitude of pressure and duration of compression to be considered. The literature does not seem to provide support for the view that emergency surgery influences the outcome of acute CES, but decompression should be performed as rapidly as possible after adequate examinations, preferably with some degree of urgency (7,15).

CONCLUSIONS

Incomplete chronic CES may occur more frequently in spinal stenosis than currently recognized. Adequately designed prospective studies are needed in this area. Acute postoperative CES is a potential complication after decompressive surgery. Regular postoperative neurologic examinations should always be performed to detect any signs of a developing CES as early as possible. In case of established acute postoperative CES, surgical decompression should be performed without undue delay, after adequate examination of the patient.

REFERENCES

1. Baba H, Maezawa Y, Furusawa N, Kawahara N, Tomita K. Lumbar spinal stenosis causing intermittent priapism. *Paraplegia* 1995;33:6:338–345.
2. Boccanera L, Laus M. Cauda equina syndrome following lumbar spinal stenosis surgery. *Spine* 1987;12;7: 712–715.
3. Deburge A, Bitan F, Lassale B, Vaquin G. Syndrome de la queue de cheval par migration d un greffon graisseux après laminoarthrectomie. Cauda equina compression after migration of a free fat graft used at the end of a lamino arthrectomy. *Rev Chir Orthop* 1988;74:677–678.
4. Deen HG Jr, Zimmerman RS, Swanson SK, Larson TR. Assessment of bladder function after lumbar decompressive laminectomy for spinal stenosis: a prospective study. *J Neurosurg* 1994;80:6:971–974.
5. Delamarter RB, Sherman JE, Carr JB. 1991 Volvo Award in Experimental Studies, cauda equina syndrome: neurologic recovery following immediate, early or late decompression. *Spine* 1991;16:1022–1029.

6. Foster OJ, Harrison MJ, Crockard HA. Exercise provoked faecal incontinence in spinal stenosis. *J Neurol Neurosurg Psychiatry* 1987;50:3:362–363.

7. Gleave JRW, MacFarlane R. Prognosis for recovery of bladder function following lumbar central disc prolapse. *Br J Neurosurg* 1990;76:205–210.

8. Hidalgo Ovejero AM, Garcia Mata S, Sauras Herranz MA, Maravi Petri E, Martinez Grande M. Intermittent priapism in spinal stenosis. *Acta Orthop Belg* 1991;57:2:192–194.

9. Hiraizumi Y, Transfeldt EE, Fujimaki E, Nakabayashi H, Ishikawa T, Sato H. Electrophysiologic evaluation of intermittent saceral nerve dysfunction in lumbar spinal canal stenosis. *Spine* 1993;18:1355–1360.

10. Hopkins A, Clarke C, Brindley G. Erections on walking as a symptom of spinal canal stenosis. *J Neurol Neurosurg Psychiatry* 1987;50:1371–1374.

11. Johnsson K-E. Lumbar spinal stenosis. A retrospective study of 163 cases in southern Sweden. *Acta Orthop Scand* 1995;66:403–405.

12. Jönsson B, Strömqvist B. Symptoms and signs in degeneration of the lumbar spine. A prospective consecutive study of 300 patients. *J Bone Joint Surg* 1993;75B:381–385.

13. Jönsson B, Strömqvist B. Lumbar spine surgery in the elderly. Complications and surgical results. *Spine* 1994; 19:13:1431–1435.

14. Kikuchi S, Konno S, Kayama S, Sato K, Olmarker K. Increased resistance to acute compression injury in chronically compressed spinal nerve roots. An experimental study. *Spine* 1996;21:2544–2550.

15. Kostuik JP, Harrington I, Alexander D, et al. Cauda equina syndrome and lumbar disc herniation. *J Bone Joint Surg* 1986;68A:386–391.

16. Laus M, Pignatti G, Alfonso C, Ferrari D, De Cristofaro R, Giunti A. Complications in the surgical treatment of lumbar stenosis. *Chir Organi Mov* 1992;77:65–71.

17. Mayer PJ, Jacobsen FS. Cauda equina syndrome after surgical treatment of lumbar spinal stenosis with application of free autogenous fat graft. A report of two cases. *J Bone Joint Surg Am* 1989;71:1090–1093.

18. McNeill TW. Pelvic visceral dysfunction cauda equina syndrome. In: Wiesel SW, Weinstein JN, Herkowitz HN, Dvorak J, Bell GR, eds. *The lumbar spine, volume I*, 2nd ed. Philadelphia: WB Saunders, 1996:569–582.

19. Olmarker K, Rydevik B, Holm S, Bagge U. Effects of experimental, graded compression on blood flow in spinal nerve roots. A vital microscopic study on the porcine cauda equina. *J Orthop Res* 1989;7:817–823.

20. Olmarker K, Rydevik B, Holm S. Edema formation in spinal nerve roots induced by experimental, graded compression. An experimental study on the pig cauda equina with special reference to differences in effects between rapid and slow onset of compression. *Spine* 1989;14:569–573.

21. Olmarker K, Rydevik B, Hansson T, Holm S. Compression-induced changes of the nutritional supply to the porcine cauda equina. *J Spinal Disord* 1990;3:25–29.

22. Olmarker K, Holm S, Rydevik B. Importance of compression onset rate for the degree of impairment of impulse propagation in experimental compression injury of the porcine cauda equina. *Spine* 1990;15:416–419.

23. Olmarker K. Spinal nerve root compression. Nutrition and function of the porcine cauda equina compressed in vivo. *Acta Orthop Scand Suppl* 1991;62:5–15.

24. Olmarker K, Takahashi K, Rydevik B. Anatomy and compression pathophysiology of the nerve roots of the lumbar spine. In: Andersson GBJ, MacNeill T, eds. *Spinal stenosis*. St. Louis: Mosby-Year Book, 1992:77–90.

25. Perner A, Andersen JT, Juhler M. Lower urinary tract symptoms in lumbar root compression syndromes: a prospective survey. *Spine* 1997;22:2693–269.

26. Ram Z, Finder G, Spiegelman R, Schacked I, Tadmor R, Sahar A. Intermittent priapism in spinal canal stenosis. *Spine* 1987;12:377–378.

27. Rydevik BL, Pedowitz RA, Hargens AR, Swenson MR, Myers RR, Garfin SR. Effects of acute, graded compression on spinal nerve root function and structure. An experimental study of the pig cauda equina. *Spine* 1991; 16:487–493.

28. Scott PJ. Bladder paralysis in cauda equina lesions from disc prolapse. *J Bone Joint Surg* 1965;47B:224–235.

29. Smith AY, Woodside JR. Urodynamic evaluation of patients with spinal stenosis. *Urology* 1988;32:474–477.

30. Spangfort EV. The lumbar disc herniation: a computer-aided analysis of 2,504 operations. *Acta Orthop Scand Suppl* 1972;43:38–39.

31. Strömqvist B, Jönsson B, Annertz M, Holtås S. Cauda equina syndrome caused by migrating fat graft after lumbar spinal decompression. A case report demonstrated with magnetic resonance imaging. *Spine* 1991;16: 100–101.

32. Tay ECK, Chacha PB. Midline prolapse of a lumbar intervertebral disc with compression of the cauda equina. *J Bone Joint Surg* 1979;41B:43–46.

33. Valls PL, Naul LG, Kanter SL. Paraplegia after a routine lumbar laminectomy: report of a rare complication and successful management. *Neurosurgery* 1990;27:638–640.

34. Willen JG, Griffiths ER, Mastaglia FL, Beaver R. Intermittent parasympathetic symptoms in lumbar spinal stenosis. *Spinal Disord* 1989;2:109–113.

35. Woods DA, Wilson-MacDonald J. A complication of spinal decompression. A case report. *Spine* 1995;20: 2467–2469.

Lumbar Spinal Stenosis
edited by Robert Gunzburg and Marek Szpalski
Lippincott Williams & Wilkins, Philadelphia, © 2000.

10

Iatrogenic Stenosis

Robert C. Mulholland

Department of Orthopaedics and Trauma, University Hospital Nottingham, and Spinal Disorders Unit, University Hospital, Queens Medical Center, Nottingham NG7 2RD, United Kingdom

Iatrogenic diseases are those produced by doctors in the course of treating a patient. Iatrogenic stenosis therefore could be restricted to stenosis clearly due to a particular treatment, or it could be widened to include stenosis occurring after treatment that is not necessarily due directly to the treatment. I shall deal with the anatomic or pathologic state of stenosis, which may not always produce the clinical syndrome, although the syndrome is always associated with the pathologic disorder.

It would be appropriate if the pathologic nature of spinal stenosis was briefly described.

Central canal stenosis refers to stenosis produced in the central part of the canal, usually by redundant flavum, or in a patient who had prior laminectomy and flavectomy. The compressing factor may be bone that either is put there as part of a fusion or represents regrowth of bone from the removed lamina. The anterior constricting factor is the disc, which as a consequence perhaps of disc narrowing is bulging backward, producing further reduction of the area of the central canal.

Lateral canal stenosis is related to a number of different factors.

Subarticular stenosis due to osteophytes and joint arthritic change reduce the space between the joint and the back of the vertebrae. If there is segmental failure and forward translation, the superior facet on the lower vertebrae actually migrates down the pedicle and narrows the space between itself and the back of the vertebrae, crushing the underlying nerve. Associated flaval calcification, where the flavum is medially attached to the articular process and blends with its capsule, is another important factor in compressing the root. At the foramen, bulging disc and upward migration of the superior articular process (so-called up-down stenosis) may occur, combined with narrowing of the exit foramen due to disc space narrowing.

It will become clear that the pathology of acquired spinal stenosis is disc space narrowing, facet arthritis, and flaval infolding. The clinical syndrome produced is immensely variable, and, as we know, vascular factors play a vital role.

LATE-ONSET STENOSIS AFTER DISCECTOMY OR CHYMOPAPAINE FOR UNCOMPLICATED PROLAPSED INTERVERTEBRAL DISC

Disc space narrowing is a variable consequence of the surgical treatment of a herniated disc. However, the degree of disc narrowing bears no relation to clinical outcome (3,6). One would anticipate that such narrowing would be more likely to be associated with mechanical disturbance of the back, i.e., a greater incidence of back pain, that such narrowing would narrow the exit foramina, and that facet degenerative changes would produce subfacetal root pain. In patients who had a disc protrusion, a proportion inevitably returns with a relapse. The differential diagnosis is that they have developed a further protrusion or have some stenosis. The poor results achieved by reexploration in those patients who have not had a further disc protrusion is good evidence that stenosis is seldom an important clinical factor. Surgeons should be wary of being enticed into a further wide decompression to deal with postlaminectomy stenosis in the absence of a further disc herniation.

An exception to this is if a patient develops spondylolisthesis after an overgenerous operation for a disc protrusion, perhaps associated with a pars fracture, when the patient may present with stenosis, which will present as the typical clinical stenotic syndrome seen in degenerative spondylolisthesis.

Chymopapaine is one of the most critically evaluated therapies for disc protrusion. There have been many long-term follow-up series (5,7,14,17,18). When we began to use chymopapaine in the mid 1970s, we were concerned that the biologic effects of mucopolysaccharide destruction, i.e., the disc space narrowing that followed, would in time be associated with the development of lateral canal stenosis. However, late-onset stenotic syndromes have not developed in any of the reported series. There have been recurrent disc protrusions (about 4%), which is slightly lower than is seen in the surgically treated patient. In our own long-term follow-up comparing surgically treated patients with those treated with chymopapaine, the surgically treated patients, if they had symptoms, tended to have back pain, whereas the chymopapaine patients tended to have leg pain, which often had been a persistent symptom since treatment. In this regard, we are all aware that most reported series of early failure of surgical or chymopapaine treatment of a herniated disc ascribe such failure to the coincident presence of spinal stenosis. As we are aware from the epidemiologic work of Porter et al. (15), patients with smaller spinal diameters are more likely to have symptoms from a herniated disc than those with large canals. Whenever we deal surgically with a herniation, we inevitably tend to deal with any real or perceived stenosis. Chymopapaine clearly cannot address this. Coincident spinal stenosis is a factor in the 30% primary failure rate, and is not produced by chymopapaine; this is early failure before disc space narrowing has occurred.

SPINAL STENOSIS AFTER SPINAL FUSION

Prior to intertransverse fusion, spinal fusion was a posterior operation. Bone was laid posteriorly over the lamina and the interlaminar space. It was suggested that, on occasion, such bone grew into the interlaminar space and produced spinal stenosis. The evidence for this is anecdotal, and I suspect very questionable now that we know more about remodeling of the spinal canal after fracture. However, there are two situations where stenosis does occur after spinal fusion.

It will be appreciated that, after a fusion, particularly after a two- or three-level fusion, spinal movement is concentrated at the level above the fusion. Curiously, the work of Luk et al. (10) established that hypermobility does not necessarily occur, and if it does, others have established that the next level up may be more mobile. I presume this is because inevitably the tissues immediately above a fusion are somewhat scarred and restrict movement. The study of Luk et al. dealt with anterior fusion only, so that surgical injury to the facet joints above a posterior fusion may have a confounding effect is possible. In some patients, if segmental failure develops immediately above a fusion, then the degenerative process described occurs, and they present with a stenotic problem. Although their back pain may be mechanical and provide a mandate for extending the fusion, in many patients it is stenotic back pain. Decompression is an essential part of any surgical treatment, although it usually is accompanied by fusion if there is established actual or potential translation.

A popular device used for spinal fusion is the Hartshill rectangle (2). The wires of the device obtrude into the canal at the upper margin of the solid fusion and lie posterior to the still mobile disc. The dura therefore is moved below them, and granulation and fibrous tissue can produce a stenotic situation at the upper level of the fusion.

POSTERIOR BONE GROWTH AFTER DECOMPRESSION IN SPINAL STENOSIS

It is well recognized that there is a late failure rate in patients who have decompression for spinal stenosis (8). Although the reasons for this are varied, one factor is the regrowth of bone over the decompression area. Postachinni and Cinotti (16) showed a clear relationship between the long-term result and the amount of bone that grows over the decompressed area. What is of interest is that if a fusion is done at the same time, the amount of bone regrowth is less. This would certainly give support to those who advocate routine fusion when stenosis is dealt with. I suspect that in those patients who have spondylolisthesis or incipient spondylolisthesis as shown by preoperative flexion films under load, they are mobile and fusion is indicated. If the spine is stiff and immobile and remains so after decompression, I do not believe that fusion is required. I presume that the bone formed over the decompression is a consequence of underlying spinal movement—nature's attempt to stabilize the spine. The study by Chen et al. (1) strongly supports the view of Postachinni et al. In a review of 48 patients after 4 to 7 years, mild growth of bone was seen in 50%, moderate in 29%, and marked in 15%. They noted that spinal instability accelerated bone growth and that patients with moderate or severe bone growth had a less satisfactory clinical result. It was clear this was a time-related phenomenon; the longer the follow-up, the greater the clinical significance of bone regrowth.

The clinical significance of these studies is that perhaps one should be cautious about generous decompression immediately above a fusion. This is sometimes clinically indicated, i.e., stenosis extending up to L2–3, with a degenerative spondylolisthesis at L4–5, and no abnormal translation above, so that a fusion of L4–5 is all that is clinically indicated. Decompression above this if one elects only to fuse L4–5 should perhaps be an interlaminar decompression rather than a total laminectomy. Although not clearly stated, one gets the impression from both studies that total laminectomy was the method of decompression. One suspects that interlaminar decompression by maintaining at least the continuity of the lamina over the decompression may result in bone growth over the decompression at the level of the retained lamina rather than directly onto the dural sac. However, I would emphasize that in doing this procedure, especially in the upper lumbar spine, more than two thirds of the lamina has to be removed to satisfactorily remove the flavum lying deep to the trailing edge.

The procedure of laminoplasty, which re-covers the decompressed canal with the lamina and a structurally placed bone graft supporting it in place, as well as fusing the segments, would appear to be an appropriate operation that might be expected to make impossible the subsequent development of spinal stenosis due to bone growing over the laminectomy defect (11,12,19). The procedure applied to the lumbar spine was described in the late 1980s by Tsuji, and there were further reports by Matsui from the same unit in 1992 and 1997 (11,12). Some 80% of patients achieved good or excellent results, but the only comment they make in the 1997 article is that preoperative and postoperative radiologic changes showed no significant correlation with JOA (Japanese Orthopedic Association) score changes and repeat surgery. Laminoplasty is a more complex procedure than either interlaminar decompression or full laminectomy and intertransverse fusion. As described, I would be concerned that decompression of the lateral recesses may be less than optimal. A prospective trial comparing the two techniques would be required, but as the meta-analysis by Niggemeyer et al. (13) and Turner et al. (20) showed, studies of the efficacy of surgery for spinal stenosis are flawed.

SPINAL STENOSIS AND CAGES

If the 1980s were the era of the spinal screw, then the 1990s are the era of the cage. At a recent symposium on cages, elegantly entitled ''Cages are for Monkeys'' (Eisenstein), we learned much about the great variety of cages and the enthusiasm for their use by surgeons and manufacturers, but little about their problems or biologic performance. One problem we have experienced with their use, and which has now been reported by others, is the creation of root entrapment or root irritation in the foramen and lateral canal. This may be related to actual intrusion of the canal posterolaterally, or inadequate disc clearance posterolaterally caused the cage to push disc material into the foramen. This is a particular problem with two cages, as if the first one is placed too close to the midline, the second cage is forced laterally and protrudes into the foramen.

It is perhaps wrong to describe this as a spinal stenosis, because although there is stenosis of the foramen, the clinical picture is one of acute radiculopathy. If computed tomography demonstrates that the cage is the compressing factor, then it is essential that it be removed, reopening the anterior approach. If the problem is disc material that has been pushed out, then posterior decompression is probably satisfactory. However, in our own two patients who had this complication, despite posterior decompression and pedicle fixation the patients were left with a chronic radiculopathy. Glassman et al. (4) reported a similar case and found it necessary to do a partial vertebral body resection to deal satisfactorily with the problem.

In a report of the Bak cage from a United States multicenter study, the complication is not alluded to (9). However, Kuslich (personal communication) does report the experience of radicular pain after use of the cages. In some patients this is ascribed to a traction effect due to distraction of the disc space, but there is no firm evidence that this is the case. I suspect that such cases on occasion are due to root compression by the cage if it is misplaced, or due to extruded disc material if cage position appears satisfactory.

I believe this potential complication associated with the use of two anterior cages is sufficiently important, such that if one is using a cage anteriorly, a single cage should be used. After all, one reason for the use of the double cage was manufacturer convenience; they could market a cage that could be used from the back and front. In the posterior approach, two cages clearly are necessary for safe insertion without risk of neurologic damage. However, in this situation one is in control of the spinal diameters, as one can ensure that there is no canal compromise at the end of the procedure.

In most patients who develop serious disability after spinal surgery, often referred to (erroneously in my view) as failed back surgery, symptoms are more likely due to disturbances of the mechanical function of the back or irreversible ischemic damage to nerve roots than developing spinal stenosis. It is surprising that in the long-term follow-up of operation for disc herniation, late stenosis associated with disc space narrowing is not a problem encountered more frequently.

REFERENCES

1. Chen Q, Baba H, Kamitani K, Furusawa N Imura S. Postoperative bone re-growth in lumbar spinal stenosis. A multivariate analysis of 48 patients. *Spine* 1994;19:2144–2149.

2. Dove J. Internal fixation of the lumbar spine. The Hartshill rectangle. *Clin Orthop* 1986;203:135–140.
3. Frymoyer JW, Matteri RE, Hanley EN, Kuhlmann D, Howe J. Failed lumbar disc surgery requiring a second operation. A long-term follow-up study. *Spine* 1978;3:7–11.
4. Glassman SD, Johnson JR, Raque G, Puno RM, Dimar JR. Management of iatrogenic spinal stenosis complicating placement of a fusion cage: a case report. *Spine* 1996;21:2383–2386.
5. Gogan WJ, Fraser RD. Chymopapaine. A 10-year, double-blind study. *Spine* 1992;17:388–394.
6. Hanley EN, Scapiro DE. The development of low-back pain after excision of a lumbar disc. *J Bone Joint Surg Am* 1989;71:719–721.
7. Javid MJ. Efficacy of chemonucleolysis. A long-term review of 105 patients. *J Neurosurg* 1985;62:662–666.
8. Jonsson B, Annertz M, Sjoberg C, Stromquist B. A prospective and consecutive study of surgically treated lumbar spinal stenosis. Part 11: Five-year follow-up by an independant observor. *Spine* 1997;22:2938–2944.
9. Kuslich SD, Ulstrom CL, Griffith SL, Ahere JW, Dowdle JD. The Bagby and Kuslich method of lumbar interbody fusion. History, techniques, and 2-year follow-up results of a United States prospective multicenter trial. *Spine* 1998;23:1267–1278; discussion 1279.
10. Luk KD, Chow DH, Evans JH, Leong JC. Lumbar spinal mobility after short anterior interbody fusion. *Spine* 1995;20:813–818.
11. Matsui H, Kanamori M, Ishihara H, Hirano N, Tsuji H. Expansive lumbar laminoplasty for degenerative spinal stenosis in patients below 70 years of age. *Eur Spine J* 1997;6:191–196.
12. Matsui H, Tsuji H, Sekido H, Hirano N, Katoh Y, Makiyama N. Results of expansive laminoplasty for lumbar spinal stenosis in active manual workers. *Spine* 1992;17[Suppl]:S37–S40.
13. Niggemeyer O, Strauss JM, Schulitz KP. Comparison of surgical procedures for degenerative lumbar spinal stenosis: a meta-analysis of the literature from 1975 to 1995. *Eur Spine J* 1997;6:423–429.
14. Nordby EJ. Eight to 13 year follow-up evaluation of chemonucleolysis patients. *Clin Orthop* 1986;206:18–23.
15. Porter RW, Hibbert CS, Wicks M. The spinal canal in symptomatic lumbar disc lesions. *J Bone Joint Surg Br* 1978;60B:485–487.
16. Postacchini F, Cinotti G. Bone Regrowth after surgical decompression for Lumbar spinal stenosis. *J Bone Joint Surg Br* 1992;74:862–869.
17. Thomas JC Jr, Wiltse LL, Widell EH Jr, Spencer CW 3rd, Zindrick MR, Field BT. Chemonucleolysis. A ten-year retrospective study. *Clin Orthop* 1986;206:61–66.
18. Tregonning GD, Transfeldt EE, McCulloch JA, Macnab I, Nachemson A. Chymopapaine versus conventional surgery for lumbar disc herniation. 10-year results of treatment. *J Bone Joint Surg Br* 1991;73:481–486.
19. Tsuji H, Itoh T, Sekido H, et al. Expansive laminoplasty for lumbar spinal stenosis. *Int Orthop* 1990;14:309–314.
20. Turner JA, Ersek M, Herron L, Deyo R. Surgery for lumbar spinal stenosis. Attempted meta-analysis of the literature. *Spine* 1992;17:1–8.

SECTION III

Imaging

Lumbar Spinal Stenosis
edited by Robert Gunzburg and Marek Szpalski
Lippincott Williams & Wilkins, Philadelphia, © 2000.

11

Conventional X-Rays and Computed Tomographic Scan in Lumbar Spinal Stenosis

Jacques Widelec, Christian Bacq, and Philippe Peetrons

*Department of Medical Imaging, Centre Hospitalier Molière Longchamps,
1190 Brussels, Belgium*

In 1954, Verbiest (17) first described the clinical syndrome caused by lumbar spine stenosis. Spinal stenosis involves a narrowing of the central spinal canal and/or the lateral recesses and the neural foramina. Central stenosis covers anteroposterior (AP) and/or transverse narrowing. Lateral stenosis includes compromise of the recess and/or neural foramen. Central stenosis may be responsible for symptoms by compressing the dural sac (cauda equina syndrome); lateral stenosis can compress a single nerve root (radiculitis) in a narrowed lateral recess.

Before the advent of computed tomography (CT), the diagnosis was suggested by conventional plain films, and myelography was more accurate in making the final diagnosis (13).

The main etiologies of lumbar spine stenosis are listed in Table 1.

DEVELOPMENTAL LUMBAR SPINE STENOSIS

The borderline between developmental lumbar spine stenosis and acquired spinal stenosis is theoretical. Both entities usually coexist to provoke symptoms. Symptoms do not appear until after the age of 40 years, when degenerative changes are superimposed on the already narrowed spinal canal. These changes include hypertrophy, which may be associated with spurs of the facets (14), laminae, and posterior vertebral body. Thickening of the ligamentum flavum and diffuse bulging disc also may be responsible for a spinal stenosis. The origin of developmental lumbar spine stenosis usually is unknown. Men are more affected than women. Developmental lumbar spine stenosis may be associated (in 10% to 20% of cases) with cervical spine stenosis (9,10) and with several rare dysplasic and dysostosic syndromes such as achondroplasia, acrosomelic dysplasia, arteriohepatic dysplasia, and Gorlin's syndrome (8).

CONVENTIONAL X-RAYS IN DEVELOPMENTAL SPINAL STENOSIS

The AP, lateral, and oblique views are necessary to make an accurate diagnosis. With these views, concomitant bony pathology can be ruled out. The entire lumbar spine often is

TABLE 1. *Etiologies of spinal stenosis*

Congenital spinal stenosis (developmental)
    Idiopathic
    Achondroplasia
    Morquio's disease
    Gorlin's syndrome
Acquired spinal stenosis (degenerative spondylolysis)
    Spondylolisthesis (degenerative form)
    Surgery: spinal fusion and laminectomy
    Calcification of the posterior longitudinal ligament
    Ossification or calcification of the ligamentum flavum
    Burst fractures
    Soft tissue: diffuse bulging disc, hypertrophy of the ligamentum flavum
    Epidural lipomatosis: circumferential or focal

involved. In case of segmental lumbar spine stenosis, L3–L4 and L4–L5 are affected more frequently (Fig. 1).

The AP view often demonstrates a decrease of the interpedicular distance mainly due to pedicular hypertrophy. This distance can easily be evaluated on plain film. On a normal posterior arch, two virtual pedicles may be interposed between both native pedicles. The distance between two adjacent posterior arches also is decreased. This sign reliably indicates developmental spinal stenosis (7).

This narrowing is the consequence of a verticalization of the laminae, with hypertrophy of the laminae and facet joints. These observations lead to the so-called cloth-peg sign (Fig. 2) (2).

Three major abnormalities may be detected on the lateral view. The first sign is platyspondility with an increased AP diameter of the vertebral body. Platyspondility can be found in

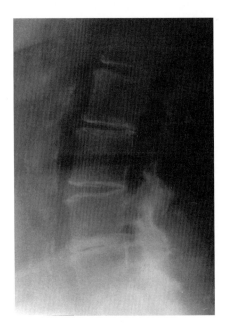

FIG. 1. Lateral conventional plain film of an acquired lumbar spine stenosis. The L4–L5 disc is severely degenerated. The posterior interapophyseal joints are hypertrophied and sclerotic, leading to a foraminal stenosis mainly at L4–L5. Note the calcification of the abdominal aorta. In this patient, several other examinations are necessary to make the differential diagnosis between an acquired lumbar spinal stenosis and a lower limb arterial insufficiency, both of which lead to a decrease in the ability to walk.

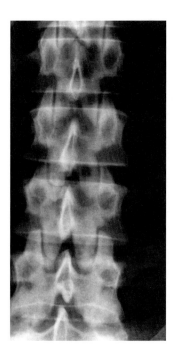

FIG. 2. Anteroposterior conventional plain film of a congenital lumbar spine stenosis. This view illustrates the cloth-peg sign characterized by a decrease of interpedicular distance, which is a result of a verticalization of the interapophyseal joint space. The interapophyseal joint space is oriented upward instead of downward.

several other pathologies such as dysostosis or dysplasia. Shortening and hypertrophy of the pedicles also are signs of developmental spinal stenosis. Platyspondilly and shortening and hypertrophy of the pedicles lead to narrowing of the neural foramina; therefore, a normal neural foramen seen on the lateral view rules out developmental spinal stenosis.

The more frequently affected levels are L4–L5 and L3–L4, but occasionally L2–L3 and L1–L2 are involved. An L5–S1 stenosis is very uncommon; when such a stenosis exists, it usually is associated with hypoplasia of the laminae (13).

COMPUTED TOMOGRAPHIC SCAN IN DEVELOPMENTAL SPINAL STENOSIS

Computed tomographic scan is an efficient tool for studying developmental spinal stenosis. The different variations of the canal shape are well illustrated. The stenotic canal can be circular, triangular, or treefold shaped.

Sagittal reconstructions are useful to recognize platyspondilly; however, transverse slices demonstrate clearly the hypertrophy and shortening of the pedicles and the decreased interpedicular distance. The posterior epidural fat extends to the junction of the two laminae. Pedicular level slices allow measurement of several spinal distances and calculation of the Jones-Thompson and Babin indexes (2).

The transverse slice through the disc will be the most informative because it illustrates which part of the stenosis deals with developmental and acquired stenosis.

The diagnostic value of spiral CT of the lumbar spine is still under discussion.

When degenerative changes are superimposed, the spinal canal becomes smaller. Narrowing of the recesses and foramina may add radiculopathies to the clinical presentation. The ligamenta flava frequently are hypertrophied.

DEGENERATIVE STENOSIS

Degenerative stenosis is probably the most frequent form of stenosis. It occurs mainly in older patients (starting at age 45 to 50 years). L4–L5 and L5–S1 usually are more affected. Hypertrophic overgrowth of the facets can be extended medially and anteriorly, leading to narrowing of the spinal canal and recesses. In the same way, posterior osteophytes of the vertebral body can narrow the canal. Lateral spurs can compress the emerging nerve and produce a radiculopathy.

Frequently, the stenotic effect is the consequence of a bulging annulus caused by a degenerated disc.

In many cases, the two kinds of stenosis will coexist. In these individuals, symptoms are more frequent and usually occur earlier in life. Complaints are more severe than in those who develop degenerative stenosis in a previously normal canal.

Calcification of the ligamenta flava is not uncommon (1,4,16,18). In most cases it is idiopathic (degenerative), or it is seen in diffuse idiopathic skeletal hyperostosis, chondrocalcinosis, and ankylosing spondylitis. It occurs more frequently in the elderly. Calcification of a hypertrophied ligamentum flavum can severely compress the dural sac and sometimes be responsible for radiculopathy.

Focal stenosis can occur with a hypertrophied ligamentum flavum or in spondylolisthesis, especially in the degenerative form. In this latter form, the stenosis is quite focal and always begins at the pseudobulging annulus level.

Epidural lipomatosis is an infrequent form of central spinal stenosis (3,5,15). The main etiologies are chronic steroid use and severe obesity. However, in a number of cases, no etiologic factor can be found. The excess of fatty tissue is located in the epidural space. Multiple contiguous levels may be involved. The most affected spinal segments are the thoracic spine and the lumbar spine. This excessive fatty deposit around the thecal sac may induce chronic myelopathy and radiculopathy. Epidural lipomatosis is easily recognizable on CT scan. The fat deposits mainly are posterior to the sac and narrow the thecal sac anteroposteriorly.

STENOSIS OF THE NEURAL FORAMEN AND LATERAL RECESS

Stenosis of the neural foramen and lateral recess probably is the second most frequent cause of radiculopathy after herniated disc. The lateral recess may be compromised or obliterated by degenerative spurs arising from the vertebral body and pedicles and by bone hypertrophy and/or osteophytes of the superior articular facet, which is the most common etiology.

Congenital stenosis of the lateral recess mainly is associated with congenital stenosis of the central canal. In this case the spinal canal is usually trefoil shape. This morphology frequently is observed in African patients. Lateral recesses often are asymmetric. A wide lateral recess may coexist with a contralateral narrow recess (12). More frequently a narrow lateral recess may be found with a normal spinal canal (12).

Three different types of acquired lateral stenosis can be distinguished.

Anterior stenosis usually is consecutive to a bulging disc associated or not with an osteophyte. This kind of stenosis becomes symptomatic when the recess is narrowed by an anterior osteophyte arising from the vertebral plate. Computed tomographic scan is better than MRI at displaying lateral recess morphology.

Lateral stenosis is consecutive to an osteophyte of the superior articular joint or to its hypertrophy. In this form, the whole joint usually is hypertrophied. Hypertrophy mainly affects the superior facet of the underlying vertebra, which progressively narrows the lateral recess. This conformation of lateral recess narrowing often is associated with anterior osteo-phytes, bulging disc, degenerative spondylolisthesis, and synovial cyst, but it also can be isolated (11). Computed tomographic scan is superior to MRI in visualizing the degenerative changes of the posterior elements.

Degenerative spondylolisthesis is consecutive to arthrosis of the posterior joint. The upper vertebra slides forward and downward on the plate of the underlying vertebra. This slip frequently leads to a lateral recess stenosis.

Stenosis can affect the neural foramen. Constitutional narrowing of the neural foramen mainly is associated with congenital stenosis. This feature easily can observed on conventional lateral X-ray view of the lumbar spine. The foramen appears flattened instead of oval shaped in the lateral view.

Acquired foraminal stenosis can be divided into three groups. Crock's syndrome (6) is defined by radicular compression between the inferior border of the pedicle and the tip of the upper articular facet due to a severe decrease of the height of the intervertebral disc pushing the pedicle downward. The foraminal morphology is well appreciated by MRI parasagittal acquisitions.

Stenosis due to hypertrophic arthrosis of the upper articular facet frequently leads to radicu-lar compression in the foramen. It is observed mainly in hyperlordotic patient in whom the discs are spared while the posterior elements are overloaded.

Spondylolisthesis can be the source of a foraminal stenosis. Both types of spondylolisthesis (isthmic lysis and degenerative) can be responsible for foraminal stenosis. In both cases, a decrease of the height and AP diameter of the foramen is seen. In the isthmic lysis, the presence of Gill's nodules can contribute to narrowing of the foramen. The degenerative form is caused by hypertrophic stenosis of the posterior element (upper facet joint) associated with intervertebral arthrosis. Magnetic resonance imaging clearly depicts foraminal stenosis in case of spondylolisthesis.

REFERENCES

1. Avrahami E, Wigler I, Stern D, et al. Computed tomography demonstrated of the calcification of the ligamenta flava of the lumbosacral spine associated with protrusion of the intervertebral disc. *Spine* 1990;15:21–23.
2. Babin E, Capesius P, Maitrot D. Signes radiologiques osseux des variétés morphologiques de canaux lombaires étroits. *Ann Radiol* 1977;20:491–499.
3. Bednar DA, Esses SI, Kucharczyk W. Symptomatic lumbar epidural lipomatosis in a normal male. *Spine* 1990; 15:52.
4. Brown TR, Quinn SF, D'Agostino AN. Deposition of calcium pyrophosphate dehydrate crystals in the ligamen-tum flavum: evaluation with MR imaging and CT. *Radiology* 1991;178:871–873.
5. Buthiau D, Piette MN, Ducerveau MN, Robert G, Godeau P, Heitz F. Steroid-induced spinal epidural lipomatosis: CT-survey. *J Comput Assist Tomogr* 1988;12:501–503.
6. Crock HV. Normal and pathological anatomy of the lumbar spinal canal nerve root canal. *J Bone Joint Surg Br* 1981;63:487–490.
7. Dietemann J-L. *Imagerie du rachis lombaire.* Paris: Masson, 1995
8. Dietemann J-L, Rimmelin A, Zöllner G, Durckel J. Imagerie des sténoses du canal lombaire. *Rev Rhum* 1996; 2:153–160.
9. Edwards WC, La Rocca S-H. The developmental segmental diameter in combined cervical and lumbar spondylo-listhesis. *Spine* 1985;10:42–49.
10. Epstein N-E, Epstein J-A, Carras R, Murthy V-S, Hyman R-A. Coexisting cervical and lumbar spinal stenosis: diagnosis and management. *Neurosurgery* 1984;15:489–496.
11. Lassale B, Benoist M, Morvan G, Massare C, Deburge A, Cauchoix J. Sténose du canal lombaire. Etude nosologique et sémiologique. A propos de 163 cas opérés. *Rev Rhum* 1983;50:39–45.
12. Lassale B, Morvan G, Gottin M. Anatomy and radiological anatomy of the lumbar radicular canals. *Anat Clin* 1984;6:195–201.
13. Lin JP, Shao SF. Radiographic detection of spinal stenosis. *Appl Radiol* 1988;Jan:43–49, March:29–33.
14. Penning L, Wilmink JT. Posture dependent bilateral compression of L4 or L5 nerve roots in facet hypertrophy. *Spine* 1987;12:488–500.

15. Quint DJ, Boulos RS, Sanders WP, Mehta BA, Patel SC, Tiel RL. Epidural lipomatosis. *Radiology* 1988;169: 485–490.
16. Stollman A, Pinto R, Kricheff I. Radiologic imaging of symptomatic ligamentum flavum with and without ossification. *AJNR* 1987;8:991–994.
17. Verbiest H. A radicular syndrome from developmental narrowing of the lumbar vertebral canal. *J Bone Joint Surg* 1954;36B:230–237.
18. Williams DM, Gabrielsen TO, Latack JT. Ossification in the caudal attachments of the ligamentum flavum. *Radiology* 1982;154:693–697.

Lumbar Spinal Stenosis
edited by Robert Gunzburg and Marek Szpalski
Lippincott Williams & Wilkins, Philadelphia, © 2000.

12

Diagnostic Imaging in Lumbar Spinal Stenosis

Dynamic Myelography, Computed Tomographic Myelography, Magnetic Resonance Imaging, and Magnetic Resonance Myelography

Jan T. Wilmink

Department of Radiology, University Hospital, 6202 AZ Maastricht, The Netherlands

Dynamic or flexion/extension studies of the lumbar spine help us to understand the effects of postural changes on the structures of the spinal column and the contents of the normal spinal canal, as well as the production in spinal stenosis of symptoms such as neurogenic claudication and posture-dependent sciatica. In addition, pitfalls in diagnostic imaging can be avoided by using the biomechanic insights provided by dynamic studies. Imaging techniques most frequently used for these studies are lumbar myelography (radiculography, caudography) and computed tomographic (CT) myelography. Dynamic lumbar studies are not feasible in most magnetic resonance imaging (MRI) scanners because of the lack of room inside the magnet.

The second part of this chapter deals with MRI in spinal stenosis. Although MRI does not provide the bright signal intensity of densely calcified bony structures that CT does, spinal dimensions can be easily and accurately assessed. Bony invasion of the spinal canal by facet arthrosis is demonstrated, and the role of soft tissue encroachment by bulging disc and flaval hypertrophy is better evaluated by MRI than by CT. Finally, high-resolution images of intradural nerve roots can be produced using specialized pulse sequences (MR myelography), which are useful for confirming nerve root involvement in cases of marginal stenosis.

DYNAMIC STUDIES IN NORMALS

When the lumbar spine moves from flexion (kyphosis) to extension (lordosis), several things happen (Fig. 1) (2,10).

- The posterior disc surface bulges backward into the spinal canal and indents the anterior dural surface.

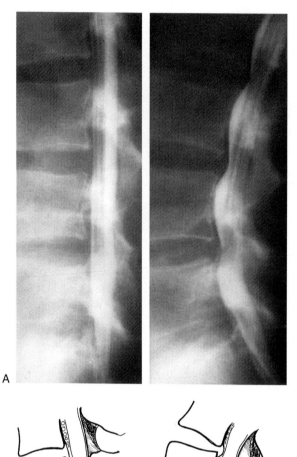

A   B

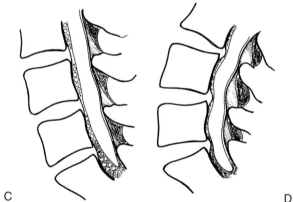

C   D

FIG. 1. Lumbar myelogram in flexion **(A,C)** and extension **(B,D)**. In extension the annulus fibrosus bulges backward whereas the posterior ligaments and fat pads bulge forward. The dural sac is compressed at the disc level and compensates by bulging forward into the space behind the vertebral body, which contains a compressible epidural venous plexus. (Diagram by L. Penning.)

- The fat pad normally present dorsal to the dural sac at the interspinous level is compressed by the spinous processes approaching one another. It bulges forward, thus indenting the dorsal dural surface (7).
- The flaval ligaments dorsolateral to the dural sac shorten and bulge inward slightly against the dorsolateral surface of the dural sac (7).
- The net effect of these events is that the transverse area of the dural sac at the disc level may be decreased by up to 30% in normal individuals (Fig. 2). This waisting of the dural sac at the disc level is compensated by anterior dural bulging into the space behind the vertebral body, where there is a rich and compressible epidural venous plexus. This venous plexus acts as a pressure regulator within the spinal canal, compensating for posture-induced

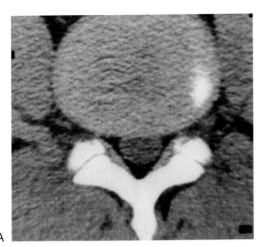 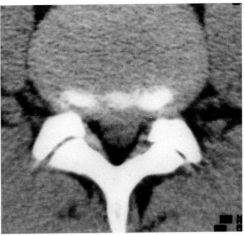

A B

FIG. 2. Computed tomographic sections at L4–5 in an asymptomatic volunteer. **A:** In flexion the transverse area of dural sac amounts to 166 mm². **B:** In extension the area is reduced to 116 mm². Note slight posterior bulging of the disc, inward bulging of flaval ligaments, and thickening of epidural fat.

space reduction by ejecting blood from the epidural veins to the paravertebral veins. In this way, changes in cerebrospinal fluid pressure in the lumbar dural sac (and ultimately the intracranial cavity) caused by flexion/extension movements are prevented.

These posture-induced changes occur in normal individuals and do not lead to complaints, because the spinal canal and dural sac are roomy enough to accommodate the space reduction occurring in lumbar extension.

FLEXION/EXTENSION IN SPINAL STENOSIS

When the lumbar spinal canal is abnormally narrow, the effects of spinal extension as described may exceed physiologic limits and cause compression, either of the entire cauda equina in concentric stenosis or of single nerve roots sleeves in lateral recess narrowing.

Concentric Stenosis

Developmental shallowness of the spinal canal and acquired transverse narrowing due to degenerative hypertrophy of the facets and flaval ligaments usually combine in varying degrees to produce concentric stenosis of the lumbar spinal canal, most frequently at the L4–5 level, less frequently at L3–4 and L2–3, and very rarely at L5–S1 (10).

Clear-cut borderlines between normal and pathologic values for transverse area of dural sac are hard to give, because there is considerable overlap between symptomatic and asymptomatic individuals. In a CT myelographic study, we found a mean surface area of the dural sac at L4–5 of 145 mm² (range 86 to 230 mm²) in lumbar extension in a control group of 30 young individuals (7). Another study comparing CT and the myelographic root image indicated that a myelographic block occurs at L4–5 or L3–4 when the transverse area of the dural sac decreases below 40 mm² (8). At this point, the walls of the spinal canal compress the bunched cauda equina fibers and the surrounding cerebrospinal fluid is driven from the level of compression. In spinal stenosis this will occur in the lordotic or extended spinal

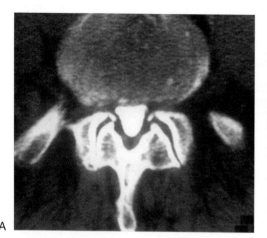
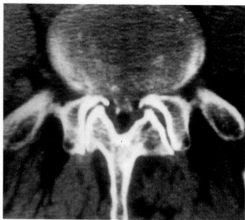

A   B

FIG. 3. Computed tomographic sections at L4–5 in a patient suffering from transverse spinal narrowing due to facet hypertrophy and neurogenic claudication. **A:** Flexion presents a seemingly normal picture. **B:** In extension there is almost total collapse of dural sac.

posture (subject standing erect or walking) and the clinical symptom of neurogenic claudication occurs: paresthetic nonsciatic pain often described as numbness, coldness, cramping, or weakness. Patients usually find that they can relieve the symptoms by reducing lumbar lordosis (sitting or squatting with flexed lumbar spine). This is an important point of distinction with regard to ischemic intermittent claudication, in which symptoms are relieved by cessation of muscular effort in the legs instead of postural change (4,12). Figure 3 illustrates the effect of lumbar flexion/extension movements on the dural sac in an individual with lumbar spinal narrowing.

These observations have some practical consequences. When imaging patients with irradiating low back complaints, especially when these complaints are posture dependent, an effort should be made to maintain lumbar lordosis (myelography in prone position, CT and MRI supine with the legs stretched out flat). If lordosis is reduced by performing lumbar myelography with the patient sitting on a stool in a flexed spinal posture or by performing CT with the knees drawn up, spinal narrowing may be mitigated, and the diagnosis missed in cases with marginal stenosis. In MRI the latter problem is less severe because of the lack of room inside the magnet.

One can ask if it is necessary to perform flexion/extension studies in every spinal imaging procedure. As long as care is taken to image these patients in extension (lordosis), additional flexion (kyphosis) studies are necessary only when one wishes to demonstrate the posture-dependent nature of the spinal narrowing. Spinal surgeons sometimes are struck by the apparent discrepancy between severe spinal narrowing seen on diagnostic images produced in lordosis and the much less marked narrowing seen at operation with the patient positioned in kyphosis. Preoperative dynamic studies can explain the discrepancy.

Lateral Recess Narrowing

In these cases there is localized narrowing of the spinal canal only in the region of the lateral recess. The bony lateral recess is bordered anteriorly by the dorsal surface of the superior part of the vertebral body, laterally by the pedicle, and posteriorly by the superior articular process. The critical area in lateral recess narrowing is not at this level; it is located

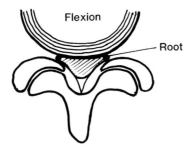

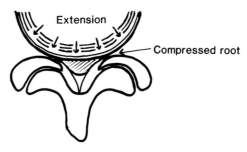

FIG. 4. Mechanism of nerve root compression.

some millimeters more cranially where there is a ligamentous lateral recess formed by the dorsal surface of the disc anteriorly and the facet capsule and flaval ligament dorsolaterally. Dysplastic or degenerative hypertrophy of the articular process and the covering ligaments may result in formation of a buttress behind the emerging nerve root and root sleeve entering the lateral recess. This does not in itself compress the nerve root, but fixes it in place so that the root is unable to move away when the disc bulges backward in lumbar extension (Fig. 4) (6).

This mechanism does not cause neurogenic claudication but rather posture-dependent sciatica irradiating into the dermatome of the compressed nerve root (5). The pain often is bilateral.

Spinal measurements are of limited value in assessing this type of nerve root compression. The anteroposterior diameter of the bony lateral recess is not relevant. Measuring the transverse diameter of the spinal canal between the inner surfaces of the ligaments covering the facets appears to enable a rough subdivision between symptomatic and asymptomatic individuals, with a cut-off value at 11 mm (9). One should keep in mind, however, that narrowing of the lateral recess can only cause symptoms when a nerve root is entrapped (Fig. 5). In addition to imaging the potential cause (interfacet narrowing combined with bulging disc), one should seek to verify the effect (nerve root compression). The cause is best brought to view by CT or MRI, but the state of the intradural root and root sleeve often is difficult to assess with these techniques, especially in cases with some degree of spinal narrowing. The effect of such narrowing on the root is best studied by water-soluble x-ray myelography or MR myelography (see following).

MAGNETIC RESONANCE IMAGING IN SPINAL STENOSIS

Although conclusive proof based on a well-designed large-scale comparative study is not yet available, anecdotal evidence strongly suggests that MRI performed with modern machines and techniques is superior to CT for imaging degenerative spinal disease.

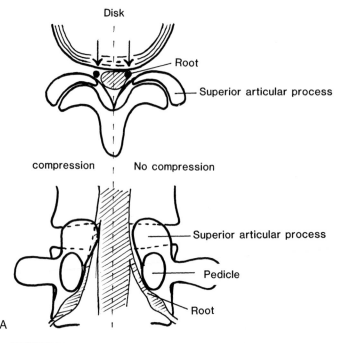

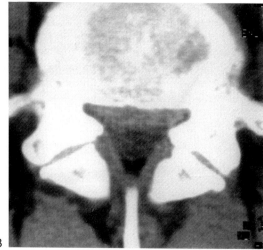

FIG. 5. Position of the nerve root in the lateral recess is crucial for production of symptoms. **A:** The nerve root on the **left** emerges from dural sac at the disc level and is laterally positioned, thus making it vulnerable to compression. The nerve root on the **right** emerges below disc level, courses medial to the lateral recess, and is not compressed. **B:** L4–5 disc filling in the entrance to the lateral recesses of L5 bilaterally. The position and condition of the nerve roots are difficult to ascertain. Left oblique lumbar myelogram shows high emergence of the L5 root sleeve. *(Figure continues.)*

Especially in the more complex cases, the superior soft tissue resolution of MRI combined with its versatility in choice of image contrast (T1-, T2-, or proton density-weighted) and imaging planes (axial, sagittal, coronal, or oblique) make it the technique of choice for diagnostic imaging of lumbar disc herniation. In spinal stenosis there is some disagreement, with some still preferring CT. The reason usually given for this preference is the bright image of calcified bony structures produced by CT, which provides a clearer view of the borders of the spinal canal and of densely calcified hypertrophic spurring in spondylosis and spondylarthrosis.

With some experience, bony structures can be clearly identified as bone marrow generally

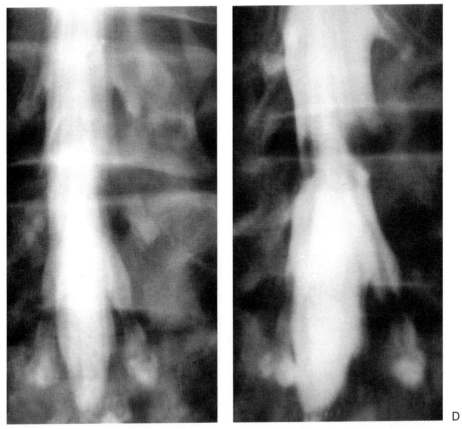

C   D

FIG. 5. *Continued.* **C:** In flexion there is no root compression. **D:** In extension there is clear compression of the root, root sleeve, and adjacent dural sac. There is similar compression of the contralateral L5 root (not shown).

produces a bright signal on T1-weighted images, whereas cortical bone shows up as a dark line. Densely calcified degenerative structures may present confusing dark areas on some images, but the problem usually is resolved by studying MR sequences with different contrast weighting. Magnetic resonance imaging has a significant advantage in its better soft tissue resolution, as encroachment on the spinal canal of inward bulging discs and flaval ligaments usually plays a significant incremental role in narrowing of the bony spinal canal (Fig. 6). A disadvantage of MRI is that lumbar flexion/extension studies are not possible because of the limited room within the scanner. Studies performed in lordosis (patient supine, legs stretched out flat) will provide good diagnostic images with little risk of false-negative results.

Magnetic Resonance Myelography

The earlier discussion hopefully made it clear that MRI is excellent at demonstrating potential causes of nerve root compression, including spinal stenosis. In the previous section the point was stressed that these potential causes do not always produce the result of nerve

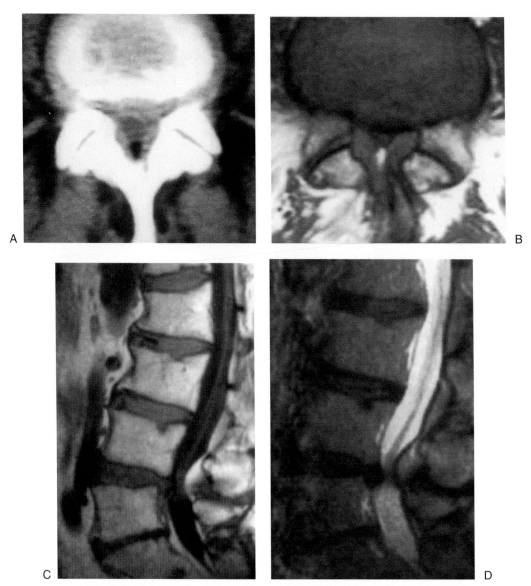

FIG. 6. A: Computed tomographic section through L4–5 showing disc bulging with localized protrusion, and facet and flaval hypertrophy producing narrowing of the spinal canal. **B:** Magnetic resonance study of similar case shows the same features well on transverse T1-weighted image. Sagittal T1-weighted **(C)** and T2-weighted **(D)** images provide information on the type and extent of narrowing.

root compression. This has been demonstrated in a number of MRI studies in asymptomatic volunteers. The problem of deciding whether or not the nerve root is compressed is especially vexing in lateral recess narrowing, where it often is difficult to identify the nerve root on standard MR images. In these cases we previously had been obliged to perform confirmatory lumbar myelography in a number of cases. When a technique for producing good-quality MR myelograms was reported in 1992 (3), we found it to be useful in reducing uncertainly with respect to nerve root involvement (1). The image quality of these MR myelograms is impressive when performed in a high-field (1.5-T) state-of-the-art system (Fig. 7), but diagnostically adequate images can be produced in a mid-field (0.5-T) scanner (Fig. 8).

It should be stressed that MR myelography can never replace the standard MR examination. By its technical nature, the MR myelogram can image only the cerebrospinal fluid within the dural sac and the root sleeves, and the intradural nerve roots. Magnetic resonance myelography shares with conventional myelography the disadvantage of nondepiction of foraminal and sacral lesions compressing the distal root segment. Although anatomic root involvement itself is clearly depicted, the cause of such involvement (disc herniation, stenosis, or other) is poorly identified. Magnetic resonance myelography does not improve the sensitivity of the MR examination in degenerative spinal disease, but rather it could be said to improve specificity by helping to identify degenerative lesions not causing nerve root compression. It should be performed only in cases where there is doubt about nerve root involvement. It provides no additional benefit in cases where the routine MR examination is convincingly normal or in those in whom a clearly symptomatic lesion is seen.

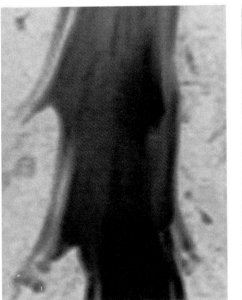 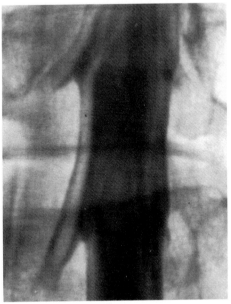

A   B

FIG. 7. High-resolution right oblique magnetic resonance myelogram acquired at 1.5 T **(A)**, with conventional water-soluble x-ray myelogram for comparison **(B)**. Note comparable depiction of nerve root and root sleeve. Bony vertebral details are not appreciated on the magnetic resonance myelogram.

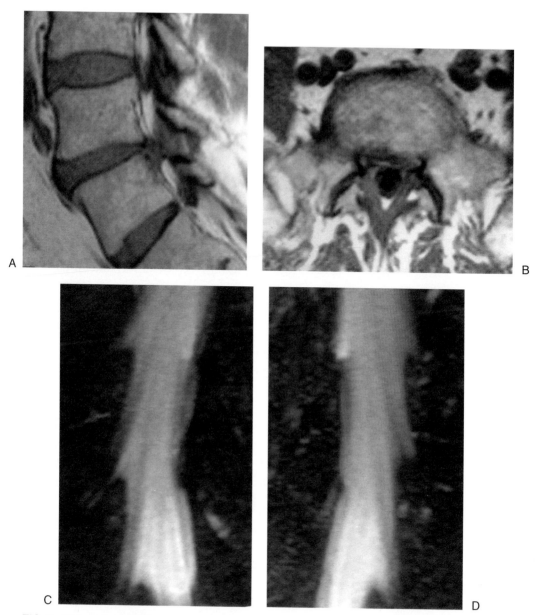

FIG. 8. Value of magnetic resonance myelography. **A:** Sagittal image shows L4–5 disc protrusion. **B:** Transverse image shows narrow lateral recesses at L5 with some indication of disc encroachment on the *left*. Root involvement is not clearly demonstrated or excluded. **C,D:** Magnetic resonance myelogram shows compression of the left L5 root and root sleeve normal aspect of these structures on the *right*. System was operating at 0.5 T.

CONCLUSION

Dynamic imaging studies of the lumbar spine can provide insight into mechanisms of nerve root compression and pain production, and they can explain posture-related anatomic changes in diagnostic images. Magnetic resonance imaging is proving to be a highly sensitive method for detecting developmental as well as degenerative spinal pathology. It has the disadvantage that irrelevant features may be detected that are not responsible for symptoms. Improved MR myelographic imaging of the nerve root is useful in difficult or marginal cases of root involvement. In addition to improved anatomic depiction, however, future efforts could be directed toward better assessment of the functional state of the nerve root and its medullary entry zone.

REFERENCES

1. Hofman PAM, Wilmink JT. Optimising the image of the intradural nerve root: the value of MR radiculography. *Neuroradiology* 1996;38:654–657.
2. Knuttson F. Volum und formvariationen das wirbelkanals bei lordosierung un kyphosierung und ihre bedeutung fur die myelographische diagnostik. *Acta Radiol* 1942;23:441–443.
3. Krudy AG. MR myelography using heavily T_2-weighted fast spin-echo pulse sequence with fat presaturation. *AJR* 1992;159:1315–1320.
4. Paine KWE. Clinical features of lumbar spinal stenosis. *Clin Orthop* 1976;115:77–84.
5. Paine KWE, Haung PWH. Lumbar disc syndrome. *J Neurosurg* 1972;37:75–82.
6. Penning L. Functional pathology of lumbar spinal stenosis. *Clin Biomech* 1992;7:3–17.
7. Penning L, Wilmink JT. Posture-dependent bilateral compression of L4 or L5 nerve roots in facet hypertrophy. A dynamic CT-myelographic study. *Spine* 1987;12:488–500.
8. Wilmink JT. CT Morphology of intrathecal lumbosacral nerve-root compression. *AJNR* 1989;10:233–248.
9. Wilmink JT, Korte JH, Penning L. Dimensions of the spinal canal in individuals symptomatic and non-symptomatic for sciatica: a CT study. *Neuroradiology* 1988;30:547–550.
10. Wilmink JT, Penning L. Biomechanics of lumbosacral dural sac. A study of flexion-extension myelography. *Spine* 1981;6:398–408.
11. Wilmink JT, Penning L, van der Burg W. Role of stenosis of spinal canal in L4-5 nerve root compression assessed by flexion-extension myelography. *Neuroradiology* 1984;26:173–181.
12. Yamada H, Ohya M, Okada T, Shiozawa Z. Intermittent cauda equina compression due to narrow spinal canal. *J Neurosurg* 1972;37:83–88.

SECTION IV

Clinical Presentation and Physiopathology

Lumbar Spinal Stenosis
edited by Robert Gunzburg and Marek Szpalski
Lippincott Williams & Wilkins, Philadelphia, © 2000.

13

Neurologic Symptoms of Lumbar Spinal Stenosis

Gordon F.G. Findlay

Walton Centre for Neurology and Neurosurgery, NHS Trust, Liverpool L9 7LJ, United Kingdom

The recognition that narrowing of the lumbar spinal canal could result in neurologic symptoms was recognized many years ago. In 1893, Lane (6) reported a patient with bilateral neurologic deficit that he correctly related to a lumbar spondylolisthesis. DeJerine (3) described the syndrome of intermittent claudication of the spinal cord in 1911. However, it was Verbiest (11,12) who related such neurologic symptoms to the presence of lumbar canal stenosis initially in French in 1949 and then in English in 1954.

Lumbar canal stenosis may be a constitutional phenomenon in cases of achondroplasia or, more commonly, is due to the development of degenerative processes in the lumbar canal. Lumbar stenosis may exist without causing any clinical symptoms. Patients with a congenitally narrow canal may have no symptoms but then present acutely with major neurologic deficit due to the occurrence of a disc protrusion. Degenerative stenosis may cause radicular pain similar to the sciatica caused by lumbar disc herniation if the stenosis affects the lateral recess and causes bony entrapment of the nerve root (7). Other cases of lumbar stenosis will present with neurogenic claudication. Turner et al. (9) found that bilateral symptoms were more common in males than females at a ratio of 8:1, whereas unilateral symptoms occurred at a male-to-female ratio of only 3:1.

Patients with bony entrapment of a lumbar nerve root present with radicular pain—and sometimes neurologic deficit—in the area of the affected nerve root. The pain is similar to that encountered in lumbar disc herniation, except that the pain is less likely to be exacerbated by coughing or sneezing and more frequently is associated with normal straight-leg raising. The difference probably is due to the slightly more distal entrapment of the nerve root.

Neurogenic claudication is a syndrome associated with pain or neurologic symptoms that become more evident with walking or prolonged standing. The symptoms may be unilateral but more frequently are bilateral. A long history of low back pain is common, although often the patient will not have sought medical treatment and merely coped with the back pain as a fact of life. It is the development of lower limb symptoms that prompts the request for medical assistance.

When these patients walk, they will develop the onset of radicular pain or neurologic symptoms after a defined distance. The distance required to develop these symptoms may vary on a daily basis and typically will occur at lesser distances if walking downhill due to the increased lumbar lordosis associated with that activity. The initial neurologic symptoms always commence with sensory problems long before motor symptoms appear. They feel unnatural heaviness or deadness of the limbs and a sense that their legs are going to give way. Most cases will describe these symptoms as commencing in the feet and spreading up the legs, although some will describe the opposite. Severe cases may describe the onset of perineal numbness as they walk or even the development of priapism. In some cases the sensory symptoms may ascend to a clinical level significantly higher than the radiologic level, almost certainly due to a vascular effect on the cauda equina. In some cases, as the patients walk they will become aware of weakness of dorsiflexion of the ankle and describe that their feet slap on the ground as they walk further or that they start to trip up.

In all cases these neurologic symptoms are promptly relieved by sitting down or by leaning forward, whereas merely standing still affords no relief at all. Typically, they will develop the symptoms at a regular distance (the threshold) but be able to continue walking for a further similar distance before having to flex forward for relief (the tolerance). Symptoms of sphincteric disturbance are rare, but some patients may describe a sensation of urgency of micturition as they walk further. At rest the patients usually complain of little other than backache on prolonged sitting, although some will complain of cramp or a sensation of "restless legs," especially at night.

Neurologic examination of a patient with lumbar spinal stenosis often is remarkably normal. Loss of ankle jerks and distal vibration sense may be present, but in any case are common in the age group of affected patients. A voluntary decrease in the range of lumbar extension often is seen, because it may precipitate symptoms. Straight-leg raising usually is normal. Dermatomal sensory loss and muscle weakness are uncommon at rest, although they may appear if the patient is reexamined after walking to their tolerance limit. In view of the age range of the typical patient, diminished peripheral pulses or limitation of hip movement may be found. Signs of a cervical myelopathy may be seen, because lumbar stenosis is associated with cervical canal narrowing in 5% of cases (4).

The most common differential diagnosis of neurogenic claudication is intermittent ischemic claudication due to peripheral vascular disease. This originally was described in horses and then in humans by Charcot (2). The clinical differentiation of intermittent and neurogenic claudication is discussed in Chapter 14.

Other differential diagnoses are less frequent. The low back pain and referred pain associated with nonstenotic lumbar degenerative disease may mimic neurogenic claudication. Venner and Crock (10) found that 18% of their cases of isolated disc resorption described increasing leg pain and sensory disturbance on walking. Lamerton et al. (5) described the clinical symptoms associated with claudication affecting the peripheral sciatic nerve with atherosclerotic disease of the inferior gluteal artery. Baum and Hanley (1) described neurogenic claudication in association with synovial cysts of the lumbar facet joints, although this commonly is associated with degenerative stenotic changes. Tumors of the cauda equina usually do not produce claudicating symptoms, although McGuire et al. (8) reported two cases where the tumor was associated with spinal stenosis. Neurogenic claudication has been described due to a spinal arteriovenous malformation, but such presentation is rare. Patients with severe osteoarthritis of the hips may complain primarily of increasing gait difficulty as they walk further. Routine examination of the hip joints should alert the examiner to the diagnosis. Also, patients with peripheral neuropathy may complain of exercise-related symptoms, although typically they also will have symptoms at rest and characteristic sensory and reflex changes.

The clinical presentation of a patient with lumbar canal stenosis with either radicular pain from bony entrapment or neurogenic claudication normally will pose little difficulty to the alert examiner. However, the typical elderly age group of these cases means that they frequently will have associated vascular or hip disease that can confuse the situation. Clinical examination often reveals relatively little, and the best guide to accurate diagnosis remains the careful clinical history accompanied by the most careful interpretation of appropriate neuroradiologic investigation.

REFERENCES

1. Baum JA, Hanley EN. Intraspinal synovial cysts simulating spinal stenosis. *Spine* 1986;11:487–492.
2. Charcot JM. Sur la claudication intermittente observee dans un cas d'obliteration complete de l'une des arteres iliaques primitives. *CR Seances Soc Biol Fil* 1858;10:225–238.
3. DeJerine J. La claudication intermittente de la moelle epiniere. *Presse Med* 1911;19:981.
4. Epstein N, Epstein JA. Individual and coexistent lumbar and cervical spinal stenosis. In: Hopp E, ed. *Spine: state of the art reviews, volume 1.* Philadelphia: Hanley & Belfus, 1978:401.
5. Lamerton AJ, Bannister J, Withrington R, et al. Claudication of the sciatic nerve. *Br Med J* 1983;286:1785–1786.
6. Lane WA. Case of spondylolisthesis associated with progressive paraplegia. *Lancet* 1893;1:991.
7. MacNab I. Negative disc exploration. An analysis of the causes of nerve-root involvement in sixty-eight patients. *J Bone Joint Surg* 1971;53A:891–903.
8. McGuire RA, Brown MD, Green BA. Intradural spinal tumours and spinal stenosis: a report of two cases. *Spine* 1987;12:1062–1066.
9. Turner JA, Ersek M, Herron L, et al. Surgery for lumbar spinal stenosis. Attempted meta analysis of the literature. *Spine* 1992;17:1–8.
10. Venner RM, Crock HV. Clinical studies of isolated disc resorption in the lumbar spine. *J Bone Joint Surg* 1981; 63B:491–494.
11. Verbiest H. Sur certaines formes rare de compression de la quene de cheval. In: *Hommage a Clovis Vincent.* Paris: Maline, 1949:161–174.
12. Verbiest H. A radicular syndrome from developmental narrowing of the lumbar vertebral canal. *J Bone Joint Surg* 1954;36B:230–237.

Lumbar Spinal Stenosis
edited by Robert Gunzburg and Marek Szpalski
Lippincott Williams & Wilkins, Philadelphia, © 2000.

14

Distinguishing Vascular Disease from Lumbar Spinal Stenosis

Philippe Gutwirth

Department of Vascular Surgery, Antwerp Blood Vessel Centre, Centenary Clinic, 2018 Antwerp, Belgium

Symptoms of lumbar spinal origin and complaints due to vascular disease sometimes may be confused. Turning to objective signs and applying sound physiopathologic reasoning generally will enable the dedicated physician to reach the correct diagnosis on clinical grounds alone. A few difficult cases remain where diagnostic technology is needed.

The nature and mechanisms of lumbar spinal stenosis and vascular disease are completely different. In the former, pain and nervous function alterations arise from nervous tissue suffering within or at the outlets of the lumbar spinal canal and, in some cases, from painful signals originating in diseased bone and articulations of the spine itself. With vascular problems, pain and malfunction are initiated in tissues (internal organs, muscles, skin) inadequately irrigated or drained by the defective vessels, with an exception for the acute aortic dissection and the rupturing aneurysm where nociceptive signals also arise from the vessel wall itself and from the possible effects of acute expansion in the surrounding retroperitoneal space.

The clinical picture is likely to be blurred in patients suffering from both vascular and spinal conditions. Reaching a precise and complete diagnosis in such circumstances can be more challenging.

In this chapter, acute and chronic vascular problems possibly offering difficulties in the differential diagnosis with lumbar spinal disease are briefly reviewed. The distinction between intermittent claudication and spinal claudication is, in our opinion, an issue really worth attention within the frame of this book and therefore is discussed in more detail.

ACUTE CONDITIONS

Acute pain episodes can reasonably be expected in people suffering from acquired lumbar spinal stenosis. Acute back pain may be due to a muscular spasm, a worsened hernial prolapse, or a bout of inflammatory activity; acute sciatica may ensue from compression of a nerve root. One must take a full and detailed history on admission of the patient, who should inform, among other things, about chronic back problems. *The knowledge that such are present could be very misleading and very dangerous if one were to jump to conclusions!* After taking the patient's history, one must perform a thorough physical examination, being aware of all the different conditions that could be responsible for the clinical presentation. Among these conditions, the deep vascular catastrophes must not be overlooked. The problems to be discussed are those most likely to be seen in the emergency ward, and junior staff members should be warned about possible diagnostic pitfalls.

Ruptured Abdominal Aortic or Iliac Aneurysm

Rupture of an existing aortic or iliac aneurysm can cause excruciating back pain or pain in the lumbar region, sometimes extending to the buttocks and even the leg. According to the exact site of the rupture, the pain may be central or lateralized, with or without ventral extension. Palpation of the abdomen and pelvic fossae will, in most cases, reveal the pulsating mass. One should carefully look for signs of acute blood loss or peritoneal irritation. The suspicion of the clinician should be sharply raised by an anxious, sweaty, and pale subject. If any doubt persists, a complete vascular checkup should be performed by a fully trained staff member. Simple B-mode echography performed at bedside is conclusive in most cases. If the presence of an aneurysm is detected and the condition of the patient is stable, the vascular surgeon will probably ask for a computed tomographic scan. Once again: do not jump to conclusions. An old lumbar wreck having done a whole day of gardening can still harbor a troublesome aneurysm!

Acute Aortic Dissection

This dramatic condition occurs mainly in hypertensive subjects who on average are not that old. The dissection starts from an intimal tear (entry). A cleavage plane develops within the aortic wall, possibly extending into side branches, and either ending blindly or joining with the true lumen via a distal tear (reentry). *Signs and symptoms depend on the entry site and the extension of the cleavage.* The dissection itself can cause terrible pain in the back. Acute ischemia of internal organs or of one or more limbs is possible through the blind extension into, and therefore occlusion of, side or end branches (e.g., the iliac arteries). Immediate surgery often is aimed at creating a reentry to unlock a side branch and to stop further dissection.

One should remember acute dissection whenever a patient is admitted with acute back or leg pain. Again, the presence of lumbar spinal disease, real or suspected, should not obliterate the vascular problem.

Acute Leg Ischemia

This situation is the result of acute arterial occlusion by thrombosis, embolism, dissection, trauma, or extrinsic compression. The history may yield immediate clues to the diagnosis (risk factors such as smoking, previous arterial disease, cardiac disease, trauma). The signs and symptoms are obvious: decreased temperature and capillary fill, absent pulses, and pale or marmored skin. Pain intensity and distribution are variable, and sensorimotor disturbances can be present under profound ischemia. The clinical picture of embolism may evolve from a totally white leg to a less dramatic coloration due to the subsidence of the initial vasospasm. Acute ischemia is unilateral in most cases, and comparison with the other leg and foot is striking. Complete aortic thrombosis or a saddle embolus with bilateral acute ischemia are seen infrequently. In those cases, no femoral pulses are felt, and the general condition of the patient worsens rapidly. The presence of impressive arterial elements and the absence of typical lumbar elements in the clinical picture should clarify the diagnosis within a few minutes and preclude confusion with sciatica.

Deep Venous Thrombosis

Deep venous thrombosis (DVT) occurs as a result of a variety of causative factors, local or generalized, in all possible age groups. It can happen to the young woman taking oral contraceptives who possibly aggravates her thrombotic risk by smoking; it can happen to the middle-aged traveler who has been stuck to an airplane seat for more than 10 hours; it can happen to the old, sick, and bedridden. It is often a clue to tumoral, inflammatory, or constitutional disease hitherto undiagnosed. It should never be overlooked because of the acute danger of pulmonary embolism and the risk of late complications due to extensive and inadequately treated DVT (postthrombotic or postphlebitic condition). Many patients referred to us with the primary diagnosis of DVT turn out to have lumbar problems. The reverse will, of course, happen in orthopedic practice.

Local pain due to an inflammatory response of the thrombosing vein may be a first sign, without other clinical signs or symptoms. This pain generally will be worsened by direct pressure. Beginning parietal and subocclusive popliteal vein thrombosis may manifest itself in this way. The examiner aggravates the pain by gentle pushing the ham of the knee. Early thrombosis takes extension both longitudinally and cross sectionally, thereby increasing its occlusiveness. Swelling will occur progressively in the insufficiently drained area: perimalleolar edema, congestion of the calf muscles, and in case of proximal thrombosis (iliac vein) also the thigh. Segmental thrombosis generally is less dramatic because of collateral circulation, whereas complete thrombosis of calf, popliteal, and femoral veins leads to voluminous and painful congestion. Swelling and hardening may be decreased and even absent in the bedridden because of lack of the normal orthostatic factor and in subjects with significant occlusive arterial disease because of diminished postcapillary pressure. Local temperature and color may be influenced by DVT. The affected limb may feel warmer, but in some cases arterial spasm may be present with cooling (the latter probably will occur with striking visible effects on skin color and limb volume, e.g., phlegmasia cerulea). A local temperature effect occasionally may be seen in patients with acute sciatica; therefore, in itself this effect is not a very powerful discriminator.

Edematous calf muscles and irritated tissues around thrombotic calf veins can be very painful when they are stretched. This reaction can be used as a test (Homans's sign): dorsal flexion of the ankle will cause the pain. This maneuver should be executed with the patient's knee bent, otherwise one could inadvertently stretch distal branches of the sciatic nerve, thereby causing pain in an acute sciatalgic condition (Lasègue's sign) and possibly causing the clinician to draw a false conclusion!

Along with local signs, general elements such as accelerated heart rate, increased body temperature, and laboratory test results (ESR, FDP) can provide clues to the diagnosis of DVT.

If doubt persists as to the possible presence of DVT, especially when no other problem was positively identified (such as sciatica), one must perform a technical examination. In earlier times phlebography was considered the golden standard. Today, color duplex echography in a well-functioning and validated vascular laboratory will detect and detail DVT at all levels of the lower limbs. Even calf veins can be seen and evaluated correctly. Moreover, phlebography is an invasive and painful examination that exposes the patient to local (DVT!) and general hazard (contrast). Phlebography is operator dependent, in much the same way as is color duplex. Color duplex not only yields information about the venous lumen but also about the venous wall, and it characterizes blood flow both qualitatively and quantitatively. Therefore, a good color duplex examination is preferable over phlebography. In our opinion, other techniques such as radioisotope-labeled fibrinogen detection or scan, plethysmography, and continuous-wave Doppler are outdated.

CHRONIC CONDITIONS

Having briefly reviewed acute vascular events that occasionally suggest acute exacerbation of lumbar disease, we now turn to chronic vascular conditions. Because lumbar spinal stenosis essentially is a long-standing and slowly evolving process and its symptoms are influenced by position and exercise, it is not surprising that the distinction of lumbar spinal stenosis from chronic vascular disease may be troublesome in certain cases. The problem of intermittent claudication is certainly the most interesting.

Venous Insufficiency

Poorly localized pain and fatigue in the legs associated with simple chronic venous insufficiency may bear some resemblance to complaints due to lumbar spinal stenosis. Worsening is to be expected after a long period of standing or sitting in both conditions. The venous congestion leading to these complaints is a simple hydrostatic problem, the details resulting from the particular anatomic distribution of the malfunctioning veins, in which the valves are incompetent or absent, causing a high uninterrupted blood column to weigh hydrostatically in the leg. This can happen in superficial veins (varicose veins) or in the deep veins (deep venous reflux). The burden must vanish on relaxing with the legs elevated or when lying recumbent. The mechanisms of pain and discomfort in lumbar disease are much more complex, due to bony, articular, nervous, and even vascular elements involved within the spine. Reclining in itself is often not enough to eliminate the discomfort; rather it is the correction of a lordotic lumbar posture that eventually will bring relief. It is therefore essential to ask the patient if complaints remain after going to bed and in what position the patient generally sleeps. One must try to obtain more precise information about the schedule or conditions associated with the complaints, the pain distribution, and objective swelling of the ankles (impressions left by shoes and stockings). Neurogenic suffering makes some patients *think* that their legs or ankles are swollen.

In sexually active women the problem of venous insufficiency is most likely influenced by the menstrual cycle. Perimenstrual pelvic congestion sometimes is associated with low back pain and increased leg discomfort. Ovarian vein insufficiency is especially noteworthy in its ability to cause pelvic and one-sided leg pain (sometimes suggesting a nerve distribution.). Active questioning of the patient and attention to the distribution of varicose veins is crucial in detecting these kinds of problems.

The patient should be asked about previous occurrences of phlebitis, thrombosis, and venous surgery. Deep venous thrombosis may lead to late complications and complaints, due to deep venous reflux, unnoticed bouts of thrombosis with extension of deep occlusions, development of perforator vein insufficiency, and secondary varicose veins. This postphlebitic situation is much more complicated than the simple primary problem. In extreme cases, venous congestion may be so important that the venous pressure increase that occurs during exercise becomes intolerable (venous claudication). The context of this is rather obvious, and no diagnostic difficulty is to be expected.

In general one should be attentive to the possible presence of following signs of venous disease: varicose veins (primary or secondary), distal skin changes (brownish color, telangiectatic corona, healed leg ulcers, atrophic or sclerotic areas, hypodermic induration), pitting edema, and organized edema.

Extreme obesity often is a challenging factor in clinical work, and for the problems under discussion there is no exception to the rule. Moreover, obesity in itself is an important risk factor for both lumbar and venous disease. Should the two occur in the same patient, then a conclusive separation of complaints with respect to either cause may even be impossible.

When the patient presents with only vague complaints and few conclusive clinical elements that possibly fit with lumbar or venous disease, one must turn to technical assessment. Eliminating or confirming the presence of venous insufficiency is possible by noninvasive diagnostic methods in nearly all patients: color duplex echography is certainly the most important, and plethysmography and some other functional tests can be useful. Compression therapy with elastic stockings selectively improves venous return, and the result of such a measure occasionally can be very informative.

Chronic (Intermittent) Ischemia and the Problem of Intermittent Claudication

Intermittent Leg Pain and Discomfort

Intermittent leg pain, weakness, and limping may result from disease affecting leg arteries and veins, leg bones or joints, the lumbar spine, or the medulla itself. In many cases the exact cause will be diagnosed readily by the alert clinician. Osteoarthritic hips and knees cause or increase pain and discomfort on walking. Venous claudication was mentioned. Diseases of the medulla may cause intermittent complaints and be a source of confusion. The intermittent pain and discomfort (episodic, cyclic, in association with activity, position, or posture) may be of a truly discontinuous character or it may be superimposed on a continuous baseline complaint.

Lumbar spinal stenosis can mimic arterial intermittent claudication in such a way as to be confusing, sometimes even to experts. To describe this situation, terms such as pseudo-, lumbar, neurogenic, and spinal claudication have been used. We will be using the latter. Intermittent claudication of arterial origin may be designated as arterial claudication.

Chronic versus Intermittent Ischemia

True chronic ischemia due to arterial occlusive disease should be distinguished from purely intermittent ischemia. The former is a permanent sufferance of tissues due to a lack of arterial perfusion, with rest pain, muscular wasting, and progressive skin changes that eventually lead to gangrene. It is a devastating condition with unmistakable signs. The latter occurs in response to muscle exercise and is the topic discussed in this section. Patients with true chronic ischemia who still are able to walk have very short distance claudication in addition to their baseline complaints (rest pain, sleepless nights). To make a distinction among all these conditions, chronic arterial disease of the lower limbs has been classified in four stages (I = asymptomatic, II = intermittent claudication, III = rest pain, IV = gangrene). It is regrettable that chronic *ischemia* is often said to be classified this way. It is the occlusive *disease* that is classified with respect to its functional consequences, not the ischemia. In second-stage occlusive disease of the arteries of the lower limbs, ischemia is intermittent and not chronic, by definition.

Mechanism

Arterial claudication is a returning ischemia of leg muscles in relation to activity and due to occlusive arteriopathy. The pain is probably due to stimulation of nociceptive nerve endings by acid metabolites and mediators that are produced and released as a result of exercise-induced tissue hypoxia and sluggishly cleared by failing perfusion. On halting the muscular effort and decreasing the local metabolic demands, the normal situation is restored over a few minutes, which typically allows for a new stretch of walking, exactly as long as the previous one.

Spinal claudication is a returning neurogenic pain due to compression and possibly ischemia of nervous tissue within or at the outlets of the spinal canal. The mechanism of compression probably is rather complex (discussed elsewhere in this volume) and involves postural factors as well as movement. In most cases, regularity of the claudicating pattern will be less convincing than in the arterial case.

Presentation

Arterial claudication involves the posterior leg muscles only, sometimes the buttocks, perhaps the thigh, always the calf, never the anterior muscles, and never the groin (Fig. 1). It is most likely to be confused with S1 root suffering. Intermittent numbness of the sole of the foot may occur after exercise. Numbness (hypoesthesia) must not be confused with paresthesia (pins and needles)!

In spinal claudication, elements other than the leg pain alone often are present: sensorimotor disturbances (pain, paresthesia, numbness) in the related nerve root area and low back pain. The pain may appear or be worsened by lying supine, sitting, or walking downstairs. Bending forward often will alleviate the pain. These factors would never be seen in arterial disease. However, both arterial and spinal claudication may be absent when riding a bicycle and may be present on climbing stairs (the latter as a rule in arterial claudication).

Diagnosis

The diagnosis is to be oriented by taking a careful history (smoking, previous arterial disease, cold feet, previous lumbar problems, postural and occupational pain factors, walking distance, walking stairs) and giving a thorough physical examination, including appropriate orthopedic and neurologic tests (Table 1). A quick run through the pedal pulses before and after a simple tip-toe exercise test also should be performed. Immediately after the exercise test, remember to look at the color of the soles (the technique of vascular examination is detailed in next section). In many cases it will be possible to exclude one of the two conditions on clinical grounds alone. In the troublesome case doubt will persist. Sometimes people develop both arterial and lumbar disease! In such a case the orthopedic and vascular surgeons must cooperate in evaluating the patient. In most vascular departments, clinical arterial assess-

LEG PAIN
lumbar vs. arterial causes

Intermittent claudication: **posterior** distribution

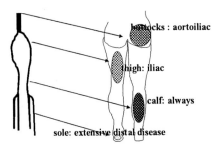

buttocks : aortoiliac

thigh: iliac

calf: always

sole: extensive distal disease

FIG. 1. Arterial claudication presents with pain in the posterior leg muscles.

TABLE 1. *History and physical examination: check for previous problems and risk factors*

Vascular	Lumbar
Color	Back pain
Volume	Radicular distribution
Temperature	Motor disturbances
Arterial lesions	Altered sensation
Capillary refill	Postural influence

ment will be complemented by functional tests (exercise, arterial pressure indexes), Doppler, and color duplex, or a combination thereof, if necessary. A clinician should never feel unhappy if his other-subspeciality colleague reaches formal conclusions through clinical means only! Multidisciplinary work goes beyond simple referral; thorough mutual consultation, the effectiveness of diagnosis and treatment will be enhanced and costs will be cut. Computed tomography and nuclear magnetic resonance, for instance, can be useful for both vascular and orthopedic purposes when a clear and motivated request is put to the radiologist.

Details of Clinical Evidence and Further Documentation of Arterial Disease

Physiopathology of Arterial Perfusion (in a Nutshell)

In the normal subject, impedance to blood flow of large- and medium-sized vessels is unimportant. The impedance is concentrated in the arteriolar part of the circulation, where, accordingly, the pressure drop along the bloodstream is steepest. Tissue perfusion is regulated mainly by the state of constriction of these very small vessels. In arterial disease, large- and medium-sized arteries may offer a significant impedance to blood flow. The arterial pressure drop is divided over the impedance due to lesions and the arteriolar impedance, in much the same way as the voltage drop is in a series impedance circuit. In stage II arterial occlusive disease, leg muscles are sufficiently perfused in the resting state, because their metabolic needs are limited. Accordingly, the arteriolar impedance is rather high (limited capillary blood flow), and the pressure in between both impedances is still high. Pulses downstream of the lesions often can be felt. Exercise increases the metabolic demand of the involved muscles, the concerned arterioles open, and the pressure downstream of the lesions drops sharply. Pulses no longer can be felt. The flow increases insufficiently due to the cumulated impedance, and the patient claudicates.

Bruits and Pulses

The simple facts outlined in the previous paragraph have two consequences of tremendous importance: (i) stage II arterial disease may present with normal distal pulses at rest; and (ii) without an exercise test, arterial occlusive lesions may remain undetected. Stenotic lesions and irregularities of a diseased arterial wall often produce turbulences with audio frequencies that can be picked up by a stethoscope. To the expert, the pitch and volume of these arterial bruits yield clues as to the occlusiveness and type of lesion. The bruits increase with increased blood flow. After an exercise test bruits that were weakly heard or went totally unnoticed at rest often become loud and audible. The exercise-related amplification and change of pitch can be highly valuable in the clinical assessment of the lesions.

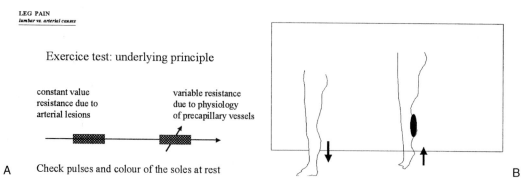

FIG. 2. Exercise test for diagnosis and classification of arterial occlusive disease of the lower limbs. Repeated heel elevation is performed for 1 minute or until severe calf pain is felt.

Exercise Test

The exercise test is designed to detect and clinically grade stage II arterial occlusive disease of the lower limbs (Fig. 2). Many variants exist. A simple and reliable test is to have the patient stand with hands against a wall and perform rhythmic heel elevation (as high as possible) for at least 1 minute or until unbearable calf pain is felt. The cardiopulmonary burden caused by this test is mild in comparison to the treadmill test. It is quick and easy, and no further equipment is needed. It is essential to examine the patient before and immediately after the test. Important diagnostic elements include the calf pain developed (claudication), pulse reduction or disappearance, and slow capillary refill (often a striking paleness of the sole of the foot is seen after the test). One should especially look for differences between both legs.

Difficult Cases

If neither lumbar nor arterial disease can be ruled out after taking a history and clinical examination, a multidisciplinary approach is needed. As noted earlier, clinical elements may be judged differently by different persons. If a technical examination can be avoided, the patient would appreciate it (even if he or she does not know).

When both lumbar and arterial pathologies are positively identified, the exact bearing of each on the daily life of the patient may be a challenging question. Some conclusions may be drawn carefully from the severity of lesions as measured by imaging techniques and functional tests. If still inconclusive, one can try to temporarily and selectively relieve one of the two conditions by medication or physical therapy. If this is effective, information of utmost practical importance is gained. Examples are antiinflammatory or analgetic drugs administered orally or by epidural injection for the lumbar condition, and rheology-based medication, hemodilution, or specific training programs for arterial occlusive disease.

CONCLUSION

Careful history taking and thorough physical examination remain the cornerstones of differential diagnosis. Well-developed clinical skills and a good understanding of the disease mechanisms involved will save time and money and avoid needless suffering of the patient. When the true limits of the bedside diagnosis have been reached, one should turn to multidisciplinary cooperation. Imaging and functional assessment must be conducted starting with the less invasive techniques, paying attention to the possible use of a single technical examination by different medical disciplines. In very difficult cases, imaginative efforts must be made to obtain practical information necessary to a rational therapeutic program.

FURTHER READING

Rutherford RB, ed. *Vascular surgery,* 3rd ed. Philadelphia: WB Saunders, Philadelphia.
The introductory chapters of this book cover the important subjects of clinical and laboratory assessment of vascular disease in a clear and synthetic style.
Giorano J, et al., eds. *The basic science of vascular surgery.* Mount Kisco, NY: Futura Publishing Co., 1988.
An excellent and concise review for those interested in the physical and physiologic background of the vascular topics discussed in this chapter.

Lumbar Spinal Stenosis
edited by Robert Gunzburg and Marek Szpalski
Lippincott Williams & Wilkins, Philadelphia, © 2000.

15

Neurophysiologic Assessment in Patients with Lumbar Spinal Stenosis

Jiri Dvorak, *Jörg Herdmann, and †Stanislav Vohanka

*Abteilung für Neurologie/Spine Unit, Schulthess Klinik, 8008 Zürich, Switzerland;
*Abteilung für Neurochirurgie, Heinrich Heine Universität, D-40001 Düsseldorf,
Germany; and †Neurologicka Klinika FN, Brno Bohunice, Zihlavska 100,
CZ-63900 Brno, Czech Republic*

Neurophysiologic examinations should help to answer the following questions about patients with lumbar spinal disorders, i.e., spinal stenosis:

- Which neural elements are involved?
- Which spinal segment is responsible for mechanical or other irritation?
- Is the lesion chronic, acute, or progressing, or has neural function improved?

Table 1 lists the different neurophysiologic tests and the neural structures they help to evaluate. Whereas somatosensory evoked potentials (SEPs) and motor evoked potentials (MEPs) are most helpful in the investigation of central nervous system pathways, electromyography (EMG), conventional neurography, F-wave, and H-reflex studies are most useful for evaluation of the peripheral segments of the sensory and motor pathways.

Sophisticated SEP techniques allow for scrutiny of the neural elements of the sensory pathways: dorsal roots, root entry zone, dorsal horns, dorsal columns, dorsal column nuclei, lemniscal fibers, thalamus, and its projections to the primary and secondary sensory areas of the cortex. Motor evoked potentials allow for assessment of lesions that affect the upper motor neuron and lesions that affect the motor root, plexus fibers, or peripheral nerve segments of the lower motor neuron. Electromyography of limb and paraspinal muscles allows for distinction between effect on motor roots and more peripheral nerve elements. Electromyography allows for a level diagnosis and evaluation of peripheral nerve disease, and it provides information on the age of the lesion. Neurography, F-wave, and H-reflex studies also allow for distinction between proximal root and peripheral nerve disease. Fractionated peripheral nerve stimulation helps to localize a circumscript peripheral lesion. Autonomic nervous system malfunction is difficult to assess. The sympathetic skin response (SSR) has proved helpful in the evaluation of autonomic peripheral neuropathy (37) and in differential diagnosis of erectile impotence (27).

SOMATOSENSORY EVOKED POTENTIALS

In the context of spinal cord and nerve root evaluation, only so-called short latency SEPS are relevant. These are potentials recorded from the lumbar spine as well as the first components of scalp recordings. Mid- and long-latency components of scalp-recorded potentials show great

TABLE 1. *Neurophysiologic techniques used for evaluation of different neural structures*

Neurophysiologic technique	Neural structures evaluated
Somatosensory evoked potentials	Sensory nerve fibers and dorsal roots, spinal cord dorsal columns
Motor evoked potentials	Corticospinal tract (lateral spinal cord), motor roots, and motor nerve fibers
Neurography	Motor and sensory nerve fibers
F-wave	Motor roots, motor nerve fibers
H-reflex	Dorsal and motor roots, sensory and motor nerve fibers
Electromyography of limb muscles	Motor roots and motor nerve fibers
Electromyography of paraspinal muscles	Motor roots

Reprinted from ref. 13.

interindividual and intraindividual variabilities that are highly dependent on alertness and psychological factors.

Stimulation and Recording Techniques

Somatosensory evoked potentials generally are recorded after electric stimulation of peripheral nerves. The posterior tibial, sural, or common peroneal nerves of the lower limbs are used. In neurourologic involvement with bladder dysfunction or erectile impotence, SEPs can be recorded after pudendal nerve stimulation. In radicular and spinal disease, several nerves, which are supplied by different segments, must be stimulated for a level diagnosis. Dermatomal stimulation and motor point stimulation have been proposed by several authors, but even in the absence of technical problems, these procedures provide inconsistent results.

For clinical purposes it is necessary to concentrate on components that can be recognized consistently in all normal subjects (4,12).

In lower limb testing (saphenous, peroneal, posterior tibial, or sural nerve), a so-called lumbar potential can be recorded with the electrode placed in the midline over the L1 spinous process. The reference electrode is preferentially placed on the iliac crest. These cauda equina and lower cord potentials are more difficult to record after sural or saphenous nerve stimulation due to a lack of muscle Ia afferents in these nerves, which contribute a large part of the lumbar potential.

In the context of lumbar spine disease, such as spinal stenosis, only SEPs from lower limb nerves can be expected to reveal disease-related pathology.

Tibial Nerve Somatosensory Evoked Potentials

The posterior tibial nerve is stimulated behind the malleolus medialis. Recordings should be obtained from the lumbar spine and from the scalp (Cz'). The lumbar potential is best recorded by an electrode placed in the midline over the L1 spinous process, with a reference electrode two or three levels away or, even better, on the iliac crest. The lumbar potential is dominated by a negative peak at 20- to 22-ms latency, which is generated in the gray matter of the root entry zone (35,36) and which sometimes is called the "spinal cord response" (S-component) (1). In the common Fz-Cz' derivation, the scalp-recorded potential, after distal stimulation of lower limb nerves, only sometimes begins with a small negative component at 32- to 36-ms latency (N1, "N33") (41). The first positive peak (P1) with latencies between 37 and 40 ms ("N/P37" = "P40" in the European literature) is more important, because it is always recordable in normal subjects.

The peroneal nerve is stimulated at the fibular head of the knee, and the sural nerve is stimulated behind the malleolus externus. Waveforms are similar to tibial nerve SEPs, but the amplitudes are smaller. Latencies of the initial components are similar to tibial SEPs in sural nerve stimulation and are about 5 to 6 ms shorter in peroneal nerve stimulation due to the shorter peripheral pathway.

Factors Influencing Somatosensory Evoked Potential Results

Somatosensory evoked potential results are influenced by several factors: body size (39), body temperature, and peripheral neuropathies, especially those of the demyelinating types.

MOTOR EVOKED POTENTIALS

The method of painless magnetoelectric transcranial stimulation of the cerebral cortex was introduced in 1985 by Barker and co-workers (6,7). They applied to the scalp short magnetic pulses that were produced by a device designed to stimulate peripheral nerves, and they recorded muscle action potentials from upper and lower limb muscles, i.e., the MEPs. Stimulating currents within the nervous tissue are induced by a time-varying magnetic field (32) generated by a brief high-voltage current pulse conducted through a copper coil (5,22).

Figure 1 shows the sites where the stimulating coil is placed to stimulate the motor cortex, the cervical nerve roots, the lumbar nerve roots, and the sciatic nerve trunk. Muscles generally used for recording MEPs are the quadriceps femoris, tibialis anterior, gastrocnemius, and abductor hallucis. Segmental innervation of these muscles is used for level diagnosis in analogy to the segmental distribution of the afferent nerves stimulated for SEPs.

During transcranial stimulation, lower limb muscles are activated more easily if the center of the coil is moved 4 to 6 cm frontally and 2 to 3 cm contralaterally to the side from which the MEP is recorded.

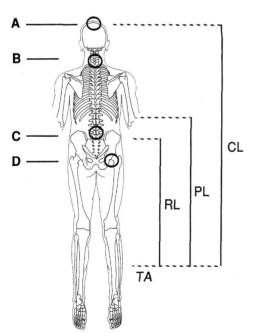

FIG. 1. Sites of magnetic stimulation. **A:** Motor cortex; **B:** cervical nerve roots; **C:** lumbar nerve roots; **D:** sciatic nerve. CL, cortical latency; PL, peripheral latency; RL, root latency.

The threshold of the resting muscle is determined by applying magnetoelectric stimuli of successively increasing strength. It has proven most practical to use magnetic stimuli of an intensity 50% above threshold for data collection. In addition, the subject is instructed to perform a slight voluntary contraction of the muscles being recorded. This procedure, referred to as facilitation (21), increases the amplitude and reduces the latency of MEPs.

For motor root stimulation over the lumbar spine, the intensity of the stimulator is adjusted so that a potential with a steep negative rise can be recorded. As such, the onset latency is not critically dependent on the positioning of the coil or the stimulation strength (10). The excitation site of the nerve root most likely is in the region of the root exit from the intervertebral foramen (10) and does not differ from that suggested for electric stimulation over the spine (31). This is probably due to "channeling" of the current flow within the foramina, which creates depolarizing currents as shown in Fig. 2 (11).

Motor evoked potentials following motor root stimulation are analyzed only for onset latency (root latency [RL]).

To judge the MEP waveform it is necessary to obtain an M-wave recording by conventional neurography.

F-wave recordings allow for determination of a total peripheral conduction time (peripheral latency [PL]) from the anterior horn cell to the muscle, which thus includes the conduction over the motor root to its exit from the intervertebral foramen. Calculation is especially important in lumbar spine disorders when motor roots measure 10 to 20 cm (20) and contribute considerably to PL, and when this procedure may help to localize the site of lesion (15).

Latencies and amplitudes of MEPs following cortical or root stimulation are measured in a manner identical to that used in peripheral nerve conduction studies. Onset latency is measured at the point of first deflection of the trace from baseline. If several sweeps have been recorded, the shortest reliable latency measurement is taken. Central motor latency (CML) is calculated in two ways:

1. Cortical latency (CL) minus RL, using MEPs following magnetoelectric stimulation only (CML-M), or
2. CL minus PL, using transcranial magnetoelectric stimulation and the F-wave technique (CML-F).

Motor evoked potentials after cortical, i.e., transcranial, stimulation also are analyzed for amplitude, duration, and number of phases. Due to the sometimes unstable baseline while performing facilitatory preinnervation for cortical stimulation, amplitudes are measured from peak to peak rather than from baseline to peak. This becomes obvious in severely pathologic MEPs. The highest reliable amplitude is used. Amplitude and duration are expressed as ratios of the M-wave amplitude and duration after supramaximal electric peripheral nerve stimulation.

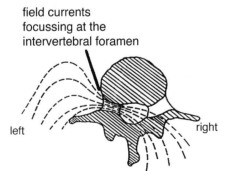

field currents
focussing at the
intervertebral foramen

left   right

FIG. 2. Channeling of currents induced by magnetoelectric stimulation around the intervertebral foramen.

Dvorak et al. (14) examined 73 patients with lumbar spinal disorders (37 women and 36 men, age range 20 to 87 years, mean 59 ± 16 [SD] years). As with normal subjects, patients were grouped according to age (young: n = 7; old: n = 66) and size (small: n = 55; tall: n = 18). According to clinical and radiologic findings, the patients were diagnosed as having spinal stenosis (n = 43) or nerve root compression syndrome (n = 30).

Twenty-eight of 43 patients (65%) with spinal stenosis showed significantly increased CML-M to at least one muscle of at least one leg. Ten of 32 patients in whom MEPs were recorded from muscles of both lower limbs showed bilaterally increased CML-M. On clinical examination, a significant motor or sensory deficit could be found in 11 lower limbs of eight patients. The CML-M to muscles of 9 of these 11 limbs (82%) were significantly increased. In 35 patients clinical examination did not reveal any significant motor or sensory deficit. In these patients MEP showed increased CML-M in 29 of 64 limbs (45%) examined. F-wave recordings were obtained from 16 muscles to which increased CML-M had been determined. The calculated CML-F values were normal in 12 cases; thus, conduction slowing could be localized within the proximal segment of the lower motor neuron, i.e., the cauda fibers, in 75% of these patients.

NEUROGRAPHY AND ELECTROMYOGRAPHY

Seddon (33,34) defined three degrees of nerve injury: neurapraxia, axonotmesis, and neurotmesis. This classification also can be applied to nerve root injuries within the lumbar spinal canal.

Neurapraxia is characterized by conduction failure without structural changes in the axon. Fibers usually regain function promptly. Short-term changes in nerve conduction within the affected nerve segment (reduced conduction velocity by as much as 30% and finally complete conduction block) probably are caused by anoxia due to ischemia. Prognosis for complete recovery is excellent, and there are generally no EMG changes. Voluntary innervation of reduced interference is temporary. There are no signs of denervation, e.g., spontaneous activity.

Axonotmesis results in loss of continuity of the axons, with immediate conduction block across the site of nerve injury. There is subsequent wallerian degeneration of the distal segment. Four to 5 days after acute interruption, the distal segment becomes inexcitable. Preceding conduction failure, there is neither change in the maximal conduction velocity of the efferent motor potential or of the afferent sensory nerve action potential, nor is it possible to distinguish axonotmesis from neurapraxia on the basis of distal nerve excitability. Recovery depends on regeneration of nerve fibers, a process that takes place at a rate of 1 to 3 mm/day, therefore taking months, perhaps years.

Neurotmesis is the state of transection of the entire nerve, including myelin sheath and connective tissue. The nerve must be sutured. Regeneration is often poorly oriented, and regenerating nerve fibers do not regain their original number or diameter. Initial neurographic findings are identical to those in axonotmesis. In axonotmesis and neurotmesis, EMG shows positive sharp waves 8 to 14 days and fibrillation potentials 14 to 20 days after nerve injury. Whereas reduced voluntary activity may be preserved in axonotmesis, this is not the case in neurotmesis.

The tibial, common and deep peroneal, superficial peroneal, and sural nerves are those commonly studied in lower limb testing. Other nerves accessible to neurography are the femoral, saphenous, and lateral femoral cutaneous nerves. The deep lying lumbosacral plexus fibers are not accessible by percutaneous electric stimulation. Measurements can be derived from indirect conduction studies, e.g., F-wave or H-reflex studies.

F-Wave

Motor conduction of cauda fibers can be assessed more directly by measurement of the F-wave first described by Magladery and McDougal (30). It is a late compound muscle action potential (CMAP) that results from backfiring of antidromically activated anterior horn cells after supramaximal peripheral stimulation of a motor nerve, which was first explored in detail in patients with Charcot-Marie-Tooth neuropathy by Kimura (25).

Recurrent activation of anterior horn cells occurs in only a minority of alpha motor neurons, preferentially in the larger motor neurons with faster conducting axons. Thus, the minimal F-wave latency is a measure of the fastest conducting fibers. However, the latency variability of consecutive F-waves is high because with successive supramaximal stimuli, recurrent discharges occur in different groups of motor neurons.

The conduction time from the spinal cord to the muscle (PL) can be calculated from the formula: PL (ms) = [minimal F-wave latency (ms) + M-wave latency (ms) − 1 (ms)]/2 (25), where 1 ms is the estimated delay for the turnaround time of the antidromic volley at the anterior horn cell.

The F-wave usually is normal in mild cases of radiculopathy. Distinct delay of the F-wave or a reduced number of clearly distinguishable F-waves after a given number of supramaximal peripheral stimuli, yet normal distal motor conduction studies, is a sign of a proximal lesion. Only in conjunction with MEPs, however, is it possible to determine conduction times for cauda fibers, i.e., motor roots, which may be affected in lumbar spinal stenosis.

H-Reflex

The H-reflex was first described by Hoffmann. The H-wave is a CMAP elicited by electric stimulation of large low threshold sensory nerve fibers (Ia muscle spindle afferents), which monosynaptically excite a motor neuron pool that innervates the muscle (from which the H-wave is recorded) via the same nerve. It is a monosynaptic reflex activity comparable to the tendon jerk, yet bypassing the muscle spindles.

In adults it is usually only recordable in a limited group of physiologic extensors, particularly in the calf muscles (S1 root). Stimulation of the tibial nerve at the knee (cathode showing proximal) with slowly increasing intensity from subthreshold to submaximal levels allows for recording of H-responses of growing amplitude from the soleus muscle. Further increase of stimulus intensity elicits M-waves of increasing size, while the H-reflex diminishes progressively and is eventually replaced by the F-wave with supramaximal stimulus intensity. H- and F-wave are of similar latency. S1 sensory or motor root affection reduces H-responses and increases their latency. Interside latency differences are a sensitive indicator of unilateral S1 radiculopathies.

In contrast to F-waves, H-reflexes are identical in response to repetitive stimuli as each stimulus transsynaptically activates the same motor neurons. H-reflex and F-wave amplitudes depend on stimulus intensity and on the excitability of the alpha motor neurons. Braddom and Aiello noted a 90-100% true positive rate and 0% true negative rate in S1 radiculopathies.

Electromyographic Studies

Electromyography must be considered an extension of the physical examination rather than simply a laboratory procedure. The muscles to be tested are selected according to clinical findings. Knowledge of the physiologic mechanisms underlying normal muscle contraction is a prerequisite for understanding the electrophysiologic abnormalities found in various disorders of the motor system. Electromyographers must be thoroughly familiar with multiple factors that can significantly affect the outcome of recordings (24).

Needle myography is not free of pain. However, the experienced examiner learns to perform this technique in a manner that is well tolerated by most patients. Care should be taken in patients with coagulopathies (bleeding tendencies) and high susceptibility to recurrent systemic infections.

Four principal steps delineate the EMG study of a muscle:

1. *Insertional activity* is evaluated with the placement and each repositioning of the needle electrode in the muscle.
2. After stationary and stable positioning of the needle electrode, the recording is evaluated at rest for detection of *spontaneous activity*.
3. *Single motor unit action potentials* (MUAPs) are recorded with a mild voluntary contraction of the muscle and examined with respect to amplitude, duration, and number of phases.
4. *Motor unit recruitment* and the *interference pattern* are recorded with a gradual increase of voluntary muscle contraction and maximal voluntary contraction, respectively.

Because a needle electrode registers (''sees'') motor unit action potentials from a limited area in the nearest vicinity of its leading-off surface only, it is necessary to record from many different areas within the muscle by repositioning the needle, moving its tip at least 2 mm perpendicular to the muscle fibers each time. Ten distinct areas should be sampled.

With lumbar spinal disorders, EMG studies are aimed at delineating damage to the lower motor neuron, i.e., axonal injury in terms of axonotmesis or neurotmesis of the motor roots with muscular denervation. Denervated muscle fibers become unstable, as they are no longer under neural control, and individual muscle fibers will fire in the absence of neural stimuli. This uncontrolled activity results in (i) increased insertional activity, (ii) increased endplate activity, and (iii) spontaneous activity. These signs of denervation in the EMG can be detected at the earliest about 8 days after the injury. Analysis of single motor unit action potentials also may reveal changes that are typical but not specific of lower motor neuron damage, e.g., radiculopathy: increased amplitude, increased number of phases, and increased duration. These changes are seen only after reinnervation or sprouting of nonaffected fibers has taken place; therefore, they are termed *chronic* signs of degeneration.

Localization of the lesion with respect to the motor roots affected is supported by examination of a variety of muscles innervated by different motor roots. If motor roots on their intraspinal course or the spinal nerve trunks within the intervertebral foramen are affected by the lesion, the paraspinal musculature, which is supplied by the posterior ramus from the spinal nerve, may show the typical EMG changes found only in limb muscles or muscles of the anterolateral body wall supplied by the anterior ramus.

The external anal sphincter is innervated from the anterior divisions of the S2 to S4 spinal nerves through the pudendal nerve. Unlike peripheral skeletal muscle, the anal sphincter always maintains a basic tonus, with isolated motor units continuously discharging at low rates. During sleep, the discharge rate is less than during consciousness. It is increased by coughing, speaking, and body movements of the trunk (18). It is therefore difficult to detect abnormal spontaneous activity in the partially denervated muscle.

In central paralysis, voluntary activity is reduced or absent, although the muscle can be activated via reflexes (simply elicited by digital examination of the anal sphincter). Reduced voluntary activity produces an incomplete interference pattern. If voluntary activity is completely lost, the basic low-frequency discharges at rest are unchanged during maximal effort to contract the muscle, and they may remain unchanged during defecation maneuvers, thereby prohibiting normal defecation.

In incomplete peripheral paralysis caused by lesions in the cauda equina, few motor units with polyphasic potentials of long duration can be volitionally activated to discharge at high frequency. If axonal degeneration occurs, fibrillation potentials, positive sharp waves, or complex repetitive discharges can be seen.

Sensitivity, Specificity, and Predictive Value

Only a few studies address these important measures of the diagnostic ability of neurophysiologic assessment of nerve root compression syndromes (19,42,43).

Electromyography performed with concentric needle electrodes is the oldest neurophysiologic method used for diagnosis of nerve root compression syndrome (38).

In this study, EMG was found to be the most sensitive of the three methods (EMG, neurography, F-wave), but the sensitivity was only 20%, which must be considered poor. This in contrast to previous studies in which the sensitivity of EMG was 54% (28), 67% (29), and even 78% (26). It must be stated, however, that the poor sensitivity of 20% was related to prediction of the exact level of a root lesion. The sensitivity of pathologic EMG findings unrelated to level was 45%, which possibly is explained by pleurisegmental innervation of the extremity muscles.

The sensitivity of F-wave in the presence of a root lesion has been found to be 35%, which is in agreement with other investigations (3,16,17,40); however, the results are poor in terms of predicting the exact level.

Dermatomal SEP in the study by Tullberg et al. (42) had a sensitivity of 40%, but the correct level was diagnosed in only 15%, a finding that corresponds to a previous study by Aminoff et al. (3). The authors concluded that of the three investigated neurophysiologic methods alone or in combination, none is a reliable predictor of anatomic level, even if diagnostic capacity is enhanced by using a number of tests.

It is recommended that neurophysiologic investigations be performed in patients with suspected lumbosacral radiculopathy or spinal stenosis, if radiologic results and clinical symptoms are conflicting or inconclusive. Patients with normal neurophysiologic tests should be considered bad candidates for surgery (24). To be predictive of surgical outcome, complete neurophysiologic investigation must be undertaken, including tests of motor and sensory function.

Vohanka and Dvorak (43) analyzed the sensitivity of neurophysiologic methods in patients with lumbar spinal disorders, such as spinal stenosis and radiculopathies due to disc herniation and/or foraminal bone stenosis. Quantitative and qualitative EMGs were performed, not only searching for denervation signs, but also analyzing the mean duration of motor action potentials (average 20 motor units per muscle). In addition, F-wave, H-reflex, (S1), MEPs obtained from the quadriceps (L4), tibialis anterior (L5), abductor hallucis (L5), and gastrocnemius muscle (S1), and dermatomal SEPs from peroneal and tibial nerve were obtained. This complex investigation required 3 to 4 hours to obtain reproducible results.

Generally accepted parameters have been accepted as criteria indicating an abnormal test. For MEP, normal values + 3 standard deviations that are adjusted to body size have been used (15,20).

Vohanka and Dvorak (43) correlated the neurophysiologic findings with computed tomographic or magnetic resonance imaging findings that were not confirmed by surgery. Quantitative analysis of motor unit potentials showed a 30% sensitivity in patients with radiculopathy but without motor deficit. The MEPs and SEPs reached sensitivities of 55%, and the MEPs had 75% false-negative findings. If all neurophysiologic tests were used, a nerve root lesion would be suspected in 73% of 29 patients with radiculopathy. Patients with objective clinical signs of nerve root compressions presented false-negative findings for SEP in 53%, denervation signs in EMG in 59%, and polyphasic reinnervation potential in 65%; for MEP, 75% of the findings were normal.

The high incidence of false-negative findings indicates that neurophysiologic tests have a low reliability to confirm clinical findings. It should be repeated that, in this study, correlation was made among clinical, neurophysiologic, and neuroradiologic assessment only, and the diagnoses were not confirmed by surgery. The specificity and sensitivity of the H-reflex in S1 radiculopathies requires further investigation in view of previously published articles by Braddom and Joynson (9) and Aiello et al. (2), who found a true-positive rate of 90% to 100%.

Haig et al. (19) performed needle EMG of paraspinal muscles in persons with and without low back pain and radiculopathy. Normal persons have few, if any, EMG abnormalities in the paraspinal musculature, which is in contrast to the high incidence of abnormalities found on computed tomography and magnetic resonance imaging (8) in asymptomatic subjects. However, persons with radiculopathy have a high degree of denervation signs on needle EMG. The authors recommend using EMG studies of paraspinal muscles to rule out false-positive imaging studies, as a second test with additional and overlapping sensitivity when results of imaging tests are normal despite high clinical suspicion for radiculopathy, or to rule out a false-negative imaging study (19). These situations are rare.

Based on available studies, it currently can be concluded that for patients with lumbar radiculopathy due to nerve root compression and/or spinal stenosis, the overall sensitivity and specificity of neurophysiologic assessment are low. Neurophysiologic assessment in patients with spinal stenosis is justified in the following situations:

- Exclusion of more distal nerve damage (neuropathy, nerve entrapment)
- Verification of subjective muscle weakness by needle EMG in patients presenting pain inhibition due to lack of cooperation
- Recurrent spinal operation, if difficult surgery is expected, to document the preoperative muscle status (medicolegal aspects)
- Need for further investigation in patients suffering from neurogenic claudication, when symptoms are presented, for example, during assessment on treadmill.

REFERENCES

1. Abbruzzese M, Favale E, Leandri M, Ratio S. Spinal components of the cerebral somatosensory evoked response in normal man: the "S wave." *Acta Neurol Scand* 1978;58:213–220.
2. Aiello I, Serra G, Migliore A. Electrophysiological findings in patients with lumbar disc prolapse. *Clin Neurophysiol* 1984;24:3313–3320.
3. Aminoff MJ, Goodin DS, Parry GJ. Electrophysiologic evaluation of lumbosacral radiculopathies: electromyography, late response, and somatosensory evoked potentials. *Neurology* 1985;35:1514–1518.
4. Anziska B, Cracco RQ. Short latency somatosensory evoked potentials: studies in patients with focal neurological disease. *Electroencephalogr Clin Neurophysiol* 1980;49:227–239.
5. Barker AT, Freeston IL, Jalinous R, Jarratt JA. Magnetic stimulation of the human brain and peripheral nervous system: an introduction and the results of an initial clinical evaluation. *Neurosurgery* 1987;20:100–109.
6. Barker AT, Freeston IL, Jalinous R, Merton PA, Morton HB. Magnetic stimulation of the human brain. *J Physiol* 1985;369:3–9.
7. Barker AT, Jalinous R, Freeston IL. Non-invasive magnetic stimulation of the human motor cortex. Lancet 1985;1:1106–1107.

8. Boden S, McCowin P, Davis D, Dina T, Mark A, Wiesel S. Abnormal magnetic-resonance scans of the cervical spine in asymptomatic subjects. J Bone Joint Surg 1990;72A:1178–1183.

9. Braddom RI, Joynson EW. Standardization of H reflex and diagnostic use in S1 radiculopathy. *Arch Phys Med Rehabil* 1974;55:1661.

10. Britton TC, Meyer BU, Herdmann J, Benecke R. Clinical use of the magnetic stimulator in the investigation of peripheral conduction time. *Muscle Nerve* 1990;13:396–406.

11. Cadwell J. Principles of magnetoelectric stimulation. In: chokroverty S, ed. *Magnetic stimulation in clinical neurophysiology.* Boston: Butterworths, 1989:13–32.

12. Chiappa KH, Choi S, Young RR. Short latency somatosensory evoked potentials following median nerve stimulation in patients with neurological lesions. In: Desmedt JE, ed. *Progress in clinical neurophysiology.* Basel: Karger, 1980:264–281.

13. Dvorak J. Neurophysiologic tests in diagnosis of nerve root compression caused by disc herniation. Spine 1996; 21(24S):39S–44S.

14. Dvorak J, Herdmann J, Janssen B, Theiler R, Grob D. Motor-evoked potentials in patients with cervical spine disorders. *Spine* 1990;15:1013–1016.

15. Dvorak J, Herdmann J, Theiler R, Grob D. Magnetic stimulation of motor cortex and motor roots for painless evaluation of central and proximal peripheral motor pathways. Normal values and clinical application in disorders of the lumbar spine. *Spine* 1991;16:955–960.

16. Eisen A, Hoirch M. The electrodiagnostic evaluation of spinal root lesions. *Spine* 1983;8:98–106.

17. Fisher MA, Shivde AJ, Teixera C, Grainer LS. Clinical and electrophysiological appraisal of the significance of radicular injury in back pain. *J Neurol Neurosurg Psychiatry* 1978;41:303–306.

18. Floyd WF, Walls EW. Electromyography of the sphincter ani externus in man. *J Physiol* 1953;122:599–609.

19. Haig AJ, LeBreck DB, Powly SG. Paraspinal mapping—quantified needle electromyography of the paraspinal muscles in persons without low back pain. *Spine* 1995;20:715–721.

20. Herdmann J, Dvorak J, Rathmer L, et al. Conduction velocities of pyramidal tract fibres and lumbar motor nerve roots: normal values. *Zentralbl Neurochir* 1991;52:197–199.

21. Hess CW, Mills KR, Murray NMF. Magnetic stimulation of the human brain: facilitation of motor responses by voluntary contraction of ipsilateral and contralateral muscles with additional observations on an amputee. *Neurosci Lett* 1986;71:235–240.

22. Hess CW, Mills KR, Murray NMF. Methodological considerations for magnetic brain stimulation. In: Barber C, Blum T, eds. *Evoked Potentials III.* London: Butterworths, 1988:456–461.

23. Hoffmann P. Ueber die Beziehung der Sehnenreflexe zur willkuerlichen Bewegung und zum Tonus. *Z Biol* 1918;68:677–694.

24. Kimura J. *Electrodiagnosis in diseases of nerve and muscle: principles and practice,* 2nd ed. Philadelphia: FA Davis Co., 1989.

25. Kimura J. F-wave velocity in the central segment of the median and ulnar nerves: a study in normal subjects and patients with Charcot-Marie-Tooth disease. *Neurology* 1974;24:539–546.

26. Knuttsson B. Comparative value of electromyographic, myelographic and clinical-neurological examinations in diagnosis of lumbar root compression syndrome. *Arch Orthop Scand Suppl* 1961;49:1–135.

27. Kunesch E, Reiners K, Müller-Mattheis V, Strohmeyer T, Ackermann R, Freud H-T. Neurological risk profile in organic erectile impotence. *J Neurol Neurosurg* 1992;55:275–281.

28. LaJoie WJ. Nerve root compression: correlation of electromyographic, myelographic and surgical findings. *Arch Phys Med Rehabil* 1972;53:390–392.

29. Lane ME, Tamhankar MN, Demopoulos JT. Discogenic radiculopathy: use of electromyography in multidisciplinary management. *N Y State J Med* 1978;78:32–36.

30. Magladery JW, McDougal DB. Electrophysiological studies of nerve and reflex activity in normal man. 1. Identification of certain reflexes in the electromyogram and the conduction velocity of peripheral nerve fibres. *Bull Johns Hopkins Hosp* 1950;86:265–290.

31. Mills KR, Murray NMF. Electrical stimulation over the human vertebral column: which neuronal elements are exited? *Electroencephalogr Clin Neurophysiol* 1986;63:582–589.

32. Polson MJR, Barker AT, Freeston IL. Stimulation of nerve trunks with time varying magnetic fields. *Med Biol Eng Comput* 1982;20:243–244.

33. Seddon HJ. *Surgical disorders of peripheral nerves,* 2nd ed. Edinburgh: Churchill Livingstone, 1975.

34. Seddon HJ. Three types of nerve injury. *Brain* 1943;66:237–288.

35. Seyal M, Gabor AJ. Generators of human spinal somatosensory evoked potentials. *J Clin Neurophysiol* 1987; 4:177–187.

36. Seyal M, Gabor AJ. The human posterior tibial somatosensory evoked potential: synapse dependent and synapse independent spinal components. *Electroencephalogr Clin Neurophysiol* 1985;62:323–331.

37. Shahani BT, Halperin JJ, Boulu P, Cohen J. Sympathetic skin response: a method of assessing unmyelinated axon dysfunction in peripheral neuropathies. *J Neurol Neurosurg Psychiatry* 1984;47:536–542.

38. Shea PA, Woods WW, Werden DH. Electromyography in diagnosis of nerve root compression syndrome. *Arch Neurol Psychiatry* 1950;64:93–104.

39. Stöhr M. Somatosensible Reizantworten von Rückenmark und Gehirn (SEP). In: Stöhr M. ed. *Evozierte potentiale.* Springer-Verlag: Berlin. 1989:112–120.

40. Tonzola RF, Ackil AA, Shahani BT, Young RR. Usefulness of electrophysiological studies in the diagnosis of lumbosacral root disease. *Ann Neurol* 1981;9:305–308.
41. Tsumoto T, Hirose N, Nonaka S, Takahashi M. Analysis of somatosensory evoked potentials to lateral popliteal nerve stimulation in man. *Electroencephalogr Clin Neurophysiol* 1972;33:379–388.
42. Tullberg T, Svanborg E, Isacsson J, Grane P. A preoperative and postoperative study of the accuracy and value of electrodiagnosis in patients with lumbosacral disc herniation. *Spine* 1993;18:837–842.
43. Vohanka S, Dvorak J. Motor and somatosensory evoked potentials in cervical spinal stenosis. In: *40th Congress of the Czech and Slovak Neurophysiology,* Brno, 1993.

Lumbar Spinal Stenosis
edited by Robert Gunzburg and Marek Szpalski
Lippincott Williams & Wilkins, Philadelphia, © 2000.

16

Stenotic Conditions in Children and Adolescents

Alvin H. Crawford

Department of Pediatric Orthopaedics, Children's Hospital, Cincinnati, Ohio 45229

Stenosis can be defined as a narrowing or constriction of a passage, duct, or opening. The term spinal stenosis has been elegantly demonstrated by Verbiest (46) to be ambiguous in that it does not identify the location, nature, or etiology of the process. In this chapter, stenosis will represent any type of narrowing of the spinal canal, nerve root canals, or intervertebral foramina. This condition may be caused by bone or soft tissue, and the narrowing may involve the bony canal, the dural sac, or both. The problem may be absolute or relative, static or dynamic. Absolute stenosis may be symptomatic in the absence of additional stimuli or compressive forces. It implies no remaining reserve capacity. Relative stenosis, on the other hand, implies that the reserve capacity is so small that minor additional compressive forces such as herniated disc, spondylolysis, neoplasia, fracture, or disc space narrowing may produce symptomatic stenosis.

Congenital stenosis results from a congenital malformation and constitutes only a small subset of patients with spinal stenosis. Most often congenital constriction of the spinal canal occurs in patients with spina bifida, failure of vertebral segmentation, congenital tumors of the lumbosacral region (most commonly lipoma), developmental disorders of the hips, knees, and feet, enuresis, and/or spastic or flaccid paralysis.

Developmental stenosis is caused by a growth disturbance of the bony walls of the vertebral canal during the prenatal and postnatal periods. Vertebral stenosis in patients with achondroplasia is an example of developmental stenosis.

Spinal stenosis can present at any age. The most common form of stenosis generally becomes symptomatic during or after the second decade of life. Cervical stenosis occasionally is seen concurrently with lumbar stenosis. These patients usually present with a history of an insidious onset of back, buttock, thigh, and calf pain. The distribution of pain in the lower extremities is dependent on the area of stenosis. It more often is bilateral than unilateral in distribution. In the classic presentation, the patient describes a syndrome of neurogenic claudication. In this situation, the back and leg pain increases with standing and walking. Sitting or lying with the hips and spine flexed substantially or completely relieves the pain. Walking becomes increasingly restricted. Patients report, however, that active activity such as pushing an object may increase walking tolerance. After walking a short distance, the patient will sit or bend forward to relieve the pain. He or she then may be able to proceed for another short distance. Pain relief is achieved by postural change that increases the size

TABLE 1. *Types of spinal stenosis*

I. Congenital stenosis
II. Developmental stenosis
  A. Idiopathic (most common)
  B. Inborn chromosomal error or mutation
    1. Achondroplasia
    2. Miscellaneous: hypochondroplasia, diastrophic dwarfism, Morquio's syndrome, hereditary multiple exostoses, cheirolumbar dysostosis
III. Acquired stenosis
  A. Degenerative
    1. Central portion of spinal canal
    2. Peripheral portion of canal, lateral recesses, and nerve root canals
    3. Degenerative spondylolisthesis
  B. Combined: any possible combination of congenital/developmental stenosis, degenerative stenosis, and herniations of the nucleus pulposus
  C. Spondylolisthetic/spondylolytic
  D. Iatrogenic
    1. Postlaminectomy
    2. Postfusion (anterior and posterior)
    3. Postchemonucleolysis
  E. Posttraumatic, late change
  F. Metabolic
    1. Paget's disease
    2. Fluorosis
    3. Epidural lipomatosis (Cushing's syndrome or long-term steroid therapy)
    4. Acromegaly
    5. Pseudogout (calcium pyrophosphate deposition)
  G. Miscellaneous
    1. Ankylosing spondylitis
    2. Ossification of the posterior longitudinal ligament
    3. Diffuse idiopathic skeletal hyperostosis
    4. Calcification or ossification of the ligamentum flavum
    5. Conjoined origin of lumbosacral nerve roots

From ref. 23.

of the spinal canal. This also explains why a patient can experience increased symptoms at night, secondary to postural increase in lordosis.

Nonsurgical management often is sufficient to control symptoms and generally consists of a physical therapy regime, judicious activity change, antiinflammatory medication, and, sometimes, spinal support with a corset or lightweight brace. Epidural steroid injection may be helpful for lower extremity symptoms. Surgery is indicated for neurologic deficit, severe intractable pain resistant to nonoperative treatment, and obvious mechanical canal compromise.

The distinction between congenital and developmental stenosis may overlap. In 1976, Verbiest (46) limited the term ''congenital stenosis'' to cases of abnormally narrow spinal canals resulting from congenital malformations. Acquired spinal stenosis occurs after birth and may be related to degenerative changes, trauma, or bone diseases; it may be even iatrogenic in nature. Schatzker and Pennall (43) suggested that spondylotic, traumatic, and iatrogenic stenosis likely represent processes occurring within a developmentally (relative) stenotic canal (Table 1).

DEVELOPMENT OF THE VERTEBRAL CANAL

Vertebral bodies enlarge circumferentially through perichondral and periosteal apposition and grow vertically through enchondral ossification. The mean interpedicular diameter in pediatric vertebra have been reported to be approximately 85% of the adult size (40). This additional increase in interpedicular distance from early childhood to adulthood occurs through membranous bone formation and internal resorption and external deposition. An unusual relative increase in interpedicular distance at a particular level should be considered a warning sign and may reflect the presence of a space-occupying underlying neoplasia, dural ectasia, or dysraphism. The spinal cord spans the length of the spinal canal in neonates. During childhood, the vertebral bodies and their accompanying discs elongate at a faster rate than the spinal cord. The spinal cord ultimately terminates in adults at the T12–L1 level (37). Unlike the midsagittal diameter of the spinal canal, the midsagittal diameter of the spinal cord varies little among individuals, depending on sex and age and not on body habitus. The achondroplastic dwarf is significant in that the length of the spinal canal does not significantly exceed that of the spinal cord and as a result subjects more of the spinal cord and its nerve roots to stenotic compromise.

RADIOGRAPHIC ANALYSIS

Multiple studies can be carried out to determine the exact dimensions of the spinal canal, including plain radiographs, tomography, computed tomography (CT), myelography, myelo-tomography, and magnetic resonance imaging (MRI), as well as ultrasound. Each imaging technique has specific advantages and disadvantages that will be explained with the particular diagnostic entity.

It is extremely difficult to evaluate the dimensions of the spinal canal by plain radiographs, unless some special grid is utilized. In the cervical spine, canal size usually is measured from the posterior aspect of the vertebral body at the midpoint between the superior and inferior endplates to the nearest point of the radiographic line marking the inner aspect of the lamina directly under the spinous process. The cervical spinal canal should be the same width as the vertebral body, with a 1:1 ratio. Measurement of plain radiographs in the lumbar spine is, for the most part, not helpful in identifying stenosis; most authors would recommend myelography, CT, or MRI. Plain films may be utilized to evaluate congenital abnormalities such as achondroplasia and other forms of dwarfism. The corollary is that CT, which primarily identifies bone and hard tissue. may not define actual narrowing of the diameter of the thecal sac as visualized with myelography (28,34). This arises from soft tissue impingement on the thecal sac caused by hypertrophied or enfolded ligaments, prominent disc, or an enlarged posterior facet capsule, all of which are radiolucent. Magnetic resonance imaging would be preferable to determine the exact dimensions of the spinal canal contents, whereas CT would be best utilized for the canal dimensions. Bolender et al. (7) reported better accuracy in the diagnosis of lumbar stenosis with myelography compared to CT without intrathecal contrast. They reported that the dimensions of the spinal canal derived from CT provided a correct diagnosis in 20% of patients, whereas myelography was accurate 83% of the time. Computed tomography is most helpful in delineating the bony shape and size of the canal, identifying deformities of the facet joints, and particularly evaluating the lateral recesses (7). Symptomatic lateral recess stenosis (defined as intense, disabling pain in one or both legs brought on by standing or walking) occurs most often at the L5–S1 level. Lateral recess depth of 3 mm or less is likely to be associated with symptoms and is considered to be stenosed (31).

There is an error in the use of CT to determine canal diameter when the beam is not directly parallel to the horizontal. Changing the angle to 20 degrees in either direction significantly and irregularly alters both the pattern and the values of the anteroposterior diameters, as well as cross-sectional area. Eubanks et al. (15) showed that transverse sections obtained from CT scans obtained at an angle did not always overestimate the canal diameter; on occasion, however, the canal was made to appear artificially stenotic. Scanning section thickness also may tend to alter the interpretation. Genant (19) reported the most useful scanning section thickness to be 4 to 5 mm.

Magnetic resonance imaging provides detailed anatomy of the spinal cord, thecal sac, nerve roots, and surrounding soft tissues. It does not demonstrate the surrounding bony structures as well as CT (41).

Although ultrasound is a noninvasive, safe, and relatively inexpensive method to evaluate spinal canal dimension, its primary advantage is its ability to be used intraoperatively. Montalvo and Quencha (32) reported that intraoperative sonography was valuable in accessing the degree of neural compression and the size of the bony or soft tissue mass causing compression in approximately 90% of patients. Intraoperative sonography can be used to diagnose calcified posterior longitudinal ligaments and spinal cord atrophy and to locate intrathecal cyst, myelomalacia, herniated disc, or an osteophyte at all levels within the spine.

Congenital and developmental stenosis manifest static forces such as basilar impression, narrowing of the foramen magnum, elevation of the dens, shortening of the clivus, invagination of the occipital condyles, and elevation of the petrous pyramids or dynamic forces such as instability associated with os odontoideum and absence of the dens. Developmental atlantoaxial instability can be found in patients with Down syndrome, spondyloepiphyseal dysplasia, Larsen's syndrome, Morquio's syndrome, osteogenesis imperfecta, and neurofibromatosis.

ACHONDROPLASIA

Achondroplasia occasionally has been noted to cause stenosis of the entire spinal canal. The foramen magnum may be narrowed through hypertrophy of its bony rim. This frequently is accompanied by hypoplasia of the clivus and basilar impression and occasionally by stenosis of the remaining cervical spine. Cervical stenosis (most frequently involving the first metameres and the cranial spinal junction) is more common in children, whereas thoracolumbar stenosis favors adults (16). These children may present in infancy with respiratory insufficiency. The central respiratory insufficiency must be differentiated from that occurring with midface dysplasia. Yamada et al. (48) reported quadraparesis and a high rate of mortality in patients with achondroplasia and stenosis of the foramen magnum. These patients usually respond to foramen magnum decompression. The most important clinical syndrome attributable to high cervical stenosis or stenosis of the cranial spinal junction is ''sudden infant death syndrome'' (5,38), which predominantly affects babies with homozygous achondroplasia in the first months of life. Other causes other than acute brainstem compression arising from a congenitally narrow occipital foramen and cranial spinal junction may contribute to respiratory failure, namely, thoracic dysmorphism, hypotonous of the pharyngeal musculature, and pulmonary hypoplasia, all of which are common in achondroplastic infants (5,21,38). There may be a less severe clinical picture of high cervical stenosis with the occipitocervical junction malformation characterized by spastic tetraparesis and deficits of the last cranial nerves. Suss et al. (44) report cervical spinal cord atrophy documented by CT in asymptomatic achondroplastic patients with cervical stenosis and point out the difficulties in accessing these findings for surgical indication or prognostic evaluation. Nelson et al. (35), studying somatosensory evoked potentials in both symptomatic and nonsymptomatic achondroplastic patients with cervical stenosis, noted abnormalities in all the patients of the former group and in as many as 44% of the latter group.

When symptomatic, both high cervical stenosis with or without occipital cervical junction malformation and diffuse cervical stenosis should be treated surgically by laminectomy, suboccipital craniectomy, and fixation, if necessary. Although at present there are no failproof criteria for assessing which patients are at greater risk for acute brainstem compression, some thoughtful pointers are provided by neurophysiologic studies (brain auditory evoked potentials, and somatosensory evoked potential) (35). Evaluation of respiratory activity during sleep and neuroradiologic investigations to assess the diameter of the occipital foramen are helpful. Children showing abnormalities on the above tests should be considered at high risk and subjected to surgical treatment. For those with normal values, the risk of sudden death is lower, but it is not to be excluded.

The prognosis of cranial spinal stenosis in homozygous achondroplasia is invariably fatal, with rare cases of survival after 3 months of age. Recently, however, several cases receiving aggressive intensive care and suboccipital cervical decompression with good results have been reported (21,33).

The abnormal spinal development of the achondroplastic dwarf can result in neurologic damage primarily due to two syndromes: lumbar spinal canal stenosis and thoracolumbar kyphosis (42). Due to changes in development of the epiphyseal plates of the vertebral body and arch in achondroplasia, the lumbar spine has a few typical abnormalities that are evident even at birth. In contrast to what is observed in the normal patient, the distance between the pedicles is either constant or decreases toward the last lumbar metameres. This radiographic finding, together with the square iliac wing, the horizontal acetabular roof, and the important decrease in muscle tone, makes diagnosis of the disease possible at birth (2). During development, the pedicles become thicker and shorter and approach the joint facets, laminae, and posterior margin of the epiphyseal plates.

A hyperplastic intervertebral disc may protrude to a greater degree into the spinal canal. When the patient stands up, the characteristic lumbar hyperlordosis appears, promoted by the horizontal sacrum, decreased muscle tone, and hip flexion, which further reduces the size of the spinal canal and the spinal root recesses (27,29,36).

Thoracolumbar kyphosis in the achondroplastic dwarf was first described by Wheeldon (47). This deformity, which is evident at birth or within the first few months of life, becomes more prominent when the nursing achondroplastic dwarf assumes the sitting position. Even though the kyphosis sometimes can reach high angular values, this deformity does not affect the vertebral bodies and usually disappears spontaneously when the child stands up. In 30% of cases, the deformity has tended to persist, if not increase, due to developmental anomalies of the vertebral metameres to compensate either for the lumbosacral hyperlordosis or the dorsal kyphosis. Most often either the child will develop a thoracolumbar hyperlordosis when he or she stands, or in as many as 30% of patients a significant thoracolumbar kyphosis persists (27).

Direct thoracolumbar radiographs still play an important role in the determination of spinal pathology. Kahanovitz et al. (24) found various clinical and radiologic correlations on the basis of plain x-ray films, i.e., distances of less than 2 cm at L1 and less than 16 mm at L5 were found only in patients with severe paraparesis. Treatment of thoracolumbar kyphosis in achondroplasia is indicated once the child is able to sit and the thoracolumbar kyphosis cannot be extended out by lateral side bending x-ray to less than 30 degrees. The treatment consists of an orthosis with a perineal sling to maintain the orthosis in place until the child is up and about walking. Most often, if the curve is flexible to less than 30 degrees on hyperextension lateral radiograph, the kyphosis is simply mechanical, related to the long trunk, and will resolve once the child is standing independently. While this may correct the kyphosis, the treatment of symptomatic thoracolumbar stenosis in achondroplasia is surgical.

In achondroplasia, coronal plane stenosis of the lumbar spine can be noted anatomically by failure of the normal cascading appearance of the interpediculate distance on a coronal

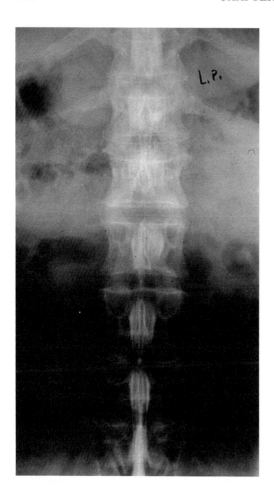

FIG. 1. Spinal stenosis in an achondro-plastic dwarf. Anteroposterior lumbar spine myelogram view shows the bony changes in achondroplasia where the interpedicular distance narrows as one descends the lumbar spine into the sacral area. Highly narrowed constriction of the spinal canal, specifically at the location of the intervertebral disc segments, is seen. The dye barely passes through.

x-ray view. The descending lumbar interpediculate distances are noted to narrow in achondroplastic patients as opposed to normal patients. The stenotic malformation of the canal reduces the spaces accommodating the nerve structures either gradually or acutely (Fig. 1). An associated lumbar disc herniation is favored by the relative increase in the volume of the intervertebral disc in relationship to the deformed bodies, which consequently tend to herniate into the canal or the foramen. In this case, the herniation occurs higher up than normal, i.e., at L1, L2, or L3. The growth of bone spurs that reduce the dimensions of the canal of the foramen even further compromises the spinal cord and nerve root in approximately 60% of cases of achondroplasia. Another stenotic factor that occurs fairly frequently (9% of cases) is hypertrophy of the ligamentum flavum, which may or not be calcified. Last, there may be a wedge-shaped deformity of one or more of the vertebral bodies, particularly between T10–L2, representing a kyphosis that has not been corrected. Compression of the conus and the roots may occur. About 23% of cases present this complication (17). The length of clinical history in these patients has been reported as less than 1 year in 36% of cases.

Prognostically, patients can be divided into two groups. The first group consists of patients with spinal stenosis combined with thoracolumbar kyphosis; the second group consists of those patients with spinal stenosis but no thoracolumbar kyphosis with or without disc herniation. Prognosis is less favorable in the first group, so any evidence of fixed thoracolumbar kyphosis in achrondroplasia must be pursued aggressively early in the child's life. The second group has a more favorable prognosis provided the symptoms are mild and the clinical history does not exceed 3 years. Patients with severe neurologic damage do not have a good prognosis even when decompressive surgery is performed within 3 years of clinical onset.

MYELODYSPLASIA

Patients with myelodysplasia more often than not have some form of occult if not absolute cord tethering resulting in an Arnold-Chiari formation and presenting with cervical spinal cord stenosis. They also may present with lower extremity problems because of lipomeningocele of the lumbar spine. These patients usually are treated by pediatric neurosurgeons.

Syringomyelia, on the other hand, most often is picked up by the orthopedic surgeon in the management of scoliosis. Most frequently this scoliosis is identified by a left-sided curve. Although left-sided idiopathic scoliosis is not necessarily indicative of some neurologic compromise, a higher incidence of neurologic compromise, however subtle, has been found in patients with left-sided curves (9). If the patient presents with a left-sided scoliosis in addition to any evidence of neurologic disorder, i.e., an absence of an abdominal reflex, a cavus foot with high arches, or intrinsic abnormalities of the hand and foot, then MRI is indicated.

SCOLIOSIS

Idiopathic scoliosis rarely presents a problem with spinal stenosis. Since the advent of school screening and earlier detection of severe deformities, rarely is the deformity in an idiopathic scoliosis significant enough to cause neurologic deficits and/or spinal stenosis. Rapidly progressing scoliosis absent congenital anomalies with evidence of progressive neurologic involvement should warrant an early MRI of the spinal canal. The MRI of the spinal canal in severe scoliotic deformities may be misleading because of a severe rotational effect. Often a high-volume CT myelogram will be more informative.

Patients with congenital scoliosis and kyphosis are at 25% risk of having associated segmental defects of the cervical spine. These patients should be screened with lateral radiographs at the cervical spine. Treatment of this condition when clinical spinal stenosis occurs is usually laminaplasty and decompression.

HERNIATED DISC

Children and adolescents may have an idiopathic spinal stenosis that only becomes clinically evident when aggravated by another primary disease process such as disc herniation. Because idiopathic spinal stenosis rarely is symptomatic, it most often is identified at the time of disc herniation. The most common physical finding in patients with a herniated nucleus pulposus is the positive straight-leg raising test (less than 60 degrees in 85% of patients). Several studies have described the relationship between developmental spinal stenosis and clinical symptomatology (20,39). The general consensus is that pure developmental spinal stenosis rarely is symptomatic. A combination of acquired and congenital processes usually is required to bring about symptoms of cord and nerve root compression. The aggravating factor may be one of many processes, with the most common being trauma and degenerative changes.

Herniated disc may be a significant component of spinal stenosis in children. Characteristic CT findings with a herniated disc include displacement of the anterior epidural fat and encroachment of the dural sac. In younger patients, there usually is a severe protrusion, with

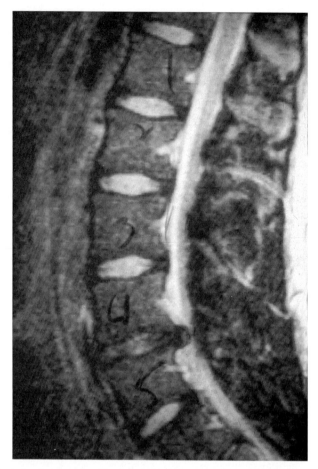

FIG. 2. Herniated disc in an older 18-year-old adolescent. Magnetic resonance image reveals a large herniation of the L4–5 disc into the spinal canal. Note the relative narrowing of the anteroposterior spinal canal diameter. Most often herniated disc problems in adolescents reveal a preexisting spinal canal stenosis. (Courtesy of Manuel Pinto, MD, Minn. Spine Center.)

prominent asymmetric and localized components (Fig. 2). In contrast, degenerative disc disease in adults often presents with diffuse angular bulging. Occasional good results have been achieved in children with physical therapy, epidural steroids, and exercise despite significant spinal canal compromise noted by CT and MRI. Physical therapy and rehabilitative efforts are indicated as long as there is no fixed neurologic component. If there is a progressive or fixed neurologic component, discectomy likely will be necessary.

Ninety-eight percent of adolescents, but only 75% to 80% of adults, do well after disc excision (14). Comparable statistics for either adults or children with spinal stenosis are not available. Because only 40% of children with herniated disc respond to conservative treatment (compared to 80% of adults), adolescents should not be subjected to protracted periods of such treatment in the presence of a neurologic deficit and persisting disability.

GROWTH PLATE INJURY

Growth plate or endplate fractures of the vertebral ring apophysis occur in adolescents. Twelve percent of children younger than 18 years of age who died of trauma were noted at autopsy to have growth or endplate fractures of the spine (1). The usual cause of these fractures had been attributed to disc material herniating into the vertebral body where the cartilaginous endplate joins the bony rim, or distraction injuries with avulsion of the growth plate from the vertebral body. The posteroinferior aspect of the L4 vertebra is one of the those most commonly involved (Fig. 3). There may be palpable or radiographic widening of the spinous processes on the lateral view. This injury may result in coincidental spinal stenosis and progressive spinal deformity, especially when accompanied by neurologic lesion. Takata et al. (45) described four types of growth plate injuries to the spine: (i) simple separation of the entire margin is defined by separation of the posterior rim of the involved vertebra and a calcified arch on CT scan with no evidence of associated large bony fracture; (ii) an avulsion fracture of some of the substance of the vertebral body, including the margin, annular rim, and cartilage; (iii) a more localized injury that included small posterior irregularities of the cartilaginous endplate; and (iv) the fracture spans the entire length of the vertebra and is not confined to the superior or the inferior margins of a disc space. Perhaps this type of lesion occurs when simultaneous avulsion of both the superior and inferior vertebral endplates occurs, splitting a shell of attached cortical bone posteriorly and spanning the entire length of the vertebral body. Later, the cavity anterior to the bony plate fills with fibrotic tissue that partially calcifies or ossifies; this accounts for the inhomogenous signal obtained on CT scan.

The clinical picture most often seen with vertebral growth plate injury with rupture of the lumbar cartilage plate into the spinal canal is similar to that of a herniated disc (10). The child usually presents after having experienced lower back pain most frequently associated with lifting a heavy weight, such as during weight lifting, but the condition has been seen in a child jumping from a height. Invariably, there is a "pop" associated with the injury at the time of trauma, followed by radiculopathy of varying degrees. There is limitation of motion in flexion, a particular short stride gait, and a limitation of straight-leg raising. There

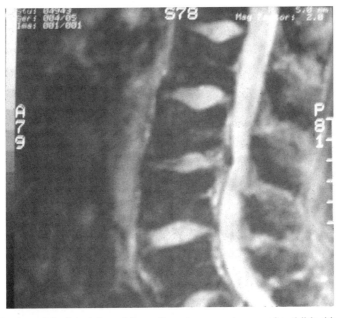

FIG. 3. Vertebral growth plate injury. Magnetic resonance image of a child with a growth plate injury off the inferoposterior rim of the L4 vertebra. Note the increased signal intensity of the osteocartilaginous segment displaced posteriorly into the canal.

are signs of stenosis, such as more pain when the child is ambulating than when he or she is sitting down and sitting still. There may or may not be dermatomal numbness, usually noted bilaterally, as well as marked weakness of the lower extremity musculature. A lumbar myelogram will reveal almost complete block of the spinal canal. The CT scan may show the retropulsed ossific rim of the osteocartilaginous endplate. The MRI shows the altered signal intensity of the posteroinferior portion of the vertebral body with the vertebral endplate projected into the spinal canal.

Once the diagnosis is confirmed, the treatment for this condition is excision of the fragment, which often is so large that it requires piecemeal removal from bilateral/lateral approaches. A good result usually can be expected with complete neurologic recovery in most cases. It is quite possible that this condition has been reported in the past as congenital lumbar ridge deformity causing spinal claudication in adolescents (4).

FRACTURES

Burst Fractures

Occasionally, fractures of the lumbar spine, specifically the burst fracture, occur in children. Nonoperative treatment of the spine usually is indicated for this injury. On occasion, these fractures cause compromise of the spinal canal because of retropulsion of bony fragments into the spinal canal. It is somewhat amazing how some of these children present with retropulsed fragments almost completely occluding the canal but who are neurologically stable. For those patients who have retropulsed fragments with neuropathy, it is important to decompress and stabilize the canal. The appropriate imaging studies, i.e., plain radiography, tomography, CT, or MRI, will help to determine the exact location of the lesion and whether or not there is any direct contusion of the thecal sac and its contents. If there is significant destruction of the vertebral body combined with obstruction of the spinal canal, surgical decompression and stabilization are mandatory (26).

Spondylolisthesis

Spondylolysis refers to a break of the pars interarticularis, and spondylolisthesis refer to a slip of the vertebra after this injury. Mild spondylolisthesis may be completely asymptomatic. Severe spondylolisthesis may result in stenosis of the lower portion of the spine, i.e., cauda equina syndrome. This disorder may occur in those patients with spondyloptosis or after destabilization of the spondylolisthetic vertebra after surgical attempts at obtaining *in situ* fusion. The clinical picture is that of localized pain in the lower back and buttocks. Symptoms are aggravated by strenuous activities that require repetitive flexion and extension of the lumbar spine. Tight hamstrings may give rise to a stiff leg gait with a short stride length. The radiographic characteristic finding of severe spondylolisthesis with stenosis is that of a myelogram showing a defect and failure of flow of the dye or an MRI with stenosis that typically identifies an outpouching of the disc of the L5–S1 junction caused by the teeter-totter effect of the L5 vertebra slipping forward on the S1 vertebra (Fig. 4). This posterior protrusion of the disc combined with anterior translation of the posterior bony and fibrous element of the L5 spondylolisthetic fragment is believed to be responsible for the stenotic condition of the lower end of the thecal sac. Decompression and fusion are indicated for this condition.

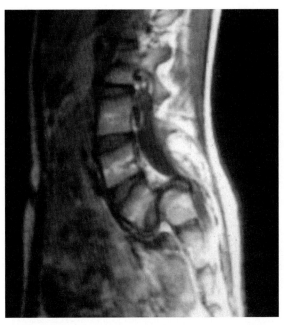

FIG. 4. Spondylolisthesis/spondyloptosis. Lateral magnetic resonance image of a child with severe spondylolisthesis reveals the intervertebral disc at L5–S1 to have been split in the transverse plane. The dorsal segment attached to the superoposterior border of S1 impinges the lower dural sac to the posterior elements, causing cauda equina syndrome.

INFLAMMATORY AND/OR INFECTIOUS CONDITIONS

Diskitis

Intervertebral diskitis has been noted to occur in young children. The symptoms often are difficult to elucidate in patients in the younger age group. It has been noted that the condition may present with symptoms of hip disorders, i.e., failure to walk in children less than 3 years of age, abdominal pain problems in those children 3 to 6 years of age, and back pain with a specific localization in children 6 to 9 years of age (11). The diskitis may or may not present as a clinical febrile condition; however, the altered gait with shortened stride length, back pain, as well as reversal of the normal lumbar lordosis are always obvious. The straight-leg raising test is markedly positive. Most often the plain lateral x-ray film will show some diminution of the height of the intervertebral disc space and a relative straightening or reversal of the normal lordosis of the lumbar spine. An MRI may show a tremendous compromise of the spinal canal with disc protrusion and stenosis possibly accounting for the child's symptoms (Fig. 5) (18). The treatment invariably is one of immobilization and broad-spectrum antibiotics initially. Rarely is operative intervention for decompression, drainage, or bacterial diagnosis indicated. Most often these children are treated with rest, antistaphylococcal antibiotics, and occasionally a cast or brace. Relief of symptoms by immobilization is the treatment of choice. Although some authors believe that diskitis represents a form of vertebral osteomyelitis, the sequela of this injury usually results in decreased intervertebral disc space and rarely fusion of the adjacent vertebra.

Epidural abscess may cause spinal stenosis with compromise of the epidural space (22). The presence of high fevers, as well as neurologic signs of meningismus, may identify this

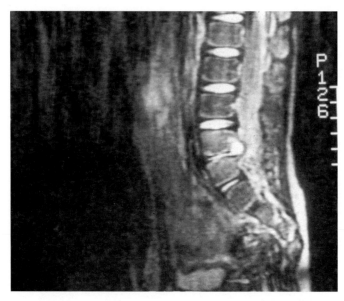

FIG. 5. Magnetic resonance image of a 4-year-old child with clinical symptoms diskitis reveals significant retropulsion of disc material into the spinal canal. This study possibly explains why the pain symptoms in a child of this age are consistent with those of a herniated disc in adults.

particular lesion. There may be marked root symptoms, muscle weakness, and decreased reflexes. Treatment most often depends on the identification of an organism. A spinal tap may reveal the bacterial etiology, and definitive antibiotic management may resolve the problem. Occasionally, an epidural cannula is necessary to drain the process.

Neonatal sepsis may occur in the intervertebral disc space possibly caused by vertebral osteomyelitis. There may be subsequent development of an angular deformity from growth plate destruction, most often kyphosis. If the diagnosis can be made early, incision and drainage will resolve the problem. Most often the diagnosis is delayed. These children usually are quite sick. There may be a flank abscess or spinal rigidity, with or without drainage. Spontaneous partial destruction may occur to the vertebral bodies, subsequently giving the appearance of a congenital deformity, most often kyphosis. If diagnosed, this problem usually can be remedied by early drainage and immobilization with cast or brace.

NEOPLASTIC CONDITIONS

Many neoplastic conditions can result in spinal canal compromise and subsequent spinal stenosis. Most pediatric spinal neoplasms are rare, and fortunately benign tumors predominate. The most frequent complaint is persistent, progressive back pain. Whereas activity back pain may be observed and treated supportively, a higher level of investigation is recommended when there is rest pain and spinal stiffness. There also may be associated weakness and bowel/bladder dysfunction. The child may be irritable, may limp, and occasionally will undergo a personality change. Spinal stiffness can be identified when the child is unable to bend forward as to touch his or her toes and the child's fingertips cannot reach between the knee and ankle. It is difficult to separate back stiffness from hamstring tightness and spasms. On occasion there is a delay in diagnosis, and permanent neuropathy results. Fortunately, most osseous neoplasms of the spinal column and canal are apparent on plain x-ray films. The use of anteroposterior, lateral, and oblique radiographs will identify 85% of the osseous lesions of the spinal column and canal on plain x-ray films. If not, a bone scan will locate the lesion. Further clarification of bony lesions highlighted by pain is best accomplished by CT. If there is a neurologic component, MRI is preferable.

Eosinophilic granuloma (Langerhans' cell histiocytosis) has been identified most frequently as a monostotic lesion of the spine. It usually is self-limiting, with 10% vertebral involvement. The term monostotic platyspondyly ("vertebra plana") or Calvé disease usually identifies the x-ray involvement of the spine as a coin-shaped density where there is significant flattening of the vertebral body involved. Spinal stenosis may occur in this condition when the soft tissue or granulomanous material enters the spinal canal. As a result of expansion of the involved vertebral segment into the canal, the symptoms are very similar to those of a herniated disc. Most frequently the eosinophilic granuloma involves the thoracic or lumbar spine and may or may not cause symptoms of stenosis. The plain film will show the flat, coin-shaped lesion, and a diagnosis can be made with confidence by needle aspiration. If there are symptoms of spinal stenosis, an MRI will determine whether or not the tumor compromises the spinal cord to the extent that it would require decompression. The lesion occasionally may heal without treatment. If there is a neurologic deficit, decompression versus low-dose irradiation is recommended. In young children in the thoracic as well as in the lumbar spine, a laminaplasty may be used to decompress the canal and maintain the stability of the vertebral segments.

Aneurysmal bone cysts occur most often in patients 5 to 20 years old; females are affected more often. The lumbar spine most commonly is involved, with the posterior elements affected 60% of the time. Aneurysmal bone cysts have been noted to present in the posterior elements with significant localized pain. Plain x-ray films are characterized by an eggshell thin cortical expansion with an osteolytic cavity. The reactive bony rim of cortical bone contains the margins of the tumor but may be absent in 30% of cases (8). The lesion is extremely vascular. Most often this pain is a result of stenosis of the spinal canal after expansion and/or disruption of the aneurysmal bone cyst fragments into the spinal canal. There may be expansion of the lamina causing direct pressure on a nerve root or limiting the canal diameter. Occasionally the process occurs very slowly, and significant compromise of the canal occurs before the condition is diagnosed. Because of the extensive vascularity, the lesion may be susceptible to selective embolization (13). Excision, curettage, and decompression of the canal and cord usually result in relief of back pain symptoms. If there has been neuropathy, the condition may not be reversed.

Osteoblastoma is identified radiographically as an osteovascular neoplasm larger than 1.3 cm in diameter when seen on radiographs. Forty percent of these lesions occur in the spine. The posterior elements of the thoracic and lumbar spine most frequently are involved. The x-ray films will reveal a destructive, expansive lesion. Osteovascular lesions of smaller dimensions are believed to be osteoid osteomas. Both lesions tend to initially present clinically as pain that occurs at rest or at night and which can be relieved by aspirin. Uncontrolled expansion may compromise the canal, thus giving rise to spinal stenosis. Excision of the lesion has tended to result in irradication of the symptoms of stenosis. There is a 10% recurrence rate. Surgical excision is the treatment of choice. Radiation should only be used when the patient is not a surgical candidate. If neuropathy has occurred, the condition may not always be reversed.

Osteoid osteoma is a smaller version of osteoblastoma; 10% will occur in the spine. It is considered to be the most common cause of painful scoliosis in adolescence. The lumbar spine is affected more than 50% of the time. The posterior elements, lamina, and pedicle are affected most frequently, rarely the body. The lesion is easily identified on bone scan. It may be seen on plain x-ray film as a radiolucent nidus with a sclerotic margin. If the pain cannot be relieved by nonsteroidal antiinflammatory drugs, surgical excision is recommended. A more perplexing problem occurs in the patient with osteoid osteoma where there has not been significant expansion and canal compromise. The lesion may be difficult to locate and persist after attempts at removal. Intraoperative bone scanning has improved the accuracy of removing the lesion. It is this author's opinion that persistence (incomplete excision) rather than recurrence is common with this lesion.

Hemangioma

Most often this lesion occurs in the vertebral body. The body is noted to be expanded and tends to compromise the anteroposterior diameter of the spinal canal. The lesion tends to grow fairly slowly, and considerable compromise of the spinal canal may have occurred before its identification. Plain anteroposterior x-ray films may show the classic coarsened, thickened, longitudinal trabecular striations and expansion of the vertebral body associated with this lesion. Magnetic resonance imaging is indicated when there is evidence of neurologic involvement (Fig. 6). Aggressive decompression of the lesion, usually by partial corpectomy, followed by structural graft stabilization and posterior instrumentation results in irradication of the symptoms of spinal stenosis. Embolization may be used preoperatively to prevent excessive intraoperative blood loss. If there is evidence of neuropathy, it may not be reversed. Recurrence is rarely a problem, even without radical excision.

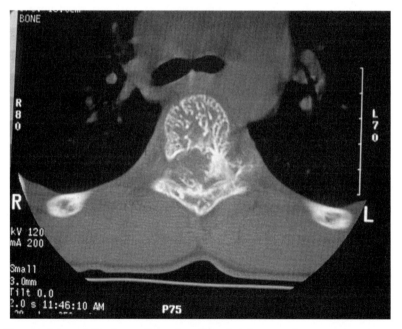

FIG. 6. Hemangioma of the lower thoracic spine. Axial magnetic resonance image reveals conscription and stenosis of the spinal canal secondary to active involvement of hemangioma in this vertebra. Note the coarsening and thickening of the trabecular in the vertebral body that is characteristic of this disorder.

Neurofibromatosis

Neurofibromatosis rarely causes direct stenosis of the spinal canal. Most often the dystrophic types of spinal deformities secondary to neurofibromatosis-1 (Von Recklinghausen) result in expansion of the spinal canal. This expansion secondary to dural ectasia is believed to be responsible for the spinal cord being relatively rarely compromised, with significant kyphoscoliotic spinal deformities caused by neurofibromatosis (12). On occasion, an intercostal neuroma, i.e., dumbbell lesion secondary to neurofibromatosis, may cause instability of the costotransverse articulation in patients with neurofibromatosis. This instability may result in the translation and projection of a rib head into the spinal canal, which leads to a relative spinal stenosis and occasionally neurologic compromise and/or paraplegia. Whereas the onset of the instability is somewhat insidious and may occur over a period of time, the final instability resulting in canal compromise more often than not is acute, and the patient presents with neurologic symptoms. Complete dislocation of the spine has been reported. Knowledge of this potential in patients with neurofibromatosis who present with symptoms of spinal stenosis may allow for immediate CT/MRI of the spinal canal and identification of this phenomenon. Rapid decompression and stabilization may lead to reversal of neurologic symptoms. Failure to identify this intracanal lesion may result in some increase in neuropathy, as well as permanency (30).

Leukemia

Leukemia is the most common cancer in children; 6% will present as back pain and vertebral collapse. Often there is extradural intracanal constriction giving rise to symptoms of stenosis. The diagnosis is very difficult to establish before the development of neurologic symptoms and signs. Kaspers et al. (25) reported a mean diagnostic delay of 5.8 months (range 1 to 18) Sometimes there is no bone involvement, and the diagnosis must be made by MRI or myelography.

Osteogenic Sarcoma

Osteogenic sarcoma may present as a primary lesion of the vertebral bodies in 0.8% to 3% of cases. It is a rare but deadly condition. Most often the presence of osteogenic sarcoma in the vertebra is a result of metastasis and, although infrequent, secondary to irradiation. A case of radiation-induced osteogenic sarcoma after treatment of a malignant schwannoma some 10 years previous by irradiation and chemotherapy resulted in a secondary osteogenic sarcoma of the twelfth vertebral body.

The signs of spinal stenosis were approached aggressively by excision of the vertebral body. After recurrence of the signs of stenosis, i.e., low back pain, a radical excision and subtotal spondylectomy with transligation of the spinal cord afforded the patient relief of his back pain symptom; however, he only survived for another 18 months and died of brain metastasis. Osteogenic sarcoma of the spine should be treated aggressively; however, results of treatment have not been encouraging.

Ewing's Sarcoma

Three and a half percent of all Ewing's sarcomas originate on the spine. It may produce a vertebra plana. The symptoms more often than not are those of spinal canal compromise, i.e., spinal stenosis (25). The condition carries an extremely poor prognosis. Aggressive surgical treatment is used to correct this stenosis; however, the primary treatment for Ewing's sarcoma is that of chemotherapy and/or irradiation.

SUMMARY

When one considers the absolute and relative causes of spinal stenosis in children, the condition is still relatively rare. Series of hospitalized children (usually in orthopedic departments) showing a high prevalence of serious disorders (sometimes potentially fatal) would certainly justify appropriate and even aggressive workup (3). This attitude seems fully justified inasmuch as low back pain is not a common psychosomatic complaint in children and teenagers. Malingering is a rare cause for back pain medical visits by adolescents. The existence of malignant disorders of the extradural space justifies the extensive investigations reported in the literature.

On the other hand, surveys identify very high numbers of recollection of nonspecific low back pain, which is in contrast to the reported prevalence of specific spinal disorders. Balaque and Nordin (3) found that 70% of ''normal'' children in some age subgroups reported previous or present low back pain. Not all of these children need extensive investigations. The cost-to-benefit ratio and the social cost would be unacceptable, and even sophisticated investigation such as MRI could show abnormal images that are nonspecific and not related to the symptomatology (6). An aggressive attitude probably would be psychologically harmful, but this factor has not been quantified.

When a child seeks medical attention for low back pain or back pain in general as the chief complaint, it is mandatory to perform an accurate and extensive medical examination. Radiologic and laboratory investigation should be based on the clinical examination. Balaque and Nordin (3) recommended the following thorough history taking: (i) family history of inflammatory bowel disease, psoriasis, episcleritis, or spinal disorders (disc herniation, ankylosis, spondylolysis, etc.); (ii) history of trauma (it is important to recognize the microtrauma); (iii) persistent pain (over a few days); (iv) disability due to pain (children unable to play or to perform sports activities that they enjoy); (v) nocturnal pain that wakens the child; (vi) general symptoms (fatigue, fever, loss of appetite, loss of weight, nocturnal sweats, etc.); and (vii) clinical signs (cutaneous changes suggesting communication with spinal cord, spinal deformity, restricted mobility, pain on palpation and/or mobilization, neurologic signs, and general signs).

Without other symptoms, if pain is limited to the low back without sciatica, a wait-and-see policy is justified. In those cases, Balaque and Nordin prefer symptomatic treatment or physical therapy and rehabilitation with careful clinical follow-up. If symptoms aggravate or persist for more than 2 weeks, then a more appropriate and clinically indicated intensive workup is mandatory.

CONCLUSIONS

Strange or stiff back movement with or without pain requires investigation. Persistent pain unrelieved by rest or worsening should be investigated. Inquire about radiculopathy, i.e., leg pain, bowel changes, or bladder changes. Imaging (ultrasound, bone scan, CT, MRI) has improved diagnostic delay. Initial management of spinal stenosis without neuropathy is nonoperative. The results of surgical intervention in children are better than in adults.

ACKNOWLEDGMENT

Kind appreciation is extended to Tiffany Whatley for preparation of this manuscript.

REFERENCES

1. Aufdermaur M. Growth plate injuries in children. *J Bone Joint Surg* 1974;56B:513–519.
2. Bailey JA II. Orthopaedic aspects of achondroplasia. *J Bone Joint Surg* 1970;52A:1285–1301.
3. Balaque F, Nordin M. Back pain in children and teen-agers. *Baillieres Clin Rheumatol* 1992;6:575–593.
4. Birkenfeld R, Kasdon DL. Congenital lumbar ridge causing spinal claudication in adolescence, report of two cases. *J Neurosurg* 1978;49:441–444.
5. Bland JD, Emery JL. Unexpected death of children with achondroplasia after the perinatal period. *Dev Med Child Neurol* 1982;24:489–492.
6. Boden SD, Davis DO, Dina TS, Patronas NJ, Weisel SW. Abnormal magnetic resonance scans of the lumbar spine in asymptomatic subjects. *J Bone Joint Surg* 1990;72A:403–408.
7. Bolender NF, Schonstrom NSR, Spengler DM. Role of computed tomography and myelography in the diagnosis of central spinal stenosis. *J Bone Joint Surg Am* 1985;67:240–246.
8. Capanna R, Albisinni U, Picci P, Calderoni P, Campanacci M, Springfield DS. Aneurysmal bone cyst of the spine. *J Bone Joint Surg* 1985;67A:527–531.
9. Coonrad R, Richardson WJ, Oakes WJ. Left thoracic curves can be different. *Orthop Trans* 1985;9:126–127.
10. Crawford AH. Operative management of spine fractures in children. *Orthop Clin North Am* 1990;21:325–339.
11. Crawford AH, Kucharzyk DW, Ruda R, Smitherman HC. Intervertebral diskitis in children. *Clin Orthop* 1991;266:70–79.
12. Crawford AH. Neurofibromatosis. In: Weinstein S, ed. *The Pediatric spine: principles and practice*. New York: Raven Press, 1994:619–649.
13. DeCristofaro R, Biagini R, Boriani S, et al. Selective arterial embolization in the treatment of aneurysmal Bone Cyst and angioma of bone. *Skeletal Radiol* 1992;21:523–527.
14. Epstein NE, Epstein JA, Carras R. Spinal stenosis and disc herniation in a 14-year-old male. *Spine* 1988;13:938–941.
15. Eubanks BA, Cann CE, Brant-Zawadzki M. CT measurement of the diameter of spinal and other bony canals: effects of section angle and thickness. *Radiology* 1985;157:243–246.
16. Ferrante L, Acqui M, Mastronardi L, Celli P, Fortuna A. Stenosis of the spinal canal in achondroplasia. *Ital J Neurol Sci* 1991;12:371–375.
17. Fortuna A, Ferrante L, Acqui M, Santoro A, Mastronardi L. Narrowing of thoracolumbar spinal canal in achondroplasia. *J Neurosurg Sci* 1989;33:185–196.
18. Gabriel KR, Crawford AH. Magnetic resonance imaging in a child who had clinical signs of diskitis: report of a case. *J Bone Joint Surg* 1988;70A:938–941.
19. Genant HK. Computer tomography of the spine: technical considerations In: Genant HK, Chafetz N, Helms CA, eds. *Computer tomography of the lumbar spine*.
20. Hasso AN, McKinney JM, Killen J, Hinshaw DB Jr, Thompson JR. Computed tomography of children and adolescents with suspected Spinal stenosis. *J Comput Assisted Tomogr* 1987;114:609–611.
21. Hecht JT, Butler IJ, Scott CI Jr. Long-term neurological sequela in achondroplasia. *Eur J Pediatr* 1984;143:58–60.
22. Jacobsen FS, Sullivan B. Spinal epidural abscess in children. *Orthopaedics* 1994;17:1131–1138.
23. Kabins MB. Congenital and development spinal stenosis. In: Weinstein SL, ed. *The pediatric spine: principles and practice*. New York: Raven Press, 1994.
24. Kahanovitz N, Rimoin DL, Sillence DO. The clinical spectrum of lumbar spine disease in achondroplasia. *Spine* 1982;7:137–140.
25. Kaspers GJL, Kamphorst W, Van de Graaff M, Van Alphen AM, Veerman AJP. Primary spinal epidural extraosseous ewings sarcoma. *Cancer* 1991;68:648–654.
26. Klassen RA. Fractures and dislocations of the thoracolumbar spine. In: Mervyn Letts R, ed. *Management of pediatric fractures*. New York: Churchill Livingstone, 1994.
27. Kopits SE. Orthopaedic complications of dwarfism. *Clin Orthop* 1976;114:153–179.
28. Ladd A, Scranton PE. Congenital cervical stenosis presenting as transient Quadriplegia in athletes. Report of two cases. *J Bone Joint Surg* 1986;68:1371–1374.
29. Lutter LD, Lonstein JE, Winter RD, Langer LO. Anatomy of the achondroplastic lumbar canal. *Clin Orthop* 1978;126:139–142.
30. Major MR, Huizenga BA. Spinal cord Compression by displaced ribs in neurofibromatosis: a report of three cases. *J Bone Joint Surg Am* 1988;70:1100–1102.
31. Mikhael MA, Ciric I, Tarkington JA, Vick NA. Neuroradiological evaluation of lateral reset syndrome. *Neuroradiology* 1981;140:97–107.
32. Montalvo BM, Quencer RM. Intraoperative sonography in spine. Current state of the art. *Neuroradiology* 1986;28:511–590.
33. Moskovitz N, Carson B, Copits S, Levitt R, Hart G. Foramen magnum decompression in an infant with homozygous achondroplasia: case report. *J Neurosurg* 1989;70:126–128.
34. Murone I. The importance of the sagittal diameter of the cervical spinal canal in relation to spondylolysis and myelopathy. *J Bone Joint Surg Br* 1974;56:30–36.
35. Nelson FW, Goldie WD, Hecht JT, Butler IJ, Scott CI. Short latency of somatosensory evoked potentials in the management of patients with achondroplasia. *Neurology* 1984;34:1053–1058.

36. Nelson MA. Spinal stenosis in achondroplasia. *Proc R Soc Med* 1972;65:1028–1029.
37. Ogden JA. Development and maturation of the neuromuscular system. In: Morrissy RT, ed. *Lovell and Winter's pediatric orthopaedics,* 3rd ed. Philadelphia: JB Lippincott, 1990:1–33.
38. Pauli RM, Scott CI, Wassman FR. Apnea and sudden unexpected death in infants with achondroplasia. *J Pediatr* 1984;104:342–348.
39. Perron O, Fassier F, Joncas J. Herniated disk and congenital spinal stenosis in the adolescent. *Rev Chir Orthop* 1996;82:29–33.
40. Porter R. Lumbar spinal stenosis. Development of the vertebral canal In: Weinstein JN, Wiesel SW, eds. *The lumbar spine*. Philadelphia: WB Saunders, 1990:589–594.
41. Ritterbusch JF, McGinty LD, Spar J, Orrison WW. Magnetic resonance imaging for stenosis and subluxation in Klippel-Feil syndrome. *Spine* 1991;16:539–541.
42. Savini R, Gargiuld G, Cevellati S, Disilvestri M. *Achondroplasia and lumbar stenosis.* The Central Scoliosis Institute of Orthopaedics. Rizzoli, Bologna, Italy.
43. Schatzker J, Pennall GF. Spinal stenosis, a cause of colloquial compression. *J Bone Joint Surg Br* 1968;50: 606–618.
44. Suss RA, Uduarhelyi GB, Wang H, Kumar AJ, Ziureich SH, Rosenbaum AE. Myelography in achondroplasia: value of lateral C1-C2 puncture and nonionic water-soluble contrast medium. *Radiology* 1983;149:159–163.
45. Takata K, Inoue S, Takahashi K, Ohtsuka Y. Fracture of the posterior margin of a lumbar vertebral body. *J Bone Joint Surg* 1988;70:589–594.
46. Verbiest H. Fallacies of the present definition, nomenclature, and classification of the stenoses of the lumbar vertebral canal. *Spine* 1976;1:217–225.
47. Wheeldon T. A study of achondroplasia. Introducing a new symptom, a wedged-shaped vertebra. *Am J Disord Child* 1920;19:1.
48. Yamada H, Nakamura S, Tajima M. Neurologic manifestations of pediatric achondroplasia. *J Neurosurg* 1981; 54:49–57.

Lumbar Spinal Stenosis
edited by Robert Gunzburg and Marek Szpalski
Lippincott Williams & Wilkins, Philadelphia, © 2000.

17

Neurologic Compression Theory

Gordon F.G. Findlay

*Walton Centre for Neurology and Neurosurgery, NHS Trust, Lower Lane,
Liverpool L9 7L3, United Kingdom*

In recent years, extensive experimental and clinical research has been conducted in an attempt to elucidate the etiologic and pathologic mechanisms that occur in lumbar spinal stenosis to produce the varied clinical symptoms and effects seen in patients. However, it is interesting to note that many authorities in the past had turned their attention to this problem. The main line of thought of these early researchers was directed to the occurrence of compression of the nerve root or cauda equina.

As long ago as 1891, Gowers (6) stated that "narrowing of the foramina may damage the nerve roots." In an eponymous lecture in 1927, Putti (20) described not only the foraminal changes caused by facetal degeneration, but he also described the clinical picture and discussed surgical therapy. By 1949, Verbiest (26) had developed the concept of differing types of spinal stenosis and their relationship to neurogenic claudication. Further work detailing the compression of lumbar nerve roots within the foraminal region was described by others, including Epstein (5) and Crock (3).

Despite these efforts and those of current researchers, many mysteries remain in the understanding of the etiopathology of lumbar spinal stenosis. Anatomically identical changes in a single motion segment may produce no clinical symptoms, persistent radicular pain, or neurogenic claudication. Possibly, patients with radicular pain and no claudication suffer from similar mechanisms as do those with disc herniation. The root may be affected by compression, stretching, and inflammation. In those who claudicate, these mechanisms may be added to by vascular changes or compression at more than one segmental level (19). Age may be a factor. Claudication is encountered more frequently in the more elderly. Are they more susceptible to the effects of vascular compromise?

Any theory regarding etiology should explain why some people with very degenerate and stenotic lumbar spines remain asymptomatic. Others will have severe impairment with only single-level disease, whereas others will have multilevel involvement with varying combinations of lateral recess and central narrowing. Why do some patients with severe narrowing or compression of the cauda equina (such as those with intradural tumors) not show features of claudication? Clearly the answer to these questions does not lie with one simple explanation. Multiple factors are at work. In this chapter, the evidence that compression of neurologic tissues is important is reviewed. Vascular theories are examined in Chapter 18.

Mechanical stimulation of an exposed and previously normal lumbar nerve root in a patient undergoing surgery under local anesthesia does not elicit radicular pain (10,24). However, compression may lead to numbness and weakness in the affected area of the limb. Prolonged compression of a peripheral nerve followed by light mechanical stimulation is known to produce abnormal electrical discharge from the nerve (7) and abnormal behavior indicating pain in experimental animals (1). However, the relevance of these facts to the clinical situation of a patient with symptoms of nerve root involvement is uncertain. Such a patient with spinal stenosis will have undergone very gradual development of the stenosis. The changes sustained by the nerve root during this period can only be speculated. The root is not only compressed but is subject to dynamic movement, vascular changes, and perhaps the effect of noxious substances from the adjacent degenerate lumbar disc or even the facet joints themselves (27). Experimental studies to elucidate the mechanisms involved are helpful to our understanding, but by necessity they normally are conducted over much shorter time periods than the true clinical situation.

There is no doubt that compression of a lumbar nerve root or the cauda equina results in morphologic change. Rydevik et al. (22) showed that compression resulted in disproportionately more displacement of the superficial part of the root, which led to shear forces and damage within the root structure. This shear effect was most marked at the edge of the compressed zone. In addition to deformation, compression results in microvascular changes and reduction in the degree of contact of the root with the cerebrospinal fluid. Rydevik et al. (23) showed that nutrition to the root was via both blood vessels and the cerebrospinal fluid, with the latter being most important. The combination of these changes eventually results in intraneural edema and fibrosis (11), which renders the neurons unable to respond to increased demand. The changes lead to abnormal ectopic neuronal firing (21) and pain and sensory disturbances, which suggests that the large-fiber sensory nerves are more susceptible to such damage.

Compression also leads to a change in the permeability of the root capillaries, which leads to edema (13). They showed that such edema would occur after only 2 hours of compression at 50 mm Hg. In a subsequent article, Olmarker et al. (15) showed that very low levels of compression impaired supply of nutrition to the root. Compression at levels of only 10 mm Hg led to a 20% to 30% reduction of methyl glucose transport. The reduction of nutritional transport was directly proportional to the applied pressure (15). It is possible that compression impedes the clearance of vasoactive peptides from the root or, more importantly, the dorsal root ganglion (2).

In an attempt to provide a model to examine the more chronic effects of stenosis, Delamarter et al. (4) constricted the cauda equina of dogs to varying degrees. They found that, by 3 months, all the roots had become atrophic in the most severely compressed animals. Distal to the zone of compression there were dystrophic axons showing wallerian degeneration. Proximal to the lesion they found evidence of blockage of axoplasmic flow and even permanent changes in the posterior columns of the cord. Yoshizawa et al. (28) constricted a single lumbar nerve root with a Silastic tube in dogs and examined the changes found at 12 months. There was thickening of the dura and arachnoid, wallerian degeneration, loss of large myelinated fibers, and reduction in the compound action potential and sensory nerve conduction velocity. They believed that the most significant factor in the root dysfunction was the development of intraradicular edema.

The development of symptoms of neurogenic claudication in humans has been highly associated with the presence of compression of the cauda equina or the nerve roots at two segmental levels (18,19). Olmarker et al. (16) showed experimentally in a pig model that compression of the cauda equina at a single level to 50 mm Hg for 2 hours did not produce any reduction in the muscle action potential (MAP). However, compression at two levels to only 10 mm Hg for the same amount of time produced a 65% reduction in MAP. However, they had previously shown that such double-level compression did not lead to complete vascular congestion (14). In single-level compression at 50 mm Hg, there was complete cessation of venular and capillary flow. Pedowitz et al. (17) showed that such compression had only minor neurophysiologic effects despite this vascular stasis. Jespersen et al. (9) showed that acute compression of the cauda equina in pigs produced impaired neural function but no acute ischemic changes, although ischemia did occur in more chronic models (8). They hypothesized that double-level compression could trap the flow of neurotransmitter agents such as vasoactive intestinal peptide (VIP), thus affecting neurophysiologic function. These factors show that vascular factors cannot totally explain the clinical effects of stenosis and that additional factors must be at work.

In vivo human studies are understandably uncommon. Takahashi et al. (25) measured the lumbar epidural pressure in patients walking on a treadmill. They found that patients with spinal stenosis had higher levels of epidural pressure than normal cases and that walking with a flexed posture reduced the pressure compared to walking normally. Magnaes (12) also examined epidural pressure in patients with central lumbar stenosis. Pathologic pressure levels were found in only 67% of the cases; in some, the pressure actually exceeded mean arterial blood pressure. Those with normal epidural pressure levels could not be distinguished clinically from those with high pressure. They believed that the only identifiable mechanism in those cases was lateral compression of multiple nerve roots.

The exact nature of the etiopathologic changes that result in either radicular pain or neurogenic claudication in patients with lumbar spinal stenosis remains uncertain. Multiple factors clearly are at work. It is likely that compression of nerve roots is a consistent and significant pathologic necessity for the production of clinical symptoms. The effect of compression is modified further by factors such as ischemia and inflammation.

REFERENCES

1. Bennett GJ, Xie Y-K A peripheral mononeuropathy in rat that produces disorders of pain sensation like those seen in man. *Pain* 1988;33:87–107.
2. Cornefjord M, Olmarker K, Farley DB, et al. Neuropeptide changes in compressed spinal nerve roots. *Spine* 1995;20:670–673.
3. Crock HV. Isolated lumbar disc resorption as a cause of nerve root canal stenosis. *Clin Orthop* 1976;115: 109–115.
4. Delamarter RB, Bohlman HH, Dodge LD, et al. Experimental lumbar spinal stenosis. Analysis of the cortical evoked potentials, microvasculature and histopathology. *J Bone Joint Surg* 1990;72A:110–120.
5. Epstein JA. Diagnosis and treatment of painful neurological disorders caused by spondylosis of the lumbar spine. *J Neurosurg* 1960;17:991–998.
6. Gowers WR. *A manual of diseases of the nervous system,* 2nd ed. Churchill: London, 1891.
7. Howe JF, Loeser JD, Calvin WH. Mechanosensitivity of dorsal root ganglia and chronically injured axons: a physiological basis for the radicular pain of nerve root compression. *Pain* 1977;3:25–41.
8. Jespersen SM, Hansen ES, Hoy K, et al. Two-level spinal stenosis in minipigs. Hemodynamic effects of exercise. *Spine* 1995;20:2765–2773.
9. Jespersen SM, Christensen K, Svenstrup L, et al. Spinal cord and nerve root blood flow in acute double level spinal stenosis. *Spine* 1997;22:2900–2910.
10. Lindahl O. Hyperalgesia of the lumbar nerve roots in sciatica. *Acta Orthop Scand* 1966;37:367–374.
11. Lundborg G. Structure and function of the intraneural microvessels as related to trauma, edema formation and nerve function. *J Bone Joint Surg* 1975;57A:938–948.
12. Magnaes B. Clinical recording of pressure on the spinal cord and cauda equina. Part 2: position changes in pressure on the cauda equina in central lumbar spinal stenosis. *J Neurosurg* 1982;57:57–63.
13. Olmarker K, Rydevik B, Holm S. Edema formation in spinal nerve roots induced by experimental, graded compression. An experimental study on the pig cauda equina with special reference to differences in effects between rapid and slow onset of compression. *Spine* 1989;14:559–563.
14. Olmarker K, Rydevik B, Holm S, et al. Effects of experimental graded compression on blood flow in spinal nerve roots. A vital microscopic study on the porcine cauda equina. *J Orthop Res* 1989;7:817–823.
15. Olmarker K, Rydevik B, Hansson T, et al. Compression-induced changes of the nutritional supply to the porcine cauda equina. *J Spinal Disord* 1990;3:25–29.
16. Olmarker K, Holm S, Rydevik B. More pronounced effects of double level compression than single level

compression on impulse propagation in the porcine cauda equina. Presented to the International Society for the Study of the Lumbar Spine, Boston, Massachusetts, 1990.

17. Pedowitz RA, Garfin SR, Massie JB, et al. Effects of magnitude and duration of compression on spinal nerve root conduction. *Spine* 1992;17:194–199.

18. Porter RW. Central spinal stenosis. Classification and pathogenesis. *Acta Orthop Scand* 1993;251[Suppl]:64–66.

19. Porter RW, Ward D. Cauda equina dysfunction. The significance of two-level pathology. *Spine* 1991;17:9–15.

20. Putti V. Lady Jones Lecture: on new conceptions in the pathogenesis of sciatic pain. *Lancet* 1927;2:53–60.

21. Rydevik B, Brown MD, Lundborg G. Pathoanatomy and pathophysiology of nerve root compression. *Spine* 1984;9:7–15.

22. Rydevik B, Lundborg G, Skalak R. Biomechanics of peripheral nerves. In: Nordin M, Frankel VH, eds. *Basic biomechanics of the musculoskeletal system*. Philadelphia: Lea & Febiger, 1989:75–87.

23. Rydevik B, Holm S, Brown MD, et al. Diffusion from the cerebrospinal fluid as a nutritional pathway for spinal nerve roots. *Acta Physiol Scand* 1990;138:247–248.

24. Smyth MJ, Wright V. Sciatica and the intervertebral disc—an experimental study. *J Bone Joint Surg* 1958; 40A:1401–1403.

25. Takahashi K, Kagechika K, Takino T, et al. Changes in epidural pressure during walking in patients with lumbar spinal stenosis. *Spine* 1995;20:2746–2749.

26. Verbiest H. Sur certaines formes rare de compression de la quene de cheval. In: *Hommage a Clovis Vincent*. Paris: Maline, 1949:161–174.

27. Wehling P, Bandara G, Evans CH. Synovial cytokines impair the function of the sciatic nerve in rats: a possible element in the pathophysiology of radicular syndromes. *NeuroOrthopaedics* 1989;7:55–59.

28. Yoshizawa H, Kobayashi S, Morita T. Chronic nerve root compression. Pathophysiologic mechanism of nerve root dysfunction. *Spine* 1995;20:397–407.

Lumbar Spinal Stenosis
edited by Robert Gunzburg and Marek Szpalski
Lippincott Williams & Wilkins, Philadelphia, © 2000.

18

Vascular Compression Theory

Richard Porter

Doncaster DN4 7AZ, United Kingdom

Spinal stenosis has pathologic effects on the blood supply of the cauda equina. When proposing a theory for neurogenic claudication, it is important to appreciate the normal vascular anatomy and how it can be compromised both passively and actively in the presence of stenosis.

ANATOMY

The veins of the roots of the cauda equina (which do not anastomose between roots) drain distally toward the foramen. There is a physiologic valve that prevents backflow from the extradural radicular veins back into the nerve root. It is probable that with high pressure occlusion of the extradural part of the root, this valve cannot compensate and that there is backflow of radicular blood in the veins toward the conus, with blood then draining into the veins of other roots. Compression of the intradural part of a root of the cauda equina, which is above venous pressure, will result in venous blood draining away on either side of the compression, distally to the foramen, and proximally toward the conus.

The arteries enter the nerve roots at the foramen, as branches of the lumbar arteries. They run toward the conus, anastomosing with other arteries at the conus. If there is compression of the roots above arterial pressure, there is a watershed, with arterial blood on one side coming from the conus and on the other side from the foramen. Only the segment of the root under the compression will be impaired of oxygenated blood.

PATHOLOGY

Venous Congestion

One of the radiologic features of neurogenic claudication is the high frequency of multiple level stenosis in the central and root canals (4). The vascular anatomy of the nerve roots makes them vulnerable to venous congestion of the intervening segment if there is multiple-level stenosis at pressures above venous pressure. The arteries will continue to feed the segment at the higher arterial pressure, but impaired drainage will reduce blood flow, oxygen supply, and nutrition, with a buildup of metabolites in the segment between the two blocks.

This hypothesis is compatible with experimental studies. A single level compression of 10 mm Hg in a porcine cauda equina model had little effect on the function, but a two-level compression of 10 mm Hg caused marked reduction of blood flow by 64%, and there was

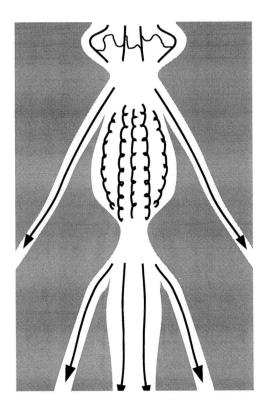

FIG. 1. Method by which two levels of central stenosis will cause congestion of all the intervening cauda equina.

significant reduction in protein transport and nerve conduction (2). This congestion also agrees with myeloscopic studies that show congested cauda equina in claudicating patients (3).

Venous congestion of the roots of the cauda equina may follow two levels of central stenosis (Fig. 1). However, if there is a single level of central stenosis and a more distal level of root canal stenosis, only one root will be congested (Fig. 2). Neurogenic claudication can affect one or both legs, perhaps depending on whether many roots or only a single root is congested.

This is compatible with the observation that 50% of patients with bilateral claudication have a degenerative spondylolisthesis, with symmetric forward displacement at L4–5 and a more proximal stenosis at L3–4 (4). However, about half the patients with unilateral claudication have a degenerative lumbar scoliosis, with asymmetric degeneration mainly on the concave side of the curve. They often have a central stenosis and a more distal root canal stenosis on the concave side of the curve.

Walking

If venous pooling of the nerve roots of the cauda equina between two levels of low-pressure stenosis is responsible for the symptoms of neurogenic claudication, one has to ask why symptoms are not usually present at rest. They occur when walking, and they are relieved by rest. One might argue that the block pressure will increase with the dynamic activity of walking. There will be increased local vasodilatation of the radicular arteries in response to exercise. Exercising a single limb of a mouse will produce vasodilatation in the ipsilateral

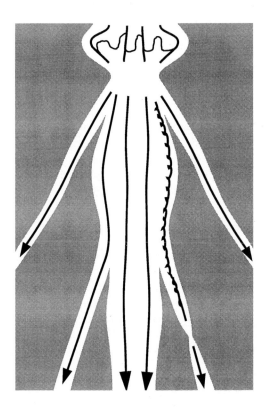

FIG. 2. Method by which one level of central stenosis and a more distal level of root canal stenosis will cause congestion of one root.

region of the spinal cord. Blood flow in the nerve root also is increased with peripheral nerve stimulation. One might expect, therefore, that the arteries of the cauda equina will dilate with exercise, and, if space is at a premium, the pressure at the site of stenosis will rise to a critical level.

Other features associated with walking will tend to increase the block pressure. Movement of the spine in the sagittal plane alters the epidural pressure at the site of stenosis, rising to a little above normal pressure in flexion (15 to 18 mm Hg) and rising greatly above venous pressure in extension (80 to 100 mm Hg). Not only is the central canal affected by motion, but segmental rotation that accompanies walking will compromise the root canal where the degenerate capsule of the facet joint limits the available space for the nerve root complex.

Increased venous return from the exercising lower limbs will be accompanied by engorgement of the pelvic veins and Batson's venous plexus, reducing the available space for the cauda equina. Extradural venous engorgement that occurs while the patient is walking will contribute to the block pressure.

Thus, there may be many patients with stenosis in whom the pressures at rest are just below venous pressure. There is no congestion at rest, but with exercise the block pressure rises, and the cauda equine becomes congested when the patient walks.

Despite this explanation, if venous congestion were the explanation, one would expect some patients to have stenosis pressure that is sufficiently high, even at rest, to cause venous congestion and, therefore, symptoms at rest.

Failed Arterial Vasodilatation

There is considerable arterial vasodilatation (200%) of the cauda equina in a porcine model, when proximal electrical stimulation initiates tail muscle activity and is maintained for at least 30 minutes (1). When applying a two-level block to the porcine cauda equina, the increased blood flow of the cauda equina in response to electrical stimulation is less pronounced and is maintained for only a few minutes. Blood flow then falls rapidly to approximately 60% *below* resting level, and there is a failure of nerve conduction.

If this acute model is analogous to the chronic situation in spinal stenosis, it may explain the symptoms of neurogenic claudication.

Failed arterial response is compatible with the observation that patients with neurogenic claudication tend to be in the arteriosclerotic age group, and that peripheral vascular disease and neurogenic claudication often coexist. Pathologic arteries may be less labile, especially in the presence of venous congestion. It also would explain why a proportion of claudicating patients will respond to injection of calcitonin, which is a potent arterial vasodilator drug.

SUMMARY

The vascular compression theory proposes that neurogenic claudication is frequently associated with multiple-level stenosis, which will result in venous congestion of the root(s) between the levels of stenosis. In arteriosclerotic subjects, if the nerve roots are congested with venous blood, the arterioles of the nerve roots fail to maintain a vasodilatation response to exercise. There is then a failure of nerve conduction that produces tiredness, weakness, heaviness, and discomfort in the lower limbs when the patient walks. If the patient stops walking, nerve function temporarily recovers to permit a further short period of walking.

REFERENCES

1. Baker AR, Collins T, Porter RW, Kidd C. Laser doppler study of porcine cauda equina blood flow: the effect of electrical stimulation of the rootlets during single and double site, low pressure compression of the cauda equina. *Spine* 1995;20:660–664
2. Olmarker K, Holm S, Rydevik B. Single versus double level nerve root compression: an experimental study of the porcine cauda equina with analyses of nerve impulse conduction properties. *Clin Orthop* 1992;6:35–39.
3. Ooi Y, Mita F, Satoh Y. Myeloscopic study on lumbar spinal canal stenosis with special reference to intermittent claudication. *Spine* 1990;15:544–549.
4. Porter RW, Ward D. Cauda equina dysfunction: the significance of multiple level pathology. *Spine* 1992;17: 9–15.

SECTION V
Conservative Treatment Modalities

Lumbar Spinal Stenosis
edited by Robert Gunzburg and Marek Szpalski
Lippincott Williams & Wilkins, Philadelphia, © 2000.

19

Pharmacologic Treatment

Malcolm I.V. Jayson

Rheumatic Diseases Centre, Hope Hospital, Salford M6 8HD, United Kingdom

Various types of pain-relieving medication commonly are prescribed for patients with spinal stenosis. However, there is little evidence that they make any difference to the long-term course of events. Drugs are helpful in controlling symptoms, and for many patients they represent the most appropriate form of treatment.

PURE ANALGESICS

Pure analgesics have central mechanisms of action and virtually no peripheral antiinflammatory activity (6).

Paracetamol (acetaminophen) is the most commonly prescribed analgesic and generally is effective as the nonsteroidal antiinflammatory drugs (NSAIDs). It is unlikely to cause peptic ulceration or renal impairment. Simple analgesics of this type are preferred in the elderly patient because of its lower risk of toxicity. Paracetamol is effective in doses of 500 to 1,000 mg given every 4 to 6 hours. Doses higher than 4 g per day can cause hepatic damage. To achieve a greater analgesic effect, paracetamol often is used in combination with weak opioids such as codeine or dextrapropoxyphene.

The use of morphine and related strong opioids in the context of back problems and spinal stenosis is controversial (3). They are very effective analgesics for patients who are in severe pain, but because of their potential for dependence, tolerance, constipation, and respiratory depression, their use should be avoided in patients with chronic back problems such as spinal stenosis. The elderly patient who suffers from spinal stenosis syndromes is at particular risk of adverse effects.

NONSTEROIDAL INFLAMMATORY DRUGS

The class of compounds possesses antiinflammatory effects due to inhibition of peripheral cyclooxygenase prostaglandin synthesis, inhibition of neutrophil activation, and aggregation and inhibition of phospholipase C in mononuclear cells (7). They also have important analgesic properties (14).

There are now more than 50 NSAIDs available, but any physician need only use a relatively small number of the different drugs.

Clinical trials have demonstrated effective pain-relieving activity in patients with low back pain (1,2). No trial has specifically addressed the issue of antiinflammatory drugs in spinal stenosis, but a systematic review found these drugs to be less effective in treating sciatica (15).

There appear to be little differences in efficacies in relieving pain between the different antiinflammatory drugs used (15); however, there are differences in their durations of actions and in their adverse effect profiles.

They may be divided into groups with either a serum half-life of less than 6 hours, such as ibuprofen, indomethacin, and diclofenac, or greater than 12 hours, such as piroxicam, naproxen, and nabumetone. To obtain prolonged duration of action of the short half-life compounds, slow-release preparations are now commonly used.

Gastrointestinal mucosal damage is the most common adverse effect. It is caused by interference by prostaglandin-mediated mucus production, mucosal blood flow, and bicarbonate production. Dyspepsia, peptic ulceration, iron deficiency anemia, and acute gastrointestinal hemorrhage are all possible adverse effects. Some NSAIDs are less harmful to the gut than others. Ibuprofen is probably the least toxic, followed by diclofenac. Azapropazone and piroxicam are more toxic (8). Prophylactic ulcer-healing drugs should be considered in patients who require an NSAID. In particular, risk factors such as older age, previous peptic ulceration, cigarette smoking, and concurrent use of anticoagulants or steroids all should be considered. H_2 receptor antagonists such as cimetidine and ranitidine, the synthetic prostaglandin analogue misoprostol, and proton pump inhibitors such as omeprazole should all be considered. Some patients who are intolerant of oral NSAIDs may be satisfactorily treated with the same agent as a suppository.

Recent evidence has identified Cox 2 antagonists as having less ulcerogenic potential than other antiinflammatory drugs. Meloxicam may possess advantages for these patients, although its true place is not yet established.

Other adverse effects of NSAIDs include renal impairment, hepatitis, blood dyscrasias, skin rashes, and central nervous system disturbance. All these drugs impair renal blood flow, and careful monitoring of renal function is important in the elderly, particularly if they have existing renal impairment or are undergoing diuretic therapy.

NSAIDs have important drug interactions with warfarin, probenecid, lithium, and antihypertensive agents. Because many elderly patients are receiving polypharmacy, care is required when prescribing these drugs.

There is a variability of response to antiinflammatory agents. When one drug is ineffective, it may be worth trying an alternative one before abandoning this class of drug.

PSYCHOTROPIC DRUGS

A significant proportion of patients are depressed. Depression amplifies a patient's perception of the severity of pain. In these circumstances, tricyclic antidepressants are effective in relieving both the pain and depression.

We now know that agents with serotonergic and noradrenergic effects have specific analgesic properties. They appear particularly helpful in patients with features suggestive of fibromyalgia.

There have been a number of clinical trials evaluating antidepressant drugs for treatment of low back pain (13). The evidence for back pain is limited, and there have not been any studies specifically directed at spinal stenosis. Nevertheless, in patients in whom there is chronic pain and in whom there appears to be an element of fibromyalgia with widespread pain, distress, poor sleep rhythm, and multiple focal tender points on investigation, it is well worth considering these agents.

Amitriptyline or related compounds are commonly used. The initial dose of amitriptyline usually is 10 to 25 mg at night, and the dose may be slowly increased at weekly intervals according to the patient's needs. A prolonged analgesic effect may be obtained (9). Patients may be maintained on these agents for the long term. Some are intolerant of adverse effects, which include drowsiness, dry mouth, postural hypotension, and urinary retention. The use of these drugs is contraindicated in patients with cardiac conduction defects.

ANTICONVULSANTS

Carbamezepine, phenytoin, or sodium valproate may be given for chronic radicular pain and may be helpful in some spinal stenosis patients. Their particular value appears to lie in patients who report a neuralgic pattern of symptoms with sharp shooting or electric shock components. There have not been any trials specifically addressing the value of anticonvulsants in spinal stenosis.

MUSCLE RELAXANTS

These drugs sometimes are used for patients with acute low back pain when there is thought to be a major element of muscle spasm. However, there is no way to reliably detect or quantify muscle spasm by clinical means, and it is uncertain whether the increased muscle tone is responsible for the severity of the pain. Some of these drugs, such as baclofen, chlormezanone, and diazepam, act centrally and frequently produce sedation as well as modest muscle relaxation. Baclofen often is given in dosages of 5 mg three times a day, and it shortens the recovery period of acute episodes of pain (4). Diazepam and the other benzodiazepines may help muscle relaxation in the short term, but dependence becomes common among chronic back sufferers and treatment should be restricted to a fixed time schedule.

The evidence for the value of muscle relaxants for chronic back pain syndromes is extremely limited, and no trials have been undertaken in spinal stenosis.

SYSTEMIC CORTICOSTEROIDS

These agents do not play any part in the management of spinal stenosis.

CALCITONIN

In Paget's disease, bony enlargement may lead to nerve root compression and the spinal stenosis syndrome. Treatment of Paget's disease with calcitonin has been reported to improve neurogenic claudication (16). These observations led Porter (11) to undertake an open study of calcitonin treatment in 11 of 41 patients with neurogenic claudication; considerable improvement in walking distance was found. Ten subjects agreed to enter a randomized, double-blind, crossover trial; eight correctly assessed subjective improvement when taking the drug. On that basis, Porter believed that the drug was useful and that it probably acted on an arterial shunt mechanism leading to improved perfusion of the cauda equina. Porter and Miller (12) then conducted a double-blind study. Although there were improvements in the calcitonin group, they could not establish that the response was an organic phenomenon. Eskola et al. (5) conducted a randomized, placebo-controlled, double-blind, crossover study of 40 spinal stenosis patients with 1-year follow-up. They found that calcitonin had beneficial effects on symptoms with a clear analgesic effect. Walking distance increased, but the crossover trend was not as good as the analgesic effect. They concluded that there was some relief of symptoms, but the effects of calcitonin seem to be poor.

The mechanisms calcitonin action in spinal stenosis are obscure. Although the original postulate was an improvement in the microcirculation, it is known that calcitonin has an analgesic effect (10), and it is possible that the modest effects observed arise for this reason.

CONCLUSION

Although there is no evidence that pharmacologic treatments will alter the course of spinal stenosis syndromes, drug therapy can be helpful in relieving symptoms. Judicious pharmacologic management and, in particular, careful choice of the type of drug, the nature of the formulation, and the timing of administration should be considered carefully to provide optimum benefit.

REFERENCES

1. Amile E, Weber H, Holm I. Treatment of acute low back pain with pyroxicam. Results of a double-blind placebo-controlled trial. *Spine* 1987;12:473–476.
2. Berry H, Bloom B, Hamilton EBD, et al. Naproxen sodium, diflunisal and placebo in the treatment of chronic back pain. *Ann Rheum Dis* 1982;41:129–132.
3. Brena SF, Sanders SH. Opioids in nonmalignant pain: questions in search of answers. *Clin J Pain* 1991;7: 342–345.
4. Dapas F, Hartman SF, Martinez L, et al. Baclofen for the treatment of acute low back pain syndrome: double-blind comparative with placebo. *Spine* 1985;10:345–349.
5. Eskola A, Pohjolainen T, Alaranta H, Soini J, Tallroth A, Slatis P. Calcitonin treatment in lumbar spinal stenosis: a randomized placebo-controlled, double-blind, cross-over study with one year follow-up. *Calcif Tissue Int* 1992;50, 400–403.
6. Flower RJ, Moncada S, Vain JR. Analgesic-antipyretics and the anti-inflammatory agents: drugs employed in the treatment of gout. In: Gilman AG, et al., eds. *The pharmacological basis of therapeutics*, 7th ed. New York: McMillan, 1985:674–715.
7. Forest MJ, Brooks PM. Mechanism of action of non-steroidal anti-inflammatory drugs. *Baillieres Clin Rheumatol* 1988;2:275–294.
8. Garcia Rodriguez LA, Jick H. Risk of upper gastro-intestinal bleeding and perforation associated with individual non-steroidal anti-inflammatory drugs. *Lancet* 1994;343:769–772.
9. Hameroff SR, Weiss JL, Lerman JC, et al. Doxepin effects on chronic pain and depression: a controlled study. *J Clin Psychiatry* 1984;45:45–52.
10. Montagnani M, Gonnelli S, Francini G, Piolini M, Gennari C. Analgesic effects of salmon calcitonin nasal spray in bone pain. *Proc Int Symp Calcitonin Rome* 1988;88:126–133.
11. Porter RW. Calcitonin treatment for neurogenic claudication. *Spine* 1983;8:585–592.
12. Porter RW, Miller CG. Neurogenic claudication and root claudication treated with calcitonin a double-blind trial. *Spine* 1988;13:1061–1064.
13. Turner JA, Denny MC. Do antidepressant medications relieve chronic low back pain? *J Fam Pract* 1993;37: 545–553.
14. Urquhart E. Central analgesic activity of non-steroidal anti-inflammatory drugs in animal and human pain models. *Semin Arthritis Rheum* 1993;23:198–205.
15. Van Tulder MW, Koes BW, Bouter LM. *Low back pain in primary care: effectiveness of diagnostic and therapeutic intervention.* Amsterdam, The Netherlands: EMGO Institute, Vrije University, 1996.
16. Walpin LA, Singer R. Paget's disease. Reversal of severe paraparesis using calcitonin. *Spine* 1979;4:214–219.

Lumbar Spinal Stenosis
edited by Robert Gunzburg and Marek Szpalski
Lippincott Williams & Wilkins, Philadelphia, © 2000.

20

Education and Exercises in Spinal Stenosis

Margareta Nordin

Occupational and Industrial Orthopedic Center, Hospital for Joint Diseases, Mount Sinai/New York University Medical Center, New York, New York 10014

Can noninvasive treatment such as exercises and education alleviate symptomatology in patients with spinal stenosis? Is there a theoretical rationale? Have clinical outcome studies or randomized control trials showed evidence of efficacy?

Spinal stenosis is grossly defined as "any type of narrowing of the spinal canal, nerve root canals, or intervertebral foramina." The detailed classification of spinal stenosis is not the aim of this chapter and can be found in Chapter 6. The symptomatology includes back pain and/or radicular pain and claudication. The goal of conservative treatment is pain alleviation and increased function for patients who chose not to have surgery. This treatment also can be indicated as a treatment before or after surgery. One comment is necessary before starting this chapter. There is no available scientific evidence on conservative treatment and its effectiveness in randomized control trials. A few outcome studies are available on conservative treatments and will be cited. Meta-analyses and surgical outcome studies have been done on patients with spinal stenosis (1,4,25). The focus of this chapter is to review a rationale for conservative treatment for patients with spinal stenosis seeking conservative treatment as an option to surgery or repeat surgery in the case of spinal stenosis.

CHOICE OF TREATMENT: CONSERVATIVE VERSUS SURGICAL

Little is known about the effectiveness of conservative treatment and the diagnosis of spinal stenosis. Little also is known about the natural history of nonsurgical spinal stenosis and patient well-being. Two recent case series demonstrated that 10% to 25% of patients worsen within 3 to 8 years, 15% to 30% improved, and the remaining patients believed that their symptoms were unchanged (11,16). These two studies are important because they demonstrate that the diagnosis of spinal stenosis does not necessarily have a somber prognosis. Patients with moderate-to-light spinal stenosis (diagnosed by imaging) who choose not to have surgery may cope well over several years. These patients may increase their function by learning about postural load and the benefit of exercises, which may lead to improved quality of life. Patients with spinal stenosis often are elderly, and a slow deterioration of functional capacity may occur for several reasons. Referring these patients to conservative treatment, such as education about spinal stenosis and an adapted exercise program, would benefit their lifestyle, increase their function, and decrease the avoidance of important activity of daily life. Also, the "baby boomer" generation is aging, is more educated, and has a great expectation of health, function, and well-being.

Atlas et al. (1) reported decreased symptoms and improved quality of life by surgery in 76% to 80% of patients surgically treated versus 35% to 50% improvement in the nonsurgical group. Unfortunately, patient outcome was evaluated by an independent observer. Patients who opted for surgery had more severe imaging findings, symptoms, and functional status compared to patients who did not have surgery. Although the groups were not comparable, some interesting findings are noteworthy. The surgically treated patients at entry of the study "were more symptomatic and had worse disability resulting from their symptoms" (1). This quote highlights the importance of discussing with patients the outcomes of choice of treatment. Patients with moderate-to-light symptoms and who are functioning at a desired level can opt for conservative treatment, and patients with severe continuous symptoms and complete block indicate a better result with surgical intervention. In a 12-year follow-up study, Hurri et al. (14) claim that choice of treatment (operative or nonoperative) is not predictive of subsequent perceived disability measured by Oswestry questionnaire (7). However the authors are cautious because of the small numbers of patients (n = 75). Only randomized controlled trials will be able to answer this question.

RATIONALE FOR CONSERVATIVE TREATMENT

The rationale for conservative treatment is to decrease pain and increase function. This can be obtained through (i) education on posture, for example, decreased load on the spinal structure and how to alleviate symptoms by posture change; (ii) specific muscle training, for example, stabilization techniques; and (iii) generic exercise program, for example, walking to improve vascularization.

Local epidural pressure measurements at the stenotic level have shown that the pressure levels decrease in lying and sitting postures (24). The pressure was increased with extension of the trunk but decreased with flexion. The highest pressure occurred in the standing posture with the trunk extended. Therefore, we can conclude that epidural pressure and perhaps symptom triggering are significantly related to posture, and that posture and position education may be of benefit.

Electromyography studies have shown that muscle recruitment and muscle activation can be compromised in patients with spine ailments. However, there are no studies directly related to patients with spinal stenosis and muscle performance. Change in trunk motion pattern has been shown in patients with spinal stenosis (23). These changes may be associated with different muscle recruitment patterns and the avoidance of high-pressure positions such as dynamic extension. In 1975, Nachemson (19) showed that hyperextension of the lumbar spine greatly increased disc pressure measurements (up to seven times body weight). In 1984, Capozzo (3) showed that fast walking (2.16 m/s) increased lumbar spine load to only two times body weight. Therefore, in patients with spinal stenosis, avoiding hyperextension and promoting walking are indicated. There is, however, a lack of understanding of the association of pain and muscle performance in patients with spinal stenosis. Nevertheless, several authors observed decreased levels of pain and increased tolerance of function in the patients who were referred to an exercise program (9,20).

Vascular insufficiency associated with lumbar spinal stenosis may lead to claudication and/or pain in the legs. Some researchers suggest that there is decreased pain and claudication in patients with spinal stenosis who are referred to a generic exercise or walking program (8,11,20,28).

BASELINE EVALUATION

Any treatment should use a baseline evaluation. Standardized clinical data are important to collect and thereby evaluate treatment outcome on a larger scale. The National Spine

Network makes such an attempt. The National Spine Network consists of 26 Centers of Excellence for spinal care at different geographic locations in the United States. This type of data collection will provide better outcomes in the future. However, the data collection structure does not allow for objective tests for functional outcome at this time. For the patient with spinal stenosis, we have mostly patient-reported functional data. In their review article, Fritz et al. (9) suggested the following patient-centered outcome measurements: treadmill walking tolerance, generic self-reported level of health status, sickness impact profile, and Medical Outcomes Survey 36-item short form (SF36) (27). Table 1 lists in full the suggested outcome measures proposed by Fritz et al. (9).

Using valid and reliable outcome measures is important. Cross-cultural health outcome assessments were summarized recently by the European Research Group on Health Outcomes. Several instruments for health outcome measures are published in several languages and tested for reliability and some for validity. This publication is most helpful for the clinician interested in patient-administered outcome measures and for the international community, because the publication describes in what languages the outcome instrument exists (15).

Treadmill and walking tests have been used to measure functional outcome in patients with spinal stenosis. These tests are functional, relatively low cost, and, if administered properly, associated with little risk. In a case series of 50 patients with lumbar spinal stenosis who underwent decompressive laminectomy, Deen et al. (5) showed that mean total preoperative ambulation time was about 7 minutes (median 5 minutes). Three months postoperatively the mean ambulating time had increased to about 13 minutes (median 15 minutes). The authors conclude that treadmill testing has become a standard test for preoperative assessment, and they intend to implement it as a postoperative follow-up assessment as well as for nonsurgical treatment options for patients with spinal stenosis. Onel et al. (20) used a walking distance test as the outcome measure for conservative inpatient treatment for patients with spinal stenosis. After 3 weeks of active exercises and salmon calcitonin injections, the improvement rate in walking distance was 89% (from 200 m to no limit). These studies indicate that a relatively safe and uncomplicated treadmill or walking test is beneficial to measure outcome. All authors stress the importance of safety and evaluation of comorbidity in this aging patient group while selecting and clearing patients for treadmill testing.

The choice of baseline data is important to develop additional treatment and outcome protocols and to give the patient an optimal treatment choice.

TABLE 1. *Potential dimensions of outcome measures for use with patients with lumbar spinal stenosis*

Pathoanatomic	Myelography
	Anterior posterior diameter of the spinal canal on computed tomography or magnetic resonance imaging scan
Physical impairment	Neurologic examination
	Straight-leg raising
	Spinal range of motion
Patient-centered outcomes	Treadmill walking tolerance (5,6)
	Sickness Impact Profile (2)
	Medical Outcomes Survey (SF36) (27)
Disease-specific self-reported level of health status	Roland Morris Index (21)
	Oswestry Low Back Pain Questionnaire (7)
	Quebec Disability Index (18)
	Wadell Disability Index (26)
Condition-specific self-reported level of health status (22)	
Self-reported expectations of treatment (17)	
Self-reported satisfaction with treatment (17)	

CONSERVATIVE TREATMENT

The theoretical rationale leads to three types of treatment individually or combined: (i) education related to posture, positioning, and daily activities; (ii) muscle training and stabilization of the spinal column; and (iii) generic exercises and improved vascularization. Accurate data about the short-term and long-term efficacy of conservative therapy are lacking. Perhaps the most important message of this chapter is to forward the concept of a more active approach in contrast to Garfin's (10) concept that patients with spinal stenosis only need aspirin and a corset. Patients with spinal stenosis who choose or who are referred to conservative treatment should have an objective evaluation that includes a treadmill walking test, postural evaluation, and functional evaluation. The evaluation should lead to a decision about the type of conservative treatment; for example, self-applied pain relief (heat or ice), education (posture, positioning), and an adapted exercise, biking, and/or walking program. The hypothesis needs to be tested in randomized controlled studies. The outcome and case studies available indicate that this type of treatment is not harmful, and, most important, it can benefit the patient's functional status and quality of life (8,13,20,28). There also seems to be an observation that patients with block or marked stenosis do not improve or show only temporary relief after conservative treatment (11,16). It is unclear if an exercise program will increase symptoms in these patients. As stated by Herno et al. (11,12), ''Obviously, the patients with block stenosis have been operated on in most cases, indicating that surgical treatment might be the method of choice of this category.''

EDUCATION

Education of the patient begins with the physician encounter, when the patient is seeking help for pain related to spinal stenosis and before referral to conservative treatment. The patient should know about treatment options and results. If the patient opts for conservative treatment, the information should include type of treatment and outcomes. The patient should be informed about expected compliance, the possible effect of conservative treatment, and the time commitment and necessary changes in lifestyle. For example, to maintain results, a daily walking program may be necessary. During the last years, we have shied away from stereotyped group therapy and focused more on individualized directed information tailored to each patient's need. A nurse, physical therapist, psychologist, or individual particularly interested in the field of educating patients can provide this education. Practical training is important, and follow-up is necessary to ensure that the patient has understood the concept and is executing the information correctly. We have found that videotapes reinforcing the concept or handouts are very welcomed by the patient. The next step will be the development of computer interactive education currently used by some clinics.

EXERCISES AND/OR WALKING PROGRAM

A stationary biking or walking program seems to be successful (5,6,8,20). Fritz et al. (8) reported on harness-supported treadmill ambulation in two patients. This is a novel approach moving in ''an unloaded position.'' This approach may be too complicated for most rehabilitation centers, but further studies will tell. As in other chronic back pain treatments, the most important objective may be to get the patient moving; the means may be less important. The rationale for walking or biking is to increase vascularization and tolerance for walking. The rationale for specific trunk exercises is to enhance the stability of the lumbar spine. Active exercise and walking or biking are mood elevators, and supervised exercises alleviate fear avoidance behaviors. Separating the effects is difficult for the researcher, but perhaps is less important in daily clinical practice for the health care provider and the patient.

CONCLUSION

Conservative management may or may not be of benefit for the patient with spinal stenosis. Patients with moderate-to-light symptoms will respond best to an active walking or exercise program. One observation is that an exercise and educational program is not harmful and yields low cost. It may benefit the patient with spinal stenosis, and it can prepare the patient better for surgery, if needed. However, randomized controlled studies are needed to compare conservative treatment and surgery in terms of quality of life and functional outcomes in patients with spinal stenosis. Improved knowledge of the natural history of patients with different classifications of spinal stenosis is needed. Studies currently are being performed that hopefully will shed light on the benefit of conservative noninvasive management for the patient with spinal stenosis.

ACKNOWLEDGMENTS

I am grateful to Jose Davila, PT student, and Helena Persson, M.D., for help with literature search. I thank Dawn Leger, Ph.D., for editorial help. This review was partially supported by Social Security Administration Disability (#SSA-RFP-97 3118) and The Hospital for Joint Diseases, Research and Development Foundation.

REFERENCES

1. Atlas SJ, Deyo RA, Keller RB, et al. The Maine Lumbar Spine Study, Part III. 1-year outcomes of surgical and nonsurgical management of lumbar spinal stenosis. *Spine* 1996;21:1787–1795.
2. Bergner M, Babbitt RA, Carter WB, Gibson BS. The Sickness Impact Profile: development and final revision of a health status measure. *Med Care* 1981;19:787–805.
3. Capozzo A. Compressive loads in the lumbar vertebral column during normal level walking. *J Orthop Res* 1984;1:292–299.
4. Ciol MA, Deyo RA, Howell E, Kreif S. An assessment of surgery for spinal stenosis: time trends, geographic variations, complications and re-operations. *J Am Geriatr Soc* 1996;44:285–290.
5. Deen HG, Zimmerman RS, Lyons MK, McPhee MC, Verheijde JL, Lemens SM. Use of the exercise treadmill to measure baseline functional status and surgical outcome in patients with severe lumbar spinal stenosis. *Spine* 1998;23:244–248.
6. Dong GX, Porter RW. Walking and cycling tests in neurogenic and intermittent claudication. *Spine* 1989;14: 965–969.
7. Fairbanks JCT, Couper J, Davies JB, O'Brien JP. The Oswestry low back pain disability questionnaire. *Physiotherapy* 1980;66:271–273.
8. Fritz JM, Delitto A, Welch WC, Erhard RE. Lumbar spinal stenosis: a review of current concepts in evaluation, management, and outcome measures. *Arch Phys Med Rehabil* 1998;79:700–708.
9. Fritz JM, Erhard RE, Delitto A, Welch WC, Nowakowski P. Preliminary results of the use of a two-stage treadmill test as a clinical diagnosis of lumbar spinal stenosis. *J Spinal Dis* 1997;10:410–416.
10. Garfin SR. Acquired spinal stenosis: making the diagnosis in the elderly. Most patients need only aspirin and corset support. *J Musculoskeletal Med* 1987;4:61–69.
11. Herno A, Airaksinen O, Saari T, Luukkonen M. Lumbar spinal stenosis: a matched-pair study of operated and non-operated patients. *Br J Neurosurg* 1996;10:461–465.
12. Herno A, Airaksinen O, Saari T, Miettinen H. The predictive value of preoperative myelography in lumbar spinal stenosis. *Spine* 1994;19:1335–1338.
13. Hirsch AT, Munnings F. Intermittent claudication: steps for evaluation and management. *Phys Ther Sports Med* 1993;21:125–138.
14. Hurri H, Slatis J, Soini J, et al. Lumbar spinal stenosis: assessment of long term outcome 12 years after operative and conservative treatment. *J Spinal Disord* 1998;11:110–115.
15. Hutchinson A, Bentzen N, Konig-Zahn C. *Cross cultural health outcome assessment: a user's guide.* European Research Group on Health Outcomes (ERGHO), 1997.

16. Johnsson K-E, Rosen I, Uden A. The natural course of lumbar spinal stenosis. *Clin Orthop* 1992;279:82–86.
17. Katz JN, Lipson SJ, Brick GW, et al. Clinical correlates of patients after laminectomy for degenerative lumbar spinal stenosis. *Spine* 1995;20:1155–1160.
18. Kopec JA, Esdaile JM, Abraamovicz M, et al. The Quebec back pain disability scale. Measurment properties. *Spine* 1995;20:341–352.
19. Nachemson A. Towards a better understanding of back pain: a review of the mechanics of the lumbar disc. *Rheumatol Rehabil* 1975;14:129–134.
20. Onel D, Hidayet S, Cigdem D. Lumbar spinal stenosis: clinical/radiologic therapeutic evaluation in 145 patients. *Spine* 1993;18:291–298.
21. Roland M, Morris R. A study of the natural history of back pain, part 1: development of a reliable and sensitive measure of disability in low back pain. *Spine* 1983;8:141–144.
22. Stucki G, Liang MH, Fossel AH, Katz JN. Relative responsivness of condition specific and generic health status measures in degenerative lumbar spinal stenosis. *J Clin Epidemiol* 1995;48:1369–1378.
23. Szpalski M, Michel F, Hayez JP. Determination of trunk motion patterns associated with permanent or transient stenosis of the lumbar spine. *Eur Spine J* 1996;5:332–337.
24. Takahashi K, Miyazaki T, Takino T, et al. Epidural pressure measurements. Relationship between epidural pressure and posture in patients with spinal stenosis. *Spine* 1995;20:650–653.
25. Turner JA, Ersek M, Herron L, Deyo R. Surgery for lumbar spinal stenosis: an attempted meta-analysis of the literature. *Spine* 1992;17:1–7.
26. Wadell G, Main CJ. Assessment of severity in low back disorders. *Spine* 1984;8:204–208.
27. Ware JE, Sherbourne CD. The MOS 36-item short form health survey (SF-36): I. Conceptual frame work and item selection. *Med Care* 1992;30:473–483.
28. Wiesel SW, Boden SD. Conservative treatment of spinal stenosis: the cornerstone. In: Andersson GBJ, McNeill TW, eds. *Lumbar spinal stenosis.* St. Louis: Mosby-Year Book, 1992:331–338.

Lumbar Spinal Stenosis
edited by Robert Gunzburg and Marek Szpalski
Lippincott Williams & Wilkins, Philadelphia, © 2000.

21

Pain Clinic Approaches

Charles Pither

*Pain Management Department and Pain Input Unit, St. Thomas Hospital,
London SE1 7EH, United Kingdom*

Traditional medical teaching hallows the diagnosis. The diagnosis is reached by taking a history, performing an examination, and then instituting special investigations to confirm or exclude hypothecated pathology. In such a formulation pain has a crucial role, not just in spinal disorders but in medicine as a whole: pain is, after all, the most common symptom reported to general practitioners. In the ideal scenario, the patient will complain of characteristic symptoms in a "classic" pattern. The tests will confirm the diagnosis and appropriate therapy will be administered.

PAIN AS A SYMPTOM

In the case of spinal stenosis, specialist investigations will conclude that there is neural compression, and surgical decompression probably will be performed. Follow-up will reveal that the patient's symptoms have resolved, and both doctor and patient leave the encounter with a glow of satisfaction.

Why is it then that pain clinics exist? More to the point, why are pain clinics full of patients who tell of long-standing spinal pain unrelieved by surgery and many other therapies and procedures?

There are a number of answers to these questions.

1. The origins and sources of spinal pain are complex (11). Frequently the clinical presentation is not "classic" and the exact source of the pain is unclear. Even complex investigations will not show the source of pain. Without a clear diagnosis, curative surgery is not feasible.
2. The functional interrelationships within the back are such that pathology in one structure can give rise to reflex or secondary dysfunction in a neighboring tissue. Thus, pain may arise from more than one source. Treatment may not address all sources.
3. As chronicity proceeds, central changes occur within the neuraxis, which has the effect of altering the sensitivity of the transduction system (23). These changes seemingly are permanent and introduce aspects of pain generation and dysfunction into the central nervous system. Thus, the pain changes from being a peripheral phenomenon related to nociception to a more central problem, effectively imprinted within the central nervous system. In this situation, no amount of peripheral manipulation, either by surgery or neural ablation, will alleviate the pain.
4. Treatment can solve one source of pain while creating others. Further interventions may not be able to rectify the ongoing pain.

5. Pain can itself have major consequences to the individual both physically and psychologically. Pain causes immobility (often through fear avoidance mechanisms), which leads to secondary stiffness weakness and deconditioning. Depression is a frequent accompaniment of pain that limits function, especially in vulnerable individuals. Altered mood has a deleterious effect on pain perception, as well as sapping energy and motivation. The effect is to set in train a vicious circle, which results in worsening physical and emotional function. Such individuals are well described as having ''a chronic pain syndrome.'' In this situation the pain is not so much a symptom but more an illness in its own right (12).

PAIN AS AN ILLNESS

Many individuals with ongoing pain somehow cope with it; they are able to maintain a good quality of life and are not overcome by poor mood and helplessness. Others will find that they enter a descending spiral of diminishing physical activity, worsening mood, poor sleep, increasing use of analgesics and other drugs, and increasing concerns for the future. These individuals experience high levels of distress and disability, and they become major consumers of health care resources. They do this because continuing to search for and cure peripheral sources of pain are ineffective in relieving the symptomatology, and such treatments fail to solve the major social and emotional dysfunction in these individuals.

Such patients are frequent attenders and often become labeled as ''difficult.'' It is now clear that the development of such problems is not related to greater degrees of tissue pathology, but is predicted by measures of psychological distress and certain social factors early in the course of the illness (1). The implication is that the pain has become a whole-person problem and can only be addressed by a holistic perspective. The pain is now an illness and needs treatment as such. Pain clinics are the most logical environments for such people to obtain the optimal therapy they require.

Treating the whole person requires that an assessment be made of the broad illness, not just the spine or low back. For this reason, interdisciplinary assessment using a biopsychosocial model is important in any person who has been troubled by pain for more than 6 months.

Ideally, pain clinics should offer an interdisciplinary approach to care. Typically pain clinic staff would include the physician, physiotherapist, psychologist, nurse, and occupational therapist.

INTERDISCIPLINARY ASSESSMENT

Assessment is unlikely to involve all staff seeing any one patient, but it is important to recognize that a physician or surgeon may not be well equipped to assess psychological issues, and neither doctors nor psychologists may be able to detect the more subtle aspects of physical dysfunction that a skilled physiotherapist may find.

Assessment should focus less on a diagnostic perspective (this should have been done previously), but rather on the nature of the pain, the limitations it causes, and the psychological effects engendered (19). The response of the family and partner, the financial and work status, and the social support are all of considerable importance. This approach has been termed ''biopsychosocial'' and is undoubtedly the most appropriate paradigm for understanding the complex interactions involved in the genesis of chronic pain.

TABLE 1. *Assessment of pain*

Pain nature
   Temporal variability
   Site
   Factors worsening and relieving
History of pain episode
Sleep
Past treatments
Current medications
Past medical history
Current limitations
Psychological function
   Concentration
   Memory
   Mood
   Past psychological or psychiatric history
Home circumstance
Employment
Relationships and support
Financial situation
   Income and benefits
   Litigation
Other life events/issues
Patient's view of cause and future

Assessment will include the factors listed in Table 1. Physical examination also will be performed.

TREATMENT

Pain clinic treatment is aimed at symptomatic relief of pain rather than disease management. Treatment is pragmatic in that the therapy with the greatest likelihood of providing benefit is initiated first. If this fails to provide benefit, other therapies are tried. The aim is not simply to cure the condition—pain clinic treatment seldom, if ever, provides a cure—but to improve the patient's quality of life.

In general, five treatment modalities are available:

1. Drugs
2. Stimulation analgesia
3. Nerve blocks and injections
4. Psychological techniques
5. Invasive implantation technologies.

This review will only briefly discuss these five modalities, with the exception of injections, particularly epidurals, which will be discussed in greater detail and specifically related to the treatment of spinal stenosis.

Drugs

Several classes of drugs are used within the pain clinic setting (5). Although analgesics of different types commonly are prescribed, antidepressants, usually in low doses, often are of value, especially for neuropathic pain. Other compounds, such as antiepileptics, also frequently are used. There is some evidence that both these classes of drugs can be of value in neuropathic pain (10).

The pain of spinal stenosis frequently is incident related (usually to walking). Such pain is difficult to treat adequately by drugs, because doses adequate to suppress the severe pain of activity cause somnolence or other side effects at rest in the absence of pain. Although most patients with persistent pain ultimately will take a variety of drugs, one has to be sanguine about their efficacy and long-term benefit. For most the effects will be minimal and the side effects problematic.

Stimulation Analgesia

Techniques such as transcutaneous electrical nerve stimulation (8) or acupuncture (17) are used frequently in pain clinics. Although there is no doubt that they do produce genuine analgesic effects in certain circumstances, they are of little benefit in spinal stenosis, except when specific radicular pain is accompanied by general back ache.

NERVE BLOCKS AND INJECTIONS
General Mechanisms

The exact mechanisms of pain generation in disc herniation and spinal stenosis are far from clear. Although it may seem self-evident that pressure on a nerve will cause pain, this is not a universal finding when this situation arises clinically. Pain-free motor weakness can be the presenting feature of herniated disc, and similar effects can occur after nerve compression in other anatomic locations. It is likely that pain arises in the acute phase not only by partial compression of the nerve, but also by inflammation and irritation. Pressure on a nerve produces an inflammatory response, which may cause secondary swelling.

In the longer term, chronic damage to the nerve may produce neuropathic pain. Initially the compression of the nerve will cause alterations in blood supply, which may have the effect of modifying the transmission of neurotransmitters and trophic substances such as nerve growth factor. These changes will not only alter the function of receptors within the dorsal horn of the spinal cord (particularly the NMDA receptor), but they also will trigger the expression of genes in the same area, which will bring about longer-term changes to the neurochemistry of the pain processing system (13). Once peripheral nerve damage has occurred, these changes can become permanent and lead to the intrusion of persistent neuropathic pain. This pain, characterized by a constant unpleasant burning sensation, is not activity-dependent (although it may be worsened by exercise) and is very difficult to treat.

In the shorter term, there is a rationale for the use of an epidural or foraminal injection of local anesthetic and steroid. Potential pain-relieving mechanisms will include the following:

1. Degenerative processes in the disc and zygapophyseal joint may produce irritant substances that contribute to inflammation and pain. Injection of a large volume of dilute solution may wash out these irritants and relieve pain.
2. Inflamed nerve roots may be swollen and worsen the effects of a narrow canal and foramen. Steroids, with their powerful antiinflammatory effects, may reduce the inflammation and thus the swelling, which in turn will reduce the compression and, hopefully, the symptoms.
3. Steroids themselves may have a long-term blocking effect on small pain nerve fibers (7).
4. Local anesthetic, by producing an absence of any neural activity for a period of time, may have an effect on reducing the hypersensitivity of the system. Although this idea of producing a long-term benefit from a short-term nerve block has not been clearly

demonstrated in controlled studies, many experienced clinicians can testify to occasions when it has been of value.

TECHNIQUE

Epidural Block

Lumbar epidural block is carried out at the level of the stenosis or one space above or below (3). Care must be taken when previous surgery has been carried out, because the ligamentum flavum will be deficient, which makes the block technically difficult. It must be acknowledged that whenever there is a compressive lesion in the spinal canal, the path of least resistance for an injected drug will not necessarily be to the damaged area. Thus, the drug may not get to the affected part; it will tend to spread up and down the epidural space to less compressed segments.

The block can be satisfactorily carried out as an outpatient procedure, without using sedation. In general, a single dose of local anesthetic and steroid is administered. A great variety of volumes and agents have been used, and there are vigorous protagonists for differing regimes. The large-volume school believes that the use of a greater volume can ensure that some of the drug does get to the affected segment. Others believe that a small volume delivered precisely to the problem area may be more effective. In general, this will entail an x-ray-guided procedure.

Caudal block is favored by some, especially for problems at the lumbosacral junction. This technique requires a high volume.

Blocks can be repeated if they are of benefit or if they are thought to be technically deficient. With repeat injections the dose of steroid must be monitored closely.

Paravertebral or Foraminal Block

If the stenosis is lateral and largely affects a single nerve root, either clinically or radiographically a local injection can be administered outside the spinal canal using x-ray guidance (22). A 22-gauge needle is inserted 5 to 6 cm from the midline toward the intervertebral foramen. Contrast medium can be injected to ascertain the spread of the injectate. This technique can be of value when the symptoms are localized to one limb or part of a limb, and it is of good anecdotal efficacy in this situation.

Efficacy of Epidural Blocks in Spinal Pain

A large number of studies have investigated the efficacy of epidural blocks in the treatment of spinal disorders, most usually disc prolapse. There is a body of literature relating to spinal stenosis specifically, but this area is less well investigated. Because of the overlap of pathology, symptomatology, and therapy, there is merit in examining the broader literature in the first instance.

It should be clearly stated at the start, however, that although the literature is extensive, much of it is of poor quality. Many of the more pertinent and specific questions are far from being answered. Three areas relating to such studies require control if meaningful data are to be produced (Table 2).

Efficacy of Epidural Steroids for Back Pain and Sciatica

Apart from numerous specific studies, there has been one recent systematic review and one meta-analysis of the benefits of lumbar epidural steroids. In a systematic review, Koes

TABLE 2. *Factors requiring control in studies of epidural steroids*

Trial design
   Randomization
   Controls, placebo
   Blinding
Patient-related factors
   Age, sex,
   Diagnosis, levels affected
   Symptomatology, duration,
   Concomitant disease or illness
Treatment
   Type of drug, carrier (local anesthetic)
   Volume of injectate
   Number of injections, times of repeats
   Certainty of accurate delivery of injectate
Assessment and follow-up
   Nature and number of measures used
      Pain
      Function
      Drug use
      Quality of life
   Time of follow-up, long-term outcome
   Other treatments

et al. (9) examined the efficacy of epidural steroid injections for low back pain. Twelve randomized studies were identified; only four scored more than 60 points on methodologic assessment. Of these four studies, two reported positive benefit and two reported negative benefit. This pattern was repeated for all 12 studies; half indicated the treatment was more effective than the reference condition, and half reported it was no better or worse. The authors concluded that there were flaws in the designs of most studies and that the efficacy of epidural steroid injection has not yet been established.

Watts and Silagy (24) undertook a meta-analysis to assess the benefit of epidural corticosteroids for the treatment of sciatica. They identified 11 trials that included 907 patients. Their analysis showed that the use of epidural steroids increased the odds ratio of short-term pain relief (more than 75%) to 2.61 (95% confidence interval 1.9 to 3.77). For longer-term relief (up to 1 year), the odds ratio fell to 1.87 (95% confidence interval 1.31 to 2.68). Their conclusion was that the epidural administration of corticosteroids is effective in the management of lumbosacral radicular pain.

It should be noted that these two studies adopt different methodologies and examine different aspects of outcome. It has long been clinical wisdom that epidural injections are more effective for radicular or limb pain than for back pain, and this picture emerges from these meta-analyses. Both studies also demonstrate the lack of serious side effects with no long-term adverse consequences.

Specific Studies in Spinal Stenosis

There have been a number of studies of the use of epidural corticosteroids in spinal stenosis. Rivest et al. (14) undertook a prospective trial of epidural injection of corticosteroid in 212 patients with either lumbar spinal stenosis or herniated disc. In general, the spinal stenosis group fared less well than the herniated disc group, with 38% of patients reporting short-term improvement. The authors concluded that more studies were needed.

Cuckler et al. (4) performed a randomized double-blind study of administration of 80 mg of methylprednisolone in 73 patients with radiographically confirmed nerve root compression. The authors failed to detect any benefit from adding the dose of steroid to the control group's injection of procaine alone. They found no long-term benefit from performing a second injection in those who had not responded to the first injection. The conclusion was that the technique was of unproven value.

Ciocon et al. (2), in a study of caudal epidural blocks in elderly patients with lumbar canal stenosis, entered 30 patients in an open uncontrolled protocol. All patients received 80 mg of methylprednisolone via the caudal route on three occasions. The authors reported worthwhile pain relief, from a mean score of 3.43 to 1.5 for up to 10 months after the injection. They concluded that caudal injection is safe, simple, and effective in elderly patients. A similar study was carried out by Rosen et al. (15). Forty patients (mean age 55 years) were given a variable number of epidural injections of 80 mg of depomedrone. Overall the authors thought the results were disappointing, with 40% of patients reporting no change from the procedures. Thirty-five percent had varying degrees of benefit, with 24% remaining asymptomatic in the longer term.

Rydevik et al. (16), in a review article on use of epidural steroids for patients with spinal stenosis, concluded that most studies do not support the use of epidural steroids, and they highlighted the potential complications. The authors go on to say, however, that epidural steroids can be considered as an alternative to surgery in elderly patients.

Finally, Fukasaki et al. (6) carried out a randomized study in 53 patients with degenerative lumbar spinal stenosis. The patients were divided into three groups that received saline, mepivacaine, or mepivacaine and 40 mg of methylprednisolone. Although there were some short-term gains in the steroid group when compared to the other groups, these benefits were not detected at 3 months. The authors concluded that there was no beneficial effect of adding steroid to the local anesthetic injection. It should be noted, however, that the protocol used a much smaller dose of steroid than that used by other workers.

CONCLUSION

Conclusive evidence from quality studies of an unequivocal benefit from epidural steroids in spinal stenosis is lacking. Given the likely mechanisms for pain generation in this condition, it is unlikely that local application of steroids or any other agent would have a specific long-term benefit. This is not the same, however, as saying that there is no place for the technique. Epidural or foraminal application of steroid can produce worthwhile relief of pain, which is a valid goal in its own right. This technique is often a valuable alternative to surgery, especially in the elderly, as there are few alternatives. It is a simple day-case procedure and has a very low risk of adverse events. The use of epidurals and nerve root blocks should be part of the armamentarium of any specialist center treating this condition.

Psychological Approaches

Patients with complex and long-standing pain problems often need psychological assessment, treatment, and ongoing support. In those cases best described by the term chronic pain syndrome, where distress is high due to long-standing psychological issues such as anxiety and depression, cognitive behavioral treatment has been shown to be effective in improving quality of life (18). Treatment usually is delivered in the form of a fixed-length interdisciplinary pain management program that incorporates a number of treatment modalities, including stretch and exercise. No specific studies have examined the outcome of such treatment in spinal stenosis.

Invasive Implantation Technologies

For individuals suffering severe and uncontrollable pain, there are options for more invasive pain management techniques that involve either implantation of long-term opioid delivery systems (25) or dorsal column stimulators (20). The former techniques can provide higher levels of pain control (21), but they are not risk free and require high levels of ongoing care. The place for their use in spinal stenosis would be limited to severe constant pain that is unrelieved by oral opioids. Application of dorsal column stimulators is best confined to pain of predominantly neuropathic origin. In cases such as failed multiple surgery, their use can improve pain control, although functional improvement does not necessarily follow.

REFERENCES

1. Burton AK, Tillotson M, Main CJ, Hollis S. Psychosocial predictors of outcome in acute and sub-chronic low back trouble. *Spine* 1995;20:722–728.
2. Ciocon JO, Galindo-Ciocon D, Amaranath L, Galindo D. Caudal epidural blocks for elderly patients with lumbar canal stenosis. *J Am Geriatr Soc* 1994;42:593–596.
3. Cousins MJ, Bridenbaugh PO. *Neural blockade in clinical anaesthesia and pain management*, 3rd ed. Philadelphia: Lippincott Raven, 1998:243.
4. Cuckler JM, Bernini PA, Wiesel SW, Booth RE Jr, Rothman RH, Pickens GT. The use of epidural steroids in the treatment of lumbar radicular pain. A prospective, randomized, double-blind study. *J Bone Joint Surg Am* 1985;67:63–66.
5. Deyo RA. Drug therapy for back pain. Which drugs help which patients? *Spine* 1996;21:2840–2899.
6. Fukasaki M, Kobayashi I, Hara T, Sumikawa K. Symptoms of spinal stenosis do not improve after epidural steroid injection. *Clin J Pain* 1998;14:148–151.
7. Johansson A, Hao J, Sjolund B. Local corticosteroid application blocks transmission in normal nociceptive C-fibres. *Acta Anaesthesiol Scand* 1990;34:335–338.
8. Johnson K. Transcutaneous nerve stimulation. In: Raj PP, ed. *The practical management of pain.* Chicago: Year-Book Medical Publishers, 1986.
9. Koes BW, Scholten RJ, Mens JM, Bouter LM. Efficacy of epidural steroid injections for low-back pain and sciatica: a systematic review of randomized clinical trials. *Pain* 1995;63:279–288.
10. McQuay HJ, Tramer M, Nye BA, Carroll D, Wiffen PJ, Moore RA. A systematic review of antidepressants in chronic pain. *Pain* 1996;68:217–227.
11. Omarker K, Myers RR. Pathogenesis of sciatic pain: role of herniated nucleus pulposus and deformation of spinal nerve root and dorsal root ganglion. *Pain* 1998;78:99–105.
12. Pinski JJ. Chronic intractable benign pain: a syndrome and its treatment with intensive short term group psychotherapy. *J Human Stress* 1978;4:17–21.
13. Price DD, Mao J, Mayer DJ. Central consequences of persistent pain states. In: Jensen TS, Turner JA, Weisenfeld-Hallin Z, eds. *Proceedings of 8th World Congress of Pain.* Seattle: IASP Press, 1997.
14. Rivest C, Katz JN, Ferrante FM, Jamison RN. Effects of epidural steroid injection on pain due to lumbar spinal stenosis or herniated disks: a prospective study. *Arthritis Care Res* 1998;11:291–297.
15. Rosen CD, Kahanovitz N, Bernstein R, Viola K. A retrospective analysis of the efficacy of epidural steroid injections. *Clin Orthop* 1988;228:270–272.
16. Rydevik BL, Cohen DB, Kostuik JP. Spine epidural steroids for patients with lumbar spinal stenosis. *Spine* 1997;22:2313–2317.
17. ter Reit G, Kleijnen J, Knipschild P. Acupuncture and chronic pain: a criteria based meta-analysis. *J Clin Epidemiol* 1990;43:1191–-1199.
18. Turk DC. Efficacy of multidisciplinary pain centres in the treatment of chronic pain. In: Cohen MJM, Campbell JN, eds. *Pain treatment centres at a crossroads. Progress in pain research and management,* volume 7. Seattle: IASP Press, 1996.
19. Turk DC, et al. Assessment of chronic pain patients. *Semin Neurol* 1994;14:206–212.
20. Turner JA, Loeser JD, Bell KB. Spinal cord stimulation for chronic low back pain: a systematic literature synthesis. *Neurosurgery* 1995;37:1088–1089.
21. Van de Kelft E, De la Porte C. Long term pain relief during spinal cord stimulation. The effect of patient selection. *Qual Life Res* 1994;3:21–27.
22. Waldeman SD. *Atlas of interventional pain management.* Philadelphia: WB Saunders, 1998:297.
23. Wall PD. Inflammatory and neurogenic pain. *Br J Anaesth* 1995;75:123–124.
24. Watts RW, Silagy CA. A meta-analysis on the efficacy of epidural corticosteroids in the treatment of sciatica. *Anaesth Intens Care* 1995;23:564–569.
25. Yoshida GM, Nelson RW, Capen DA, et al. Evaluation of continuous intraspinal narcotic analgesia for chronic pain from benign causes. *Am J Orthop* 1996;25:693–694.

Lumbar Spinal Stenosis
edited by Robert Gunzburg and Marek Szpalski
Lippincott Williams & Wilkins, Philadelphia, © 2000.

22

Spinal Cord Stimulation

Jean Pierre Van Buyten

Department of Anesthesia and Pain Management, Maria Middelares Hospital, G100 Sint-Niklaas, Belgium

Spinal cord stimulation (SCS) has been used as a more invasive method for relief of chronic pain for more than 30 years. It was Shealy et al. (12) who first implanted in 1967 an epidural electrode for electrical stimulation of the dorsal columns of the spinal cord (spinothalamic tract). The mechanism of action has not yet been elucidated, but the clinical results are considered a validation of the gate control theory of Melzack and Wall (5). Other possible mechanisms have not been proven. Spinal cord stimulation does not increase endorphins in the cerebrospinal fluid, nor is the SCS-induced analgesia reversed by naloxone. Inhibition at supraspinal levels and activation of central inhibitory mechanisms that influence sympathetic efferent neurons are other possible mechanisms.

Patients must be selected carefully for SCS by a multidisciplinary team. Examination should include psychological assessment, and all other conservative therapies must have failed. In the algorithm of pain treatment, in our center we place SCS before the use of major opioids, even those administered orally, if SCS is theoretically indicated because of the lack of side effects.

The main indication group for SCS is patients suffering from neuropathic pain. Sympathetically maintained pain is known to respond to SCS, whereas nociceptive pain responds to a lesser degree. Ischemic pain due to peripheral vascular disease or angina also is known to respond very well to SCS.

In daily practice and with growing experience and expertise, we can select some diagnostic categories that are likely to respond to SCS.

The most frequent indication in our practice is the so-called failed back treatment syndrome. Of 254 patients implanted in the last 10 years in our department, 78% were suffering from failed back treatment syndrome. Only 17% did not respond sufficiently to a trial stimulation of at least 1 month. These patients are suffering from lumbosacral fibrosis and/or arachnoiditis following multiple back operations. In these patients, the radicular pain is treated more effectively than the axial low back pain. Nevertheless, we recently reported good results on ''nociceptive'' low back pain using dual stimulation with two implanted epidural electrodes placed mostly parallel to each other (Van Buyten et al., in preparation).

Other neuropathic and deafferentation pain syndromes also respond very well:

1. Peripheral nerve and root lesions: posttraumatic neuropathy [peripheral nerve lesion, complex regional pain syndrome (CRPS), or sympathetically maintained pain (SMP), postamputation pain, plexopathies: posttraumatic, after irradiation, or due to malignancy), rhizopathy (postherpetic neuralgia)

2. Spinal cord lesions: pain after spinal cord injury, postcordotomy dysesthesia, multiple sclerosis
3. Pain due to peripheral vascular disease (7).

The outcome of SCS became better due to improvement of the expertise of the physicians and the reliability of the hardware. De La Porte and Siegfried (3) reported a 60% success rate after 4-year follow-up in failed back treatment patients.

The 5-year follow-up study by North et al. (11) on failed back surgery syndrome patients reported a success rate of 53% at 2.2 years and 47% at 5 years. Success was defined as at least 50% pain reduction and significant improvement in quality-of-life parameters. Kupers and Van den Oever (4) published an interesting study that involved Belgian health authorities. They undertook a multicenter retrospective study of nearly 700 patients, all of whom were screened by an independent third party. Fifty-two percent of the patients reported very good to good pain relief at 3.5-year follow-up. Only resumption of professional activities was disappointing (4).

Finally, North et al. (10) undertook a prospective randomized study that compared SCS with reoperation in failed back surgery syndrome patients who were candidates for reoperation. Sixty-seven percent of the patients undergoing reoperation crossed over to SCS, whereas only 17% of the patients treated with SCS crossed over to reoperation after 6 months of follow-up.

In our retrospective study (in preparation) with a mean follow-up of 3.6 years, 68% of our patients judged their therapy to be excellent, very good, or good, which is a very good result in the treatment of chronic benign pain patients. With 78% of failed back treatment syndrome patients, this indicates SCS is a good therapy for patients who underwent back surgery without good results.

The key to success of SCS (and all other invasive pain management techniques) is careful psychological assessment by a psychologist accustomed to dealing with chronic pain patients. In the Belgian study, Kupers and Van den Oever (4) reported that 36% of the patients screened were not implanted due to psychiatric contraindications. In the group with positive psychiatric advice, the success rate was 64%, whereas in the group with "some reservations" the success rate was only 18%.

Implantation can be done percutaneously using modified Tuohy needles and placing quadripolar or octapolar electrodes (one or two in dual stimulation) in the posterior epidural space. Some neurosurgeons prefer to perform a laminotomy under local anesthesia to place "resume" electrodes. No studies have proved the advantage of one technique or the other. The experience of the physician will be essential for determining the technical success rate. The most important technical goal is to provoke paresthesias with a somatotopy corresponding exactly with the somatotopy of the pain.

After implantation there should be a trial stimulation long enough for the patient to be able to judge the effect of SCS on the pain, in the patient's own environment while doing daily-life activities. After a screening period (in our country, 1 month with at least 3 weeks at home), most centers will proceed to surgical implantation of an internalized SCS if more than 50% pain reduction has been obtained.

In conclusion, SCS is a save, reversible, nondestructive therapy for treatment of chronic essentially neuropathic pain or SMP. It should be performed in patients who have been carefully selected based on physical and psychological factors. This technique has proved to be superior to all other therapies for treatment of failed back surgery syndrome.

COST EFFICACY OF SPINAL CORD STIMULATION

Although there is no doubt about the efficacy of SCS for neuropathic pain syndromes, there is still controversy regarding the cost efficacy of this therapy, especially in the long run, when the longevity of battery life, for example, will be extremely important.

A study performed by ECRI (a nonprofit agency for health technology assessment information service) in 1993 compared 100 failed back surgery syndrome patients treated with SCS to 100 failed back surgery syndrome patients treated with alternative therapies for 5-year follow-up. Spinal cord stimulation appears to be cost effective when compared to drug therapies with low efficacy and compared to repetitive surgery, with an efficacy of less than 80%.

In other studies, SCS appears to be cost effective compared to alternative therapies that cost more than $20,000 per year and have less than 78% efficacy. Examples include random care seeking patients: $20,814 per year; sympathetic bloc patients: $20,377 per year; and repeat laminectomy: $31,584 per year.

Another study from the Charles River Association (8) compared SCS to a chronic maintenance regime and found that cost savings using SCS could range from $8,000 in 5 years to more than $100,000 in 20 years.

A study at Johns Hopkins by Bell et al. (2) found that SCS pays for itself within 2.1 to 5.5 years, depending on the rate of clinical efficacy of the therapy.

The studies available are based on American data. There are no European studies. Considering these studies we need to allow for the different social security systems in those two parts of the world. In the United States, fees and hospitalization costs are significantly higher than in Europe; the cost of the hardware is the same. This makes it difficult to convince the European health authorities because the ratio of cost effectiveness is less in favor of SCS compared to alternative therapies in our countries.

No value can be placed on pain relief or improvement of quality of life. Most of the studies prove there is no significant positive effect of the therapy on the employment status of the patients.

If we consider the literature on outcome of SCS compared to alternative therapies, we see that the results are mostly better for SCS. Hardware performance (battery life, rechargeable batteries) must improve for costs to be lowered. The overall clinical outcome is slightly better, use of medication is less, quality of life parameters are better with SCS, and cost effectiveness is in favor of SCS (9).

We are still waiting for prospective studies that compare the same pain etiology with different pain treatments and exactly the same study design.

Almost as important as the technique itself is the environment in which those techniques are used. To lower costs and maximize cost efficacy of neuromodulation techniques, screening, surgical technique, and follow-up have to be performed in at least a "center of excellence" associated with a high volume of those procedures and with disease management programs. The large volume of work performed in such a center of excellence, the harmony and fluidity achieved by its team members, and the attention paid to improving the operational processes result in continual process refinements, quality improvements, and cost reduction (6).

REFERENCES

1. Bedder MD. The anesthesiologist's role in neuroaugmentative pain control techniques: spinal cord stimulation and neuraxial narcotics. *Prog Anesthesiol* 1990;4:226–236.
2. Bell GK, Kidd D, North R. *Cost-effective analysis of SCS in treatment of failed back surgery.* Charles River Association Inc., and John Hopkins, Baltimore.

3. De La Porte C, Siegfried J. Lumbosacral spinal fibrosis (spinal arachnoiditis): its diagnosis and treatment by spinal cord stimulation. *Spine* 1983;8:593–603.
4. Kupers RC, Van den Oever R. Spinal cord stimulation in Belgium: a nation-wide survey on the incidence, indications and therapeutic efficacy by the health insurer. *Pain* 1994;56:211–216.
5. Melzack R, Wall PD. Pain mechanisms: a new theory. *Science* 1965;150:971–978.
6. Herzlinger R. *Market driven health care.* Cambridge, MA: Harvard Business School.
7. Meyerson B, Linderoth B, Lind B. Spinal cord stimulation in chronic neuropathic pain. *Lakartidningen* 1991; 88:727–732.
8. Neels, Banks. *Cost-effective study of SCS treatment of FBS.* Charles River Association.
9. North R, et al. Spinal cord stimulation for chronic intractable pain experience over two decades. *Neurosurgery* 1993;32:384–395.
10. North R, Kidd DH. A prospective randomized study of spinal cord stimulation vs. reoperation for failed back surgery syndrome: initial results. *Stereotact Funct Neurosurg* 1994;62:267–272.
11. North RB, Matthew GE, Lawton MT, et al. Failed back surgery syndrome: 5 years follow-up after spinal cord stimulator implantation. *Neurosurgery* 1991;28:692–699.
12. Shealy CN, Mortimer TJ, Reswick JB. Electrical inhibition of pain by stimulation of the dorsal column. *Anesth Analg* 1967;46:489–491.

SECTION VI

Surgical Treatment Modalities

Lumbar Spinal Stenosis
edited by Robert Gunzburg and Marek Szpalski
Lippincott Williams & Wilkins, Philadelphia, © 2000.

23

Total Laminectomy

Jose A. Fernandez de Valderrama

General Rodrigo 17, 28003 Madrid, Spain

Previous lectures have reported that, in lumbar stenosis, narrowing of the spinal canal—whether central, lateral, or combined; developmental, degenerative, or iatrogenic—produces a variable degree of entrapment of nerves and vessels. This causes back and leg pain, muscle weakness, sensory and reflex changes, and a variable degree of sphincter and sexual disturbances.

When the symptoms, whether acute or progressive, correlate with radiographic abnormalities and do not respond to conservative treatment, the logical option is surgical decompression to remove pressure from the constricted neural elements within the central spinal canal or the spinal nerve canals while trying not to compromise vertebral stability.

The primary aim of decompression should be the relief of leg pain and neurogenic intermittent claudication, and not the treatment of low back pain.

Total laminectomy at one or various levels, with partial or total facetectomy, has been the classic approach used to achieve a thorough decompression of the spinal canal.

In the last decade, new advances in diagnostic imaging techniques have allowed better localization of the offending areas of neural compression. More conservative surgical approaches have been recommended with hemilaminectomies, partial laminotomies, and even multilevel interlaminar decompression to avoid postoperative instability. These usually are used in selective patients with predominantly lateral stenosis.

In central canal stenosis and mixed centrolateral stenosis, as in the trefoil-shaped central canal, wide decompression by total laminectomy with facet joint sparing technique is a relatively safe operation that has high success in the medium to long term (Fig. 1).

Age is not a limitation for this type of surgery, although comorbidity (diabetes mellitus, hip osteoarthritis, cardiovascular and pulmonary disease) contribute to poor outcome.

The patient's quality of life remains the key determinant in deciding the consideration of surgical decompression. The patient must be well informed of the operative risks and the possibility of complications. This is especially important for those in the elder age group, in which patients should not be overly optimistic about the outcome and should understand clearly that surgery may not relieve all their symptoms and that there is some possibility of an unsatisfactory result.

After elective surgical decompression has been chosen, a thorough preoperative assessment should be undertaken. Good imaging evaluation is mandatory.

The extent of surgical decompression should be planned preoperatively according to radiographs, magnetic resonance imaging, or computed tomography, but it may be modified subsequently in accordance with the surgical findings. Preoperative instability should be evaluated as well as possible by standing and flexion extension radiographs.

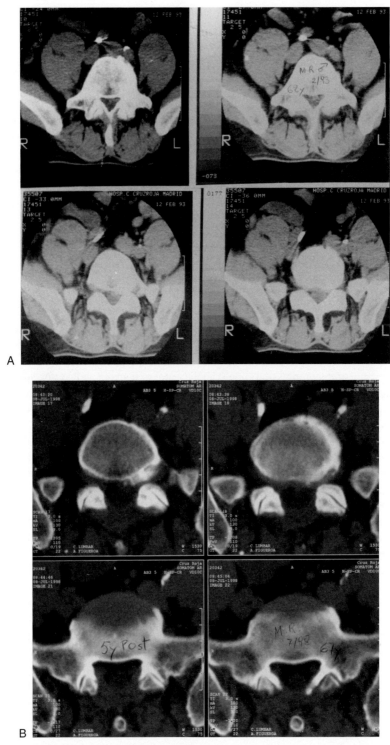

FIG. 1. A: Preoperative computed tomography of a 62-year-old man. There is severe L5–S1 degenerative stenosis. **B:** Computed tomography 5 years after total laminectomy and partial facetectomy. There is minimal bone regrowth.

SURGICAL TECHNIQUE: IMPORTANT POINTS

Proper positioning of the patient to avoid abdominal pressure will minimize blood loss during operation.

If there is no contraindication due to hip or knee osteoarthritis, the kneeling position is preferred, as it allows the abdomen to hang free, decreases lumbar lordosis, and releases tension of the distal nerve roots.

In special circumstances, as with patients who are obese or who have respiratory problems, the lateral position with a pad between the flexed knees and a pelvic restraining strap may be chosen.

Magnification with a loop and use of a fiberoptic head light afford better visualization of neural and vascular structures. Bipolar coagulation is desirable.

The appropriate level should be marked carefully and checked against the patient's x-ray films for anatomic marks or anomalies that can be easily identified. If in doubt, the appropriate level should be checked by radiograph or image intensifier. We must remember that surgical failure can occur by performing the right operation at the wrong vertebral level.

The paraspinous ligament often can be preserved to increase posterior stability. Careful segmental paraspinal muscle separation may decrease blood loss with good exposure of the posterior arch. In developmental stenosis, the laminae may be thicker and shorter than normal, whereas in degenerative stenosis the osteophytes and overgrowth of the posterior facets may give the laminae a shorter appearance. Overlapping of the laminae may make access to the spinal canal more difficult. When excising the ligamentum flavum, we may find that its consistency varies between normal elasticity and partial ossification (Fig. 2B).

In developmental stenosis, the convex laminae may produce considerable narrowing of the central canal, which carries a great risk of neural damage during surgical decompression (18). In degenerative stenosis, constriction of the central portion of the canal is produced by osteophytes and overgrowth of the inferior facet of the cephalad vertebra. Degenerative changes of the superior facet of the caudal vertebra produce narrowing of the lateral recess and the foramen.

Excision of the medial half of the facets often gives good decompression of the central and lateral recess, which allows dural reexpansion and good mobilization of the compressed root; however, complete decompression is the main object of the surgical procedure and total facetectomy should be done if it is needed. For adequate decompression, all stenosed levels must be decompressed.

As Verbiest (18) points out, with mixed stenosis there is a question of whether a part of the canal showing relative stenosis in the absence of an additional compressive agent should be decompressed prophylactically. With pure relative stenosis, the problem is how far to extend decompression beyond the level of any additional compressive agent. Bulging discs should be left undisturbed, and disc protrusions inside an area of stenosis should never be removed without previous posterior decompression. In developmental stenosis, it is a surgical dilemma whether the decompressive laminectomy should be performed over the entire area to avoid recurrence of symptoms of stenosis at other nondecompressed levels.

Any dural laceration should be repaired carefully. Safe and accurate interoperative and postoperative bleeding control is mandatory. The exposed dura should be covered by a free or pedicle fat graft, Gelfoam, or other synthetic membranes or products to isolate it from the paraspinal musculature to decrease epidural scarring.

The dorsolumbar fascia should be sutured carefully to the paraspinous ligament to maintain lordosis and to increase posterior stability. A suction drain may be placed over the fascia, but never proximal to the exposed dura.

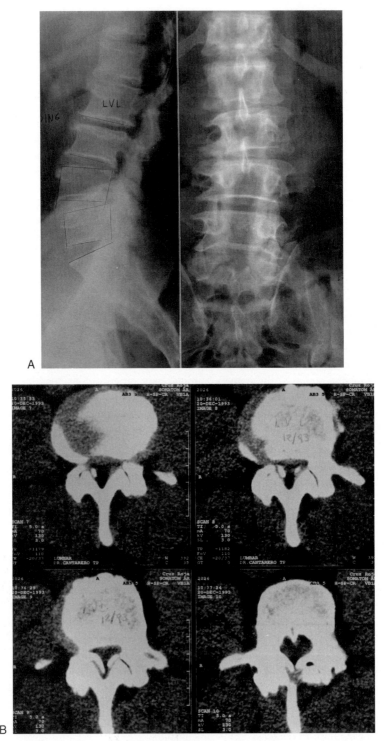

FIG. 2. A: Lateral preoperative and anteroposterior x-ray films 1 year after L3 and L4 total laminectomy in a 53-year-old man. **B:** Preoperative computed tomography. There is ossification of the ligamentum flavium. *(Figure continues.)*

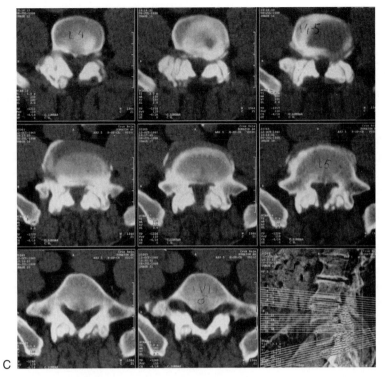

C

FIG. 2. *Continued* **C:** Computed tomography 5 years after laminectomy. There is slight bone regrowth.

Extensive decompression increases the risk of instability of the correspondent vertebral level. Preoperative instability and postoperative hypermobility following decompression is an indication for concomitant arthrodesis of the decompressed segments. Discectomy and especially preoperative lumbar scoliosis are known to increase the risk of postoperative instability and may be indications for adjunctive fixation.

With spinal instability, the best chance to regain permanent stability is a solid instrumented posterolateral arthrodesis with pedicular screws and rods. Fusion indications and techniques will be discussed extensively in the following chapters.

The problem with fusion is that it considerably increases the operative time, blood loss, and morbidity of the surgical procedure, especially in elderly patients with degenerative stenosis. There is extensive agreement that the dangers of postoperative instability and vertebral slippage due to extensive, careful decompression are much less than the consequences of insufficient decompression of the neural structures in the stenosed lumbar spinal canal. Therefore, in the absence of obvious segmental instability in elderly patients, no fusion is necessary after decompression surgery (Fig. 2).

The risk of postoperative slipping is assumed to be low in older patients with advanced degenerative changes of the disc (3). The results of local decompression for sciatica and neurogenic claudication in the elderly are good, and fusion is not indicated in older patients with degenerative stenosis (14).

Neural compression at multiple levels is a relative contraindication to surgical decompression in the elderly. The results of surgery tend to be disappointing when two or more spinal levels are involved (10,14).

The presence of postoperative slipping and its influence on the outcome have been analyzed extensively in the literature. Johnsson et al. (5) found a 65% incidence of further slipping in spinal stenosis associated with degenerative spondylolisthesis and 20% in acquired spinal stenosis without previous olisthesis. There was a good clinical outcome in 80% of patients in the nonslipping group with degenerative stenosis, whereas none of those with vertebral slipping had subjective clinical improvement. This was in contrast with the group that had associated spondylolisthesis in which further increase in slipping did not result in a good clinical outcome (5).

Turner et al. (17) attempted meta-analysis of the literature on the surgical treatment of lumbar spinal stenosis. They selected 74 of 625 articles that met the inclusion selection criteria. They found important differences in patient samples, surgical procedures, and outcome assessments, with good-to-excellent outcome in 64% (range 26% to 100%) and conflicting findings with regard to predictors of outcome. They could not find a statistically significant relationship between outcome and patient age or gender, presence of pseudoclaudication, prior back surgery, number of levels decompressed, or associated fusion. The need to demonstrate empirically the indications for, and benefits of, fusion in spinal stenosis, especially in light of its increased morbidity, is emphasized. This was in contrast with studies on degenerative spondylolisthesis that reported better outcomes for associated fusions. Despite these problems, decompressive laminectomy for lumbar spinal stenosis appears to be beneficial for many patients in reducing pain and increasing activity. It probably is associated with an acceptably low rate of complications (17).

In another recent meta-analysis, Niggemayer et al. (9) found that the duration of preoperative symptoms had an important influence on the rates of success. Decompressive laminectomy had the best result for patients with degenerative stenosis if the duration of symptoms was less than 8 years; those with symptoms for 15 years or more did better with simultaneous instrumented fusion.

Three recent reports agree that there are little data available regarding the long-term outcome of laminectomy for lumbar stenosis and that short-term results may be misleadingly favorable.

Katz et al. (6) found in a group of patient with a mean age of 69 years (range 55 to 89) that the long-term outcome was less favorable than previously reported and that comorbidity and a single interspace laminectomy were risk factors for poor outcome. Seventeen percent had a repeat operation because of instability and stenosis, and 30% had severe pain 3 to 6 years after intervention.

Herno et al. (4) analyzed a younger group of patients (mean age 49 years in men and 52 years in women) and found that a recurrence of symptomatic degenerative stenosis in patients who had previous surgery requiring a second operation was low. Sixty-six percent of the patients 7 years after laminectomy and 69% 13 years after laminectomy fit the Oswestry index category of good to excellent, which suggests that outcome continued to improve significantly with time.

A more recent article from the same institution indicates that patients who had stenosis larger than 12 mm usually had lateral and not central stenosis and had a poorer outcome after surgical intervention. Patients who had a total block on the preoperative myelogram with central stenosis had the best Oswestry scores. No previous spinal surgery, absence of comorbidity such as diabetes, hip joint arthrosis, preoperative fracture of the lumbar spine, or postoperative complications had greater chances of achieving a good outcome after decompression of lumbar spinal stenosis (1).

Diabetes mellitus has been associated with a poor outcome in all cases of lumbar spine surgery. Simpson et al. (15) compared 62 patients with diabetes to 62 nondiabetics and found that there were high rates of postoperative wound complications and prolonged hospitalization among the diabetic patients. The poorer results may have been related to coexisting diabetic neuropathy or to the failure of the nerve roots to recover after decompressive procedures.

Spivak (16) states that, in his experience, relief of activity-related symptoms after decompression has been as reliable in patients who have diabetes as in those who do not. The relief of constant pain and abnormal sensations in the lower extremity has been less reliable in patients who have diabetes, presumably because of residual symptoms of underlying diabetic neuropathy.

Postacchini and Cinotti (11) reviewed 40 patients treated surgically for spinal stenosis, 5 to 19 years (mean 8) after operation, and evaluated bone regrowth after total laminectomy and bilateral laminotomy. Their findings indicate that regrowth of the posterior arch is stimulated by abnormal vertebral motion and represents an attempt to increase vertebral stability. Regrowth of posterior facet joints may deteriorate the quality of the results with increasing time from surgery, reproducing previous pathologic conditions. On the other hand, regrowth of the laminar arch does not cause significant compression, except in degenerative spondylolisthesis. The proportion of satisfactory clinical results progressively decreased from the group with mild bone regrowth to the group with marked regrowth. Regrowth was more likely to occur after a narrow laminectomy (Fig. 3) and if the operated vertebral level was unstable (12).

Chen et al. (2) also described varying degrees of bone regrowth in surgical laminar defects as a natural postoperative repair process, with increased association with instability and in levels adjacent to spinal fusion. This association was related with poor clinical outcome in the middle and late follow-up periods.

Current trends toward more limited operative decompression with retention of the stabilizing elements and a decrease in short-term morbidity may lead to a higher rate of long-term failure due to recurrent stenosis or the development of stenosis at an adjacent level (12,16).

Another more immediate consequence of connective tissue repair following laminectomy is epidural scarring and heterotopic bone formation.

Peridural fibrosis is a natural consequence of laminectomy and surgical invasion of the spinal canal. The extent of fibrosis depends primarily on the extent of the surgical procedure and the degree of hemostasis. Peridural fibrosis can be well visualized by magnetic resonance imaging with or without gadolinium enhancement.

Scar fixation of the dura and nerve roots interferes with normal physiologic movement of these structures within the spinal canal, leading to pain and limitation of activities and simulating spinal instability (''instability catch'').

Experimental studies of LaRocca and MacNab (8) and Langenskiold and Kiviluoto (7) showed that the principal source of the scar was from the erector spinae muscle mass, which was covering the dura and extending into the canal to adhere to the dura and nerve roots. They advocated covering the dura with Gelfoam (8) and free or pedicule fat transplants (7) to prevent epidural scar formation.

Other synthetic membranes have been used, including Silastic, Dacron, and Gelfoam impregnated with methylprednisolone (19), with inconsistent results. None of these synthetic membranes covers the nerve roots and ventral areas adequately (13).

Gliatec Inc. has developed a carbohydrate polymer gel that can act as a barrier to fibroblasts responsible for scar formation.

After successful experimentation in rabbits and rats, multicenter clinical studies have been conducted in Europe and the United States, and the results were discussed in symposiums conducted in Berlin (1995) and Amsterdam (1997).

The results at single discectomy levels are very promising. The gel reabsorbs completely

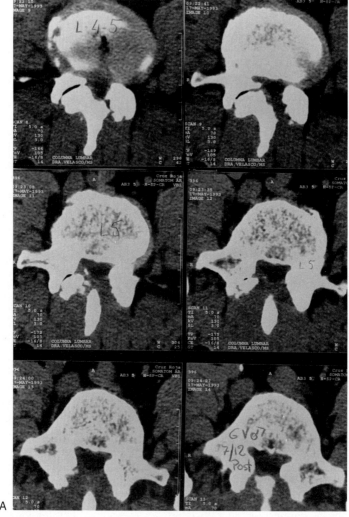

FIG. 3. A: Computed tomography 7 months after limited decompression in a 57-year-old man. There is slight bone regrowth. *(Figure continues.)*

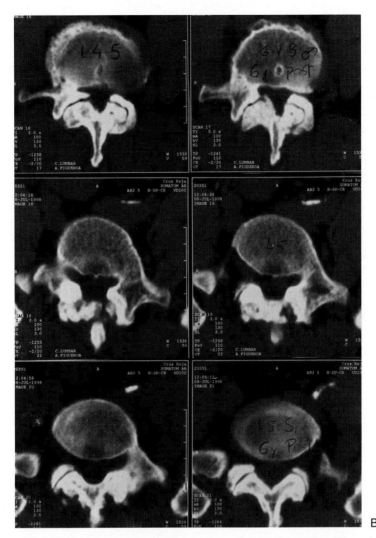

B

FIG. 3. *Continued* **B:** Computed tomography 6 years after laminotomies. There is extensive bone regrowth.

in 4 weeks without ill effects and does not appear to interfere with bone fusion. It is not clear if it interferes with healing of the annulus and dural tears, but it seems we are on the way to being able to decrease epidural scarring and perhaps bone regrowth, thus improving the outcome of spinal canal decompression procedures and avoiding or facilitating spinal reoperations.

REFERENCES

1. Airaksinen O, Herno A, Turunen V, Saari T, Suomlinen O. Surgical outcome of 438 patients treated surgically for lumbar spine stenosis. *Spine* 1996;22:2278–2282
2. Chen Q, Baba H, Kamitani K, Furusawa N, Imura S. Postoperative bone regrowth in lumbar stenosis. *Spine* 1994;19:2144–2149.
3. Grabias S. The treatment of spinal stenosis. Current concepts review. *J Bone Joint Surg* 1980;62A:308–313.
4. Herno A, Airaksinen O, Saari T. Long term results of surgical treatment of lumbar spinal stenosis. *Spine* 1993; 18:1471–1474.
5. Johnsson KE, Willner S, Johnsson K. Postoperative instability after decompression for lumbar spinal stenosis. *Spine* 1986;17:1–8.
6. Katz JN, Lipson SJ, Larson MG, McInnes JM, Fossel AH, Liang MH. The outcome of decompressive laminectomy for degenerative lumbar stenosis. *J Bone Joint Surg* 1991;73A:809–816.
7. Langenskiold A, Kiviluoto O. Prevention of epidural scar formation after operations on the lumbar spine by means of free fat transplants. *Clin Orthop* 1976;115:92–95.
8. LaRocca H, MacNab I. The laminectomy membrane: studies on its evolution, characteristics, effects and prophylaxis in dogs. *J Bone Joint Surg* 1974;56B:545–550.
9. Niggemayer O, Strauss JM, Schulitz KP. Comparison of surgical procedures for degenerative lumbar spinal stenosis: a meta-analysis of the literature from 1975 to 1995. *Eur Spine J* 1997;6:423–429.
10. Paine KWE. Results of decompression for lumbar spinal stenosis. *Clin Orthop* 1976;115:96–110.
11. Postacchini F, Cinotti G. Bone regrowth after surgical decompression for lumbar spinal stenosis. *J Bone Joint Surg* 1992;74B:862–869.
12. Postacchini F, Cinotti G, Perugia D, Gumina S. Multiple laminotomy compared with total laminectomy. *J Bone Joint Surg* 1993;75B:386–392.
13. Robertson JT. Role of peridural fibrosis in the failed lack. A review . *Eur Spine J* 1996;5[Suppl 1]:2–6.
14. Sanderson PL, Wood PLR. Surgery for lumbar spinal stenosis in old people. *J Bone Joint Surg* 1993;75B: 393–397.
15. Simpson JM, Silveri CP, Balderston RA, Simeone FA, An SH. The results of operations on the lumbar spine in patients who have diabetes mellitus. *J Bone Joint Surg* 1993;75A:1823–1829.
16. Spivak JM. Degenerative lumbar spinal stenosis. Current concepts Review. *J Bone Joint Surg* 1998;80A: 1055–1066.
17. Turner JA, Ersek M, Herron L, Deyo R. Surgery for lumbar spinal stenosis. Attempted meta-analysis of the literatures. *Spine* 1992;17:1–8.
18. Verbiest H. Results of surgical treatment of idiopathic developmental stenosis of the lumbar vertebral canal. A review of twenty seven years experience. *J Bone Joint Surg* 1977;59B:181–188.
19. Wiltse LL, Kirkaldy-Willis WH. The treatment of spinal stenosis. *Clin Orthop* 1976;115:83–91.

Lumbar Spinal Stenosis
edited by Robert Gunzburg and Marek Szpalski
Lippincott Williams & Wilkins, Philadelphia, © 2000.

24

Decompressions of the Sublaminar Central Canal, Bilateral Foramina, and Nerve Root Canals

Henry V. Crock and M. Carmel Crock

Spinal Disorders Unit, Cromwell Hospital, London W8 5JN, United Kingdom

In the literature dealing with the surgical treatment of lumbar canal stenosis, terms such as complete laminectomy, hemilaminectomy, laminotomy, and decompression of the spinal canal commonly are used. Authors rarely define the precise meanings of these various descriptive terms, nor do they provide detailed descriptions of the different techniques involved in their use. Each of these terms was used in a current concepts review on degenerative lumbar spinal canal stenosis (5), in which a distinction was drawn between wide laminectomy and other procedures designed to preserve more of the posterior osseous and ligamentous structures of the spinal canal, the latter aiming, theoretically, to diminish the problem of postoperative instability. The overriding impression that reasonably might be gained from reading this document is that, using techniques for laminectomy, decompression of the spinal canal is not very difficult, and that decompressing the canal while preserving the midline osseous and ligamentous structures is simply too time consuming.

This chapter focuses on the details of surgical techniques that will vary with the pathology encountered in different cases of spinal stenosis and on the anatomic principles that determine the safety and efficacy of the operations.

Comprehensive imaging studies should be available, including plain x-ray films of the lumbar spine, computed tomographic and magnetic resonance images, or computed tomographic radiculograms if magnetic resonance imaging is not available, and sometimes ultrasound pictures. Plain x-ray films are essential for identifying segmentation anomalies and other congenital defects such as spina bifida occulta, and to outline the bony anatomy of the spine in cases requiring operation following previous surgery. After analyzing these images, the surgeon should know whether the stenoses affect only the foramina and nerve root canals or whether the central canal also is involved. The choice of the most appropriate operation in individual cases will depend to a great extent on the interpretation of these various images but also, significantly, on the level of experience of the surgeon.

Despite the remarkable advances in the imaging techniques applied to the spine that have taken place in recent years, there is still a large gap between the pathologic changes in the spine found at operation and the radiologic interpretations of spinal imaging that traditionally focus on the dimensions of the spinal canal and common features of spondylosis. The major changes that may occur in the dimensions of the laminal arches and in their orientation in the coronal plane often lead to technical difficulties for the surgeon attempting to enter the spinal canal in the early stages of decompression. Laminal thickening up to 20 mm between the cortices is not uncommon, yet it is rarely noted in radiologic reports. The orientation of the laminal arches in the coronal plane may range from being parallel to the posterior dural surface to being almost at right angles to it.

SURGICAL TECHNIQUES

Laminectomy

Patients should be placed in the prone position, preferably with the arms by the sides and the abdomen suspended. The table should be adjusted to ensure adequate venous drainage of the head to prevent cerebral edema, which may lead to confusional states in elderly patients postoperatively.

If the spinal canal is critically narrowed, as shown in Fig. 1, decompression by excising the spinous process and central segment of the lamina is essential. In such a case, the lamina most safely is removed using a diamond-tipped high-speed drill, thinning the arch between the pars interarticularis on both sides until the anterior cortex of the lamina is eggshell thin and the ligamentum flavum has been exposed. The remnants of the lamina then can be separated from the underlying dural sac, using fine curettes or fine spatula-shaped instruments such as Kokubun's (Kokubun Instruments, Tokyo, Japan) straight or angled probes.

Lumbar Canal Decompressions with Preservation of Midline Structures of the Spine

The procedure should be considered in three phases. First, attention is focused on the paraspinal muscles and their normal anatomic relationships. The large triangle of the lumbo-dorsal aponeurosis consists of a very thin, shiny, silvery membrane that acts as the major extensor mechanism of the lumbar spine. It also encapsulates the paraspinal muscles, holding them alongside the spinous processes and laminae. Its criss-crossed fibers are largely orientated transversely in contrast to the underlying aponeurosis of the sacrospinalis muscle, which runs vertically. The lumbodorsal aponeurosis should be divided 5 mm on either side of the midline and the paraspinal muscles separated carefully using sharp scissors to sever the tendinous insertions into the spinous process and the muscular attachments along the margins of the laminae, until the muscle mass can be separated laterally and the shiny transversely

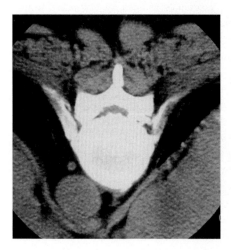

FIG. 1. Axial computed tomographic image at the thoracolumbar junction from a 45-year-old man. Spinal canal stenosis of this degree is treated most safely by excision of the midline structures of the roof of the canal.

orientated fibers of the facet joint capsules are exposed. The periosteum should be left intact on the spinous processes and laminae to reduce the risk of ectopic bone developing in the operative field at a later time. Self-retaining retractors then can be inserted. It is essential to note the times of their insertion, as these retractors act as tourniquets obstructing the blood flow in the muscles. They should be released at regular intervals of 35 to 40 minutes throughout the duration of the operation to allow revascularization of the paraspinal muscles and to prevent irreparable damage to them, which otherwise would result from prolonged retraction (2).

The normal anatomy of the interlaminar space is depicted in Fig. 2, which shows the capsular extension along the inferior margin of the superior lamina, the ligamentum flavum attachment to the undersurface of the upper lamina and to the inferior margin of the lower lamina, and the extrasynovial fat pad. This anatomy becomes grossly distorted in cases of spinal stenosis, as depicted in the lower section of the drawing. The facet joints have hypertrophied so that their inner margins lie near the midline and cover the underlying ligamentum flavum. The spinous processes abut each other and form a false joint, with gangliform tissues projecting laterally over the capsules of the facet joints. Arcuate ridges of osteophytic bone have developed around the inferior margins of the facet joints springing from the upper surface of the lower lamina.

The second phase of the operation involves opening the spinal canal. Whereas attention is drawn in the literature to changes in the facet joints particularly and to some extent to changes in the ligamentum flavum, the actual dimensions of the laminae themselves rarely are mentioned. Hypertrophy of the laminal margins can increase in depth from the normal 3 to 4 mm up to 20 mm, rendering this phase of the operation hazardous because of the possibility of dural injury, which can be inflicted when attempting to enter the spinal canal. A range of instruments should be available, including high-speed drills with diamond-tipped burrs, a sucker with a plastic tip to avoid damage from contact with the drill head, an irrigating

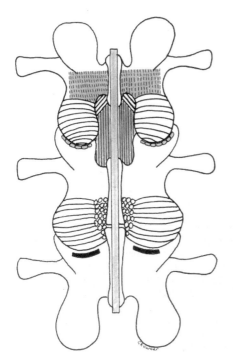

FIG. 2. Features of the normal anatomy of the roof of the lumbar canal between the upper two laminae contrasted with advanced pathologic changes often found in lumbar canal stenosis. The supraspinous and interspinous ligaments are represented in the midline. The ligamentum flavum is outlined with *parallel vertical lines.* Its upper attachment to the undersurface of the superior lamina is indicated with *dotted lines.* The transverse fibers of the facet joint capsules are shown with the capsular extensions extending along the inferior margins of the superior lamina. Extrasynovial fat pads are depicted around the inferior margins of the facet joint capsules. In the **lower section** of the drawing, the spinous processes have enlarged and abut against each other across the middle of the laminal interspace. The facet joints have enlarged enormously and obstruct view of the underlying ligamentum flavum. Gangliform tissues extending from the facet joints and the "kissing spines" cover the midline. The *black crescentic marks* adjacent to the inferior capsules of the facet joints indicate osteophytic outcrops from the upper surface of the inferior lamina.

system, long-handled angled rigid curettes with cup sizes varying between 2 and 4 mm, and fine spatula-shaped straight and angled probes. In addition, long fine osteotomes should be available, together with a range of straight and angled pituitary rongeurs with variable cup sizes.

The capsular extension is incised along the inferior margin of the upper lamina and removed. The bony margin is trimmed using the high-speed drill, from the midline along the inferior margin and medial border of the lamina, distally along the inner edge of the inferior facet until the underlying ligamentum flavum is exposed (Fig. 3). This can be accomplished with fine osteotomes or chisels (1), but better control is achieved using the high-speed drill with irrigation and suction under a well-focused light. Using this method, smooth bony margins can be achieved. The inferior margin of the upper lamina often can be trimmed further using angled curettes, starting in the midline and moving laterally, gaining some purchase against the side of the spinous process, but taking care to avoid fracturing it at its base. The instrument is used with a rotatory motion that shaves off fragments of the laminal bone until the upper attachment of the ligamentum flavum has been exposed adequately. These maneuvers are carried out on both sides of the interspace, with the surgeon moving from one side of the operating table to the other to complete the maneuvers. This is an extremely effective method of enlarging the laminar interspace, even after having commenced this phase of the operation using either osteotomes or a high-speed drill.

To complete the exposure of the ligamentum flavum, the thickened and sclerotic margins of the abutting spinous processes should be removed from beneath the interspinous ligament. Attention then is focused on the inferior lamina. The arcuate osteophytic outcrops are removed. When this lamina is thickened to between 15 and 20 mm, the high-speed drill should be used to thin the laminal margin and to penetrate it about 5 to 6 mm distal to its upper margin. The ligamentum flavum usually is grossly thickened, friable, and often calcified or ossified in cases of severe lumbar canal stenosis. It is frequently adherent to the dural sac,

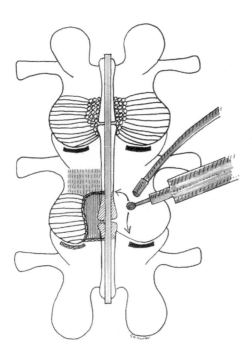

FIG. 3. Recommended method of exposing the interlaminar space in the early stages, after retraction of the paraspinal muscles. **Left:** the crescentic osteophytic bar beneath the facet joint capsule has been burred away, and the inferomedial margins of the lamina have been trimmed to expose the underlying ligamentum flavum. **Right:** position of the high-speed drill and sucker at commencement of the dissection to expose the underlying ligamentum flavum. The "kissing spines" are *cross hatched,* indicating their removal beneath the intact supraspinous and interspinous ligaments.

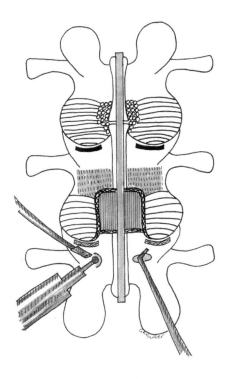

FIG. 4. Use of the high-speed drill to gain access to the spinal canal about 5 mm distal to the superior border of the inferior lamina, in cases where laminal hypertrophy is marked. **Right:** a thin spatula-shaped probe is passed into the canal to separate the underlying dural sac and epidural fat from the overlying lamina.

where it attaches to the upper margin of the inferior lamina. Once an appropriate entry point has been gained, fine probes may be inserted to separate the underlying dural sac from the lamina and ligamentum flavum, which can be removed with angled punches of appropriate dimensions (Fig. 4). This is a very safe way to enter a severely stenotic canal without damaging the dural sac. The incidence of dural injury is higher if one attempts to separate the ligamentum flavum from its inferior bony attachment using osteotomes or curettes.

The ligamentum flavum is carefully removed, retracting its free margin and inserting patties between it and the dural sac until its upper attachments have been freed along with its attachment to the medial edge of the superior facet at the interspace.

The third phase of the operation is decompression of the foramina and nerve root canals bilaterally. The medial margin of the inferior pedicle is palpated with a fine probe, and the overhanging margin of the superior facet is removed using a variety of instruments such as rigid angled curettes, narrow-bladed rongeurs, or in some cases fine osteotomes. The medial and apical margins of the superior facets at the interspace should be trimmed flush with the medial margin of the pedicle. Trimming the facet laterally by another few millimeters, just above the upper margin of the pedicle, will lead to decompression of the perineural veins, which can be seen to refill dramatically as the constricting portions of the medial and apical segments of the superior facet and the outer edge of the ligamentum flavum attachment are removed.

When the nerve root is tightly constricted in its canal, even gentle manipulation with a fine probe will result in buttock and thigh muscle twitching, which will cease as soon as satisfactory decompression has been obtained.

Where necessary, the central canal can be enlarged using angled curettes alternately on either side of the spinous processes. In some cases, the use of a 300-mm, oblique 45-degree punch may be required to enlarge the sublaminar segment of the spinal canal. Care must be

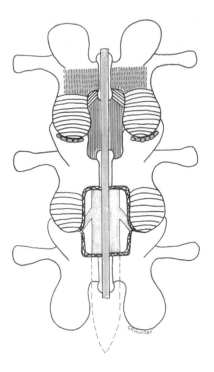

FIG. 5. Final stages of decompression of the central canal, bilateral nerve root canals, and intervertebral foramina. Epidural fat should not be removed. Perineural venous refilling should be obvious on both sides, and venous hemorrhage should only be controlled with the use of Spongistan (Ethicon Inc., Edinburgh, United Kingdom).

taken to depress the dural sac with a patty and sucker so that the instrument can be inserted without damaging the dura. At the end of these procedures, performed at either single or multiple levels, the capsules of the facet joints have been disturbed minimally and the spinous processes and interspinous ligaments remain intact. The wound then is closed simply by resuturing the lumbo dorsal aponeurosis to each side of the midline ligaments (Figs. 5 and 6).

The advantages of this method of lumbar canal decompression are far from theoretical. This is the most logical way to deal with multilevel lumbar canal decompressions, as it respects the integrity of the paraspinal muscles and re-places them in their normal anatomic relationships with the enlarged roof of the canal at the conclusion of the operation. The

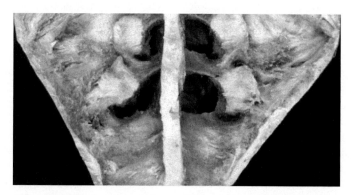

FIG. 6. Dissection depicting decompressions of the L–/5 and L5–S1 interspaces, using the operative methods described in the text.

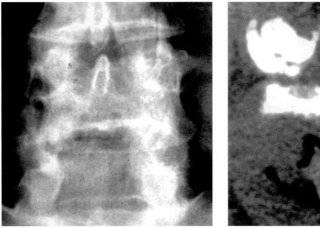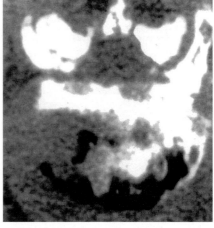

A B

FIG. 7. A: Anteroposterior x-ray film of the lumbar spine after laminectomy. The patient continued to complain of disabling leg pain. **B:** Axial computed tomographic image in the same patient, taken after laminectomy, demonstrates persistent nerve root canal stenosis on both sides. (From ref. 3, with permission.)

epidural fat should not have been disturbed during the procedure, and the fatty tissues that are present in normal paraspinal muscles subsequently will blend with the epidural fat and reduce the degree of postoperative scarring. The adequacy of decompression of the nerve root canals can be assessed most easily at operation by the demonstration of perineural venous refilling (3). Patients treated by this method report dramatic relief of their leg pain in the immediate postoperative period (4).

In contrast, patients treated with the laminectomy technique, who continue to complain of severe leg pain after operation, often will be found to have unrelieved foraminal and nerve root canal stenoses (Fig. 7). Recurrent stenosis of the lumbar canal can be predicted if, after previous surgery, further decompression is performed using that method. If, in addition to the revision laminectomy, internal fixation devices such as pedicle screws and plates are inserted—in combination with bone grafting—irreversible damage will be inflicted on the paraspinal muscles, thus heralding consequences of ectopic bone formation, restenosis, and intractable pain.

REFERENCES

1. Benini A, Magerl F. Undercutting decompression and posterior fusion with translaminar facet screw fixation in degenerative lumbar spinal stenosis: technique and results. *Neuroorthopaedics* 1995;17/18:159–172.
2. Crock HV, Crock MC. A technique for decompression of the lumbar spinal canal. *Neuroorthopaedics* 1998;5: 96–99.
3. Crock HV. Lumbar root canal decompression. Lumbar perineural venous dilation as an indicator of its efficacy. *Act Orthop Scand* 1994;65:225–227.
4. Shiraishi T, Crock HV. Lumbar perineural venous obstruction as a cause of sciatica in foraminal and nerve root canal stenosis. *Neuroorthopaedics* 1995;17/18:183–189.
5. Spivak JM. Current concepts review. Degenerative lumbar spinal stenosis. *J Bone Joint Surg Am* 1998;80: 1053–1066.

Lumbar Spinal Stenosis
edited by Robert Gunzburg and Marek Szpalski
Lippincott Williams & Wilkins, Philadelphia, © 2000.

25

Surgical Decompression of Lumbar Spinal Stenosis According to Senegas Technique

Everard Munting, *Vincent Druez, and †Dimitrios Tsoukas

Department of Surgery, Universite Catholique Louvain, 1200 Brussels, Belgium; °Evere 1140, France; and †Department of Orthopedics, Diagnostic and Therapeutic Center of Athens "Hygeia," 15123 Athens, Greece

Patients with lumbar spinal stenosis may present with neurogenic claudication, muscle weakness, sensitive disturbances, radicular pain, and low back pain. Walking disability may be caused by rapid exhaustion of the lower limbs without pain or because of radicular pain or low back pain. The latter sometimes dominate the clinical picture.

Indication for surgery is mostly dependent on functional impairment, the severity and frequency of pain, and the efficiency of conservative treatment modalities in improving the patient's daily quality of life.

Careful interrogation about function and pain localization, intensity and frequency, clinical examination, medical imaging and selective nerve blocks usually allow to determine precisely the level of symptomatic stenosis. Except in cases of obvious instability, the origin and reason of low back pain often remains unclear since there is no correlation between degenerative changes and symptoms.

After Verbiest (13), several surgical techniques have been described to decompress the neural structures. Laminectomy, laminarthrectomy, laminoplasty, and partial laminotomy of the upper or lower half of the lamina allow decompression of the neural structures.

Clinical outcome evaluated by a functional questionnaire independently filled in by the patient usually is rated excellent to good in 60% to 70% of cases (1,4–8,10,11,12). As yet, there is no consensus or proof as to whether one particular technique is better than another. Fusion with instrumentation appears to be indicated for degenerative spondylolisthesis, scoliosis, and when obvious instability is demonstrated preoperatively, for example, if arthrectomy has been performed.

The specific effect of surgery on walking disability, radicular pain, and low back pain seldom is specified. In the present study, we evaluate the outcome of each major symptom after surgical decompression according to the Senegas technique.

MATERIALS AND METHODS

Surgical Technique

The "recalibration" technique described by Senegas et al. (9) is based on the principle of removing only those parts of the anatomic structures that effectively provoke the narrowing of the spinal canal. As well documented on sagittal magnetic resonance imaging of the lumbar spine, the lamina has an oblique orientation, from anterior in the cephalad part to posterior in the caudal part. Therefore, it is the upper half of the lamina that protrudes in the spinal canal and potentially contributes to central stenosis. In the lower part of the lamina, it is the ligamentum flavum that protrudes into the canal, if it is thickened. Eventual disc protrusion, hernia, or osteophytosis of the endplates may contribute to degenerative central stenosis. The recalibration procedure consists of removing the medial part of the superior facet, the upper half of the lamina, and the medial and anterior parts of the lower facet. This is best done with a high-speed burr, particularly when the stenosis is severe. The bone is drilled until a very thin shell of bone is left and can be broken easily with a spatula or a rongeur without entering the narrowed spinal canal. The ligamentum flavum is freed from its superior insertion, allowing removal of all stenosing structures ''in one piece.'' The central canal as well as the lateral recesses are decompressed by the procedure. If the nerve roots or dural sac are still under tension because of disc protrusion, hernia, or osteophytosis of the endplates, these structures will be removed if necessary. In our practice, arthrodesis is carried out in case of obvious and focal instability, as in some cases of degenerative spondylolisthesis or if instability is demonstrated after discectomy or facetectomy. The spinous processes of the treated levels usually are removed.

Patient Description

Between 1992 and 1997, 115 patients were operated for lumbar spinal stenosis according to the Senegas technique at the Saint Luc Academic Hospital, Brussels, Belgium, by the same surgeon (EM). Before surgery, each patient was questioned regarding possible walking distance and reason for walking disability (lower limb weakness, radicular pain, paresthesia, or low back pain). The predominant symptom was identified. The preoperative score is based on this information, because it was found that when patients filled out the questionnaires, they had a tendency to worsen their preoperative status compared to the preoperative data recorded in the medical files. Past medical history, previous back surgery, associated pathology, and other relevant information were recorded. Description of the surgical procedure, number of operated levels, association of discectomy or arthrodesis, and possible incidents are noted in the operative record.

At each follow-up visit, the patient is asked for the outcome of each preoperative symptom. For the present study, a Stauffer-Coventry type questionnaire translated into French was sent to the patients. This questionnaire included a section about preoperative status, with questions and visual analogue scales (VAS) for low back pain and radicular pain, and a similar second section for the current status of the patient.

Preoperative and postoperative scores ranging from 0 to 3 were defined for walking ability, radicular pain, and low back pain as follows:

0 = severe and daily debilitating pain (8 to 10 on VAS) and a walking distance of less than 100 m

1 = responds to limiting and daily pain (5 to 7,9 on VAS) and a walking distance of less than 1,000 m

2 = nonlimiting intermittent pain or more severe but infrequent pain and a walking distance of less than 1 hour or 3 km

3 = no or almost no pain and no walking limitation.

According to this system, each patient has a total score between 0 and 9. However, one should notice that a 0 of 1 score for low back pain or radicular pain symptom means severe functional limitation or incapacitating pain for that particular patient, even with a total score of 6 or 7 of 9. On the other hand, a score of 1 for walking ability may already be appreciable for an elderly patient if he or she has no significant pain.

RESULTS

Of the 115 patients who underwent the procedure, 31 were lost to follow-up. Six patients had a long-term follow-up visit but failed to respond to the questionnaire and could not be reached by telephone. The information obtained from their medical files was compared to the group that was studied to verify that they did not constitute a worse-outcome subgroup. Sixty-five patients had a complete medical file and responded to the questionnaire; 13 had a complete medical file and had a telephone interview. The present study thus reports the clinical and functional outcome, with follow-up of more than 1 year, of 78 (68%) of 115 patients who underwent the Senegas procedure for lumbar spinal stenosis and who responded independently to a functional questionnaire.

The average age at the time of surgery was 62 years (range 16 to 90). There are 43 males and 35 females. Twelve patients had previous surgery (3 discectomies, 7 arthrodesis, 6 previous decompression procedures). All patients were severely affected: 92% had at least one "0" score, meaning severe disability, and all patients had at least a "1" score for one symptom. Figure 1 shows the total preoperative score distribution for males and females. The scores for each individual symptom are shown in Figs. 2–4. A "0" or "1" score was found in 94% of patients for walking capacity, in 85% for radicular pain, and in 74% for low back pain.

The number of operated levels was as follows: one level: 33; two levels: 21; three levels: 17; four or five levels: 7. A discectomy of one or two levels was associated with the Senegas procedure in 26% (20 of 78) and an arthrodesis in 33% (26 of 78).

According to the global postoperative score, 56% of the patients have an excellent or good result for all three symptoms. Subjectively, 67% of the patients consider their results to be excellent or good. A fair result (improvement of at least one symptom) was obtained in 17% more patients scoring both objectively and subjectively (patient's own evaluation). A poor outcome (none or minor improvement) was obtained in 27% of the patients. Subjectively, only 17% of the patients consider their results to be poor (Fig. 5 and Table 1).

The outcome of the procedure is reported for each symptom, taking into account the preoperative situation. The 78 patients are separated into three groups of "0," "1," and "2 and 3" scores, with preoperative and postoperative distributions. The outcome of the subgroups that underwent only the Senegas procedure with or without discectomy (n = 52) and decompression associated with an arthrodesis (n = 26) are shown in Fig. 6.

A severe limitation of walking ability is found in 73 patients (94%). An improvement of walking ability is obtained in 74% of the cases. In 49% the improvement is very significant.

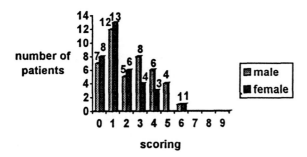

FIG. 1. Preoperative score distribution.

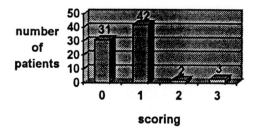

FIG. 2. Preoperative walking ability score.

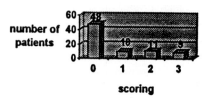

FIG. 3. Preoperative low back pain score.

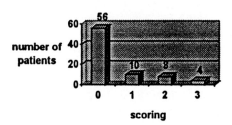

FIG. 4. Preoperative radicular pain score.

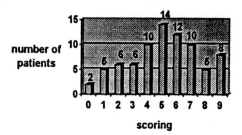

FIG. 5. Postoperative status.

TABLE 1. *Postoperative results*

Results	Objective	Subjective
Excellent or good	56%	67%
Fair	17%	17%
Poor	27%	17%

A decrease of walking ability occurred in four patients and was significant in one patient (score of 2 down to 0).

Sixty-six (85%) of 78 patients had disabling radicular pain; 65% of them improved significantly; 11% improved only slightly; and 24% remained unchanged. Two patients became very symptomatic after surgery.

Before surgery, 58 patients were severely symptomatic for low back pain (75% of the whole group). A significant improvement (score of 2 or 3) is experienced in 65% of these patients, whereas 35% remained either unchanged (n = 9) or only slightly improved (n = 11). Among the 20 patients with little or no low back pain before surgery, one became very symptomatic (score of 3 decreased to 1) and five lost one point for the low back pain score after surgery.

If the 26 patients who underwent an arthrodesis are compared to the 52 who underwent only decompression, the incidence of significant preoperative low back pain (score 0 or 1) was higher: 85% (22 of 26) versus 70% (36 of 52). The outcome for low back pain appears slightly better after surgery with arthrodesis than without arthrodesis, with 73% and 61% of the 0 and 1 scores becoming 2 and 3 scores, respectively. Increased or *de novo* low back pain after surgery occurred in one patient (4%) after arthrodesis and three patients (6%) after decompression alone, which is not significantly different.

Only 12 of the 78 patients had a previous operative procedure in the operated area. The outcome for low back pain appears similar to that of the whole group (70% significant

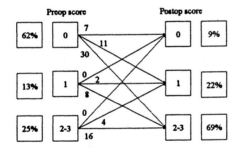

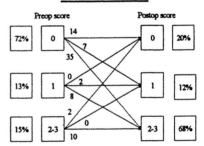

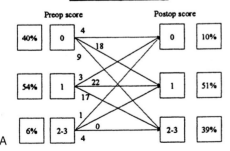

FIG. 6. Preoperative and postoperative score distribution in percent for each symptom: low back pain (LBP), radicular pain (RP), and walking ability (WA). Numbers above the *arrows* indicate the number of cases for each outcome score group originative for each preoperative score group. **A:** results for the whole group of patients. *(Figure continues.)*

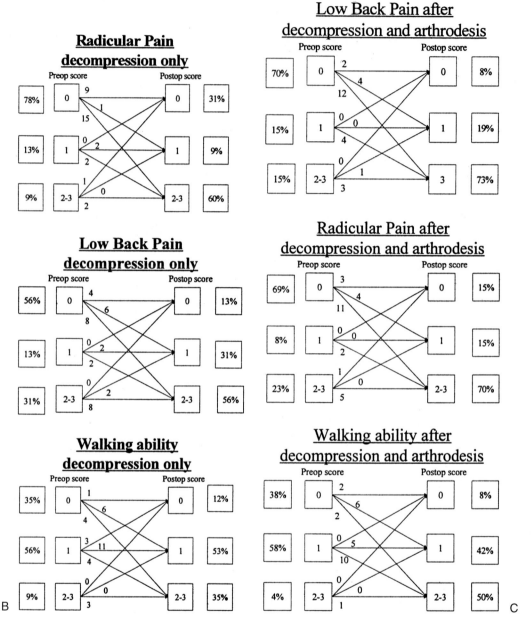

FIG. 6. *Continued* **B:** Results for patients who underwent surgical decompression only; **C:** results for patients who underwent surgical decompressions and arthrodesis.

improvement). In this group, only 2 of 8 patients with severe preoperative radicular pain are cured, but the sample is too restricted to be conclusive.

No significant postoperative complication related to the surgical technique occurred. However, a minor dural tear was made in 27% of the whole group of 115 patients, which corresponds to a total of 228 levels treated (11% per level). These were repaired without further consequences. Reoperation for a dural tear was required in one patient in whom the tear was not noticed during the index surgery. Persistent symptoms related to insufficient decompression required a second operation in two patients. Disabling low back pain led to a secondary arthrodesis in four cases. One patient had a pyogenic diskitis that was treated conservatively. One patient needed surgical drainage for hematoma with exclusion of a disc fragment.

DISCUSSION

The general conclusion of surgical treatment for lumbar spinal stenosis remains difficult to evaluate according to what is reported in the literature. The ''good-to-excellent'' results range from less than 20% to more than 90% (1,4–6,8,10,11). Obviously different problems are compared by different methods. Our group of patients is characterized by a very severe preoperative status: 92% of the patients had at least one ''0'' score and 81% had a total score of 3 or less.

The overall results of this series, based on the scoring, are slightly worse than those reported in the literature but are similar according to the patient's own evaluation (7,10,11),

Detailed reports about the initial symptoms and the outcome of specific symptoms are lacking. In our series, the functional questionnaire and the information obtained about preoperative and postoperative walking ability, radicular pain, and low back pain allow some interesting observations, particularly regarding low back pain. The indication for instrumented arthrodesis is recognized when instability is demonstrated before surgery (2,3). The patients who had an arthrodesis in this series had either a degenerative scoliosis with signs of instability or focal instability related to degenerative spondylolisthesis or disc degeneration. These patients had a demonstrated cause for low back pain and their favorable outcome (73% good to excellent) was expected. The positive effect of decompression without arthrodesis on disabling low back pain should be noted. During surgery, some of these patients had demonstrated multilevel abnormal mobility and, despite this observation, were relieved of their low back pain. On the other hand, some patients had to be reoperated because of single-level instability that become obvious postoperatively. According to our results, severe low back pain without focal instability should not be a standard indication for instrumented fusion.

Our results, as in many other reports, with a good-to-excellent outcome in only 67% of cases, stresses the need for further research and better assessment of the patient preoperatively and postoperatively. Although the patients were asked preoperatively the same questions regarding their complaints, their preoperative functional and pain status was not sufficiently detailed. No objective features such as preoperative and postoperative walking capacity evaluated on a treadmill were available.

To allow useful conclusions and valuable comparisons, all studies should be prospective and based on a precise description of the status of each patient enrolled in the study, before surgery. For lumbar spinal stenosis this assessment involves several aspects.

In addition to the classic medical information (past medical history, general and neurologic examination), the physical status of the patient should be defined by several parameters. Evaluation of the patient's general physical condition is best obtained by a submaximal effort on a bicycle ergometer. The walking capacity at a given speed on a treadmill must be recorded with the patient indicating on a VAS the pain experienced in both legs and the low back. The capacity to perform some standardized exercises (forward bending, lumbar extension, stair climbing) should be assessed, as well as the VAS results and localization of pain provoked by these exercises. Localization of pain and sensitivity disturbances can be specified further by pain drawings. Muscle strength and function can be assessed on isostatic and isometric testing devices.

The functional status can be scored by validated questionnaires such as the Oswestry low back pain disability questionnaire. Depression, anxiety, hysteria, and illness behavior are other variables that should be defined before surgery. The relevant morphologic data must be obtained and stored to allow precise description of the stenosis and eventual comparison with postoperative data.

Only with all these pieces of information, obtained preoperatively and postoperatively, will we be able to analyze objectively the results of our surgical procedures. Moreover, if a standardized methodology to describe the clinical picture of our patients before and after surgery could be installed, we will be able to compare effectively series of patients operated on by other teams using other surgical procedures. To reach these goals, a radical change of methodology is needed. Obviously, only a multidisciplinary team involving surgeons, pain specialists, physical therapists, psychologists, clinical researchers, and appropriate computer and statistical support will allow better understanding of clinical observations and improve the management of degenerative diseases of the lumbar spine.

REFERENCES

1. Airaksinen O, Herno A, Turunen V, Saari T, Suomlainen O. Surgical outcome of 438 patients treated surgically for lumbar spinal stenosis. *Spine* 1997;22:2278–2282.
2. Bridwell KH, Sedegewick TA, O'Brien MF, Lenke LQ, Baldus C. The role of fusion and instrumentation in the treatment of degenerative spondylolisthesis with spinal stenosis. *J Spinal Disord* 1993;6:461–472.
3. Herkowitz HN, Kurz LT. Degenerative lumbar spondylolisthesis with stenosis. A prospective study comparing decompression and intertransverse process arthrodesis. *J Bone Joint Surg* 1991;73A:802–808.
4. Herno A, Airaksinen O, Saari T. Long term result of surgical treatment of lumbar spinal stenosis. *Spine* 1993;18:1471–1474.
5. Herno A, Airaksinen O, Saari T, Luukkonen M. Lumbar spinal stenosis: a matched pair-study of operated and nonoperated patients. *Br J Neurosurg* 1996;10:461–465.
6. Herno A, Airaksinen O, Saari T, Sihvonen T. Surgical results of lumbar spinal stenosis. A comparison of patients with or without previous surgery. *Spine* 1995;20:964–969.
7. Postacchini F, Cinotti G, Perugia D, Gumina S. The surgical treatment of central lumbar stenosis by multiple laminotomy compared with total laminectomy. *J Bone Joint Surg* 1993;75B:386–392.
8. Postacchini F, Cinotti G, Gumina S, Perugia D. Long term results of surgery in lumbar stenosis. 8 years review of 64 patients. *Acta Orthop Scand Suppl* 1993;25:78–80.
9. Senegas J, Etchevers JP, Vital JM, Baulny D, Grenier F. Le recalibrage du canal lombaire comme alternative de la laminectomie dans le traitement de la sténose du canal lombaire. *Rev Chir Orthop* 1988;74:15–22.
10. Tuite GF, Doran SE, Stern JD, et al. Outcome after laminectomy for lumbar spinal stenosis. Part II: radiographic changes and clinical correlations. *J Neurosurg* 1994;81:707–715.
11. Tuite GF, Doran SE, Stern JD, et al. Outcome after laminectomy for lumbar spinal stenosis. Part I: clinical correlations. *J Neurosurg* 1994;81:699–706.
12. Turner JA, Ersek M, Herron L, Deyo R. Surgery for lumbar spinal stenosis. Attempted meta-analysis of the literature. *Spine* 1992;17:1–8.
13. Verbiest H. Results of surgical treatment of idiopathic developmental stenosis of the vertebral canal. *J Bone Joint Surg* 1977;59B:181–188.

Lumbar Spinal Stenosis
edited by Robert Gunzburg and Marek Szpalski
Lippincott Williams & Wilkins, Philadelphia, © 2000.

26

Endoscopic Laser Foraminoplasty

Two-year Follow-up of a Prospective Study of 200 Consecutive Patients

Martin T.N. Knight, Anukul Goswami, and Janos T. Patko

*The Spinal Foundation, Arbury Consulting Centre, Rochdale OL11 4LX,
United Kingdom*

The management of back pain has remained a source of speculation and research. Its impact on modern industrial society has been well established (36). Approximately 2% to 5% of people suffer from acute back pain every year (11,44). The majority of these patients recover fully; 10% to 25% have residual complaints. A small percentage of these patients (0.5%) have pain and neurology requiring surgery, whereas others slip into chronicity. Chronic back pain does have a significant impact on the individual, causing fear and worry, altering the perception of pain, and degrading the quality of life (44).

The available methods of treatment, such as osseous decompression, removal of discs to decompress nerve roots, and spinal fusion, have provided the standard armamentarium of the spinal surgeon. The choice has depended on the surgeon's perceptions and the information derived from the use of diagnostic tools used to identify the source of pain. Open surgical procedures for the management of spinal pain give unpredictable results and in their own right may cause additional morbidity. Widely varying claims of success are attributed to these techniques (34,35). In the quest to reduce tissue trauma and morbidity, decompressive disc procedures, such as fenestrectomy and microdiscectomy, are gaining wider acceptance and are providing encouraging results (5,32,37). The realization of the shortcomings of conventional techniques has led to the development of minimalist midline foraminal decompression with improved results (17).

The recent deployment of endoscopic techniques to the spine has allowed visual inspection of the disc to be carried out through the keyhole with the patient in the aware state and intradiscal decompression to be effected (20–22). However, these techniques could not address the foramen, epidural space, and posterior disc wall.

Laser as a tool for tissue ablation has been tried in several surgical specialties with encouraging results (12,13,31,41,42,46,48). Not only has it been effective in "precision surgery" (41), but it also has shown to reduce morbidity associated with conventional surgery (49). In 1984, laser disc decompression was introduced by Choy et al. (8) and Casper et al. (6,7). It recently was combined with endoscopy to effect intradiscal clearance (7,24,25). Its wider application as a surgical tool in spinal surgery remained underestimated until it was used to ablate bone and scar tissue (26) and so provides a means of exploring the foramen and extraforaminal zone and epidural space by the posterolateral route with the patient in the aware state.

Physical compression of nerves within the spinal canal and the foramen has dominated the conceptual perception of spinal surgeons seeking to ameliorate back pain or sciatica (2,16,57). However, additional structures in and around the spine can be the source of nociceptive stimuli (27). Recent appreciation of neural mechanisms of pain, pain mediators in and around the spinal canal, and pain modulation in the peripheral and central nervous system have cautioned us against excessive dependence on purely mechanical concepts of back pain (1,3,39,45,51,54). Importantly, the sensitivity, reliability, and predictive value of diagnostic tools such as magnetic resonance (MR) scans, computer-assisted tomograms, myelograms, and discography alone or in combination, cannot reliably establish the source and cause of back pain (4,50,55,56).

Current concepts in the management of degenerative disease of the spine are limited in concept and hampered by indirect diagnosis and operating on the unresponsive patient. The foramen as a site for compressive entrapment of the nerve root (22,43,53) and the anatomic structures that participate in its formation are established. The effect of structural variations, prior surgery, perineural scarring, facet joint and bone disease, and degenerative conditions on the dynamics of the foramen and on the contrivance of lateral recess stenosis is poorly recognized.

Posterolateral endoscopy reveals that static MR imaging (MRI) fails to demonstrate the tethering and impaction of the superior facet joint, the infolded ligamentum flavum, the facet joint capsule, the foraminal ligament, and the superior foraminal ligament on local structures. Endoscopy demonstrates that dorsal and shoulder osteophytes not only encroach on the foramen but tether to the nerves and may impinge on the posterior longitudinal ligament. Static MRI fails to demonstrate the degree of inflammation and irritation within these structures and within the disc and the precise longevity of a disc protrusion. Endoscopy reveals that the MR scan underestimates the degree of local scarring and the vascular hyperemia and thrombosis occurring within. The mechanism of defining local and referred pain is obfuscated further because the local structures, when irritated or sensitized, produce distributions of pain otherwise deemed atypical. The function of the foramen is a delicate balance between the size of the foraminal boundaries and the status of their contents. This balance is easily compromised by pathology, irritation, or sensitization of tethered tissues and abnormal motion.

In this prospective study, we present the results of the management of back pain using the ''viviprudence'' system of ''aware state'' and endoscopic diagnosis of the causes of pain followed by pain source ablation in the epidural, foraminal, and extraforaminal zones combined with lateral recess and intradiscal decompression achieved by endoscopic laser foraminoplasty.

MATERIALS AND METHODS

Study Construct

The study was designed prospectively and consisted of 200 consecutive patients treated between March 1994 and November 1996.

Data Acquisition

Full details of history and symptoms were recorded by questionnaire, which included a pain manikin, visual analogue pain scores (VAPS), Oswestry disability scores, patient satisfaction scores (PSS), patient target achievement scores (PTAS), and psychological indexes. The latter are not a part of this report. Patients were evaluated at 6 and 12 weeks and 6 months after surgery. They were reviewed at yearly intervals unless clinical symptoms required closer supervision. The data were input by bar coding and computerized for comparison with follow-up data.

Oswestry Disability Index

Oswestry disability scores were substratified for back, buttock, and leg pain. Computerized comparison calculated the postoperative index as the final score divided by the initial score as a percentage, where 100% was deemed an excellent result, greater than 50% was good, greater than 20% was improved, less than 20% was poor, and negative values were deemed a worse result.

Visual Analogue Pain Scores

Visual analogue pain scores were substratified for back, buttock, and leg pain. Preoperative and follow-up visual analogue pain levels were measured using a visual analogue pain scale with the following guidelines to patients: pain level 10 = excruciating pain, unbearable for any time; 9 = horrible pain bearable for only a short time; 6 = distressing pain bearable for some time; 3 = mild pain; 0 = no pain.

Computerized comparison calculated the postoperative index as the final pain score divided by the initial pain score as a percentage. A patient who was pain free was deemed excellent result. An index greater than 50% was deemed good, greater than 20% was improved, less than 20% was poor, and negative values were deemed a worse result.

Clinical Evaluation

Full clinical neurologic and postural analysis was performed together with plain anteroposterior and neutral weight-bearing x-ray films and a dynamic series of digitized instability radiographs in flexion and extension during both sitting and standing.

Patients were prescribed muscle balance physiotherapy for a period of 3 months. If pain intensity remained high and the response to physiotherapy remained inadequate, the patients were referred for MR scan. Gadolinium enhancement was added where prior spinal surgery had been involved or perineural scarring was suspected.

Inclusion Criteria

Inclusion criteria included the presence of back, buttock, or leg pain or combination thereof persisting despite advanced muscle balancing physiotherapy and a failure of other conservative methods.

The presence of the following conditions was included:

- Compressive radiculopathy with sensorimotor impairment
- Disc extrusion or sequestration and predominantly back pain
- Disc extrusion or sequestration and predominantly leg pain
- Degeneration and settlement and predominantly back pain
- Degeneration and settlement and predominantly buttock pain
- Degeneration and settlement and predominantly leg pain
- Positive tension signs radiating below the knee

- Nonradicular pain persisting despite facet joint injection
- Lateral recess stenosis with dynamic compressive radiculopathy
- Lateral recess stenosis with dynamic noncompressive radiculopathy
- The above conditions with previous conventional surgery at the index level
- The above conditions with perineural scarring at the index level
- Spondylolytic spondylolisthesis
- Failed back syndrome
- Patients with bilateral or multiple level pathology were analyzed for contribution arising from adjacent sides or levels.

Exclusions

- Cauda equina syndrome
- Painless motor deficit
- Tumors.

Definitions

If the MR scan clearly identified loss of foraminal space and loss of perineural fat and a foraminal dimension less than 5 mm, the patients were diagnosed with lateral recess stenosis.

Surgical Protocol

Patients were consented for a staged procedure consisting of:

- Spinal probing and discography on two segments or more approached on the side of maximal symptoms
- Endoscopic laser foraminoplasty and flexible endoscopic intradiscal discectomy, neurolysis, undercutting, and osteophytectomy as required. However, the final decision for the second stage (endoscopic laser foraminoplasty) was made only after spinal probing and discography reproduced the type, intensity, and distribution of pain similar to that which the patient had experienced and of significant intensity.

Spinal probing and discography was done at suspected levels that demonstrated degenerative changes and clinically reproduced the site of back pain and neurologic radiation.

Spinal probing differs from discography in that it relies on specific probing of the anterior margin of the facet joint, perineural structures, and disc wall at several points. Discography defines the distribution of degeneration within the disc and the acceptance volume and the presence of annular leaks.

Operative Technique

Neurolept (aware state) analgesia was performed using a 2- to 5-mg bolus of hypnoval at the onset of the operation, 2 to 5 μ/kg fentanyl, and 30 to 70 μ/kg droperidol. Patient feedback is essential in these cases where the presence of perineural scarring is often unexpectedly dense and masks the neural structures. A bolus dose of 1.5 g of cefuroxime was given at onset of operation. The skin and subcutis were infiltrated with the local anesthetic xylocaine 0.25% 0.75 to 1.5 mg/kg with 1:400,000 adrenaline. During advancement of the cannulated probe under x-ray control, continuous doses of local anesthetic were injected into the surrounding musculature.

The distribution and intensity of the evoked sensations were recorded on a data sheet that described the patient response to facet joint probing, annulus probing, and during discography. The pattern of the discography, disc wall bulging, integrity and thickness of the posterior wall, and acceptance volume were recorded.

Push-up Test

The push-up test consisted of extending the arms and hyperextending the lumbar spine while encouraging the abdomen to sag in the prone position. If this maneuver evoked the patient's leg or back pain prior to surgery, then clearance of same at the end of the procedure denoted sufficient clearance of the cause of the pain and a positive push-up test.

Lasing Technique

The probe was replaced with a guidewire, and a 4.6-mm dilator tube under biplanar x-ray control was railroaded to the exit root foramen. During the entire procedure, an image intensifier was used to ensure the correct position of the endoscope and the laser probe. The trocar was removed, and a Richard Wolf (Richard Wolf GmbH, Knittlingen, Baden Wurttenburg, Germany) endoscope with an eccentrically placed 2.5-mm working channel and two irrigation channels was inserted. A side-firing, 2.1-mm-diameter laser probe with internal irrigation was inserted through the endoscope. The extraforaminal zone and margin of the foramen were cleared. The ascending and descending facet joint surfaces were excavated and undercut to allow admission of the endoscope beyond the isthmus of the foramen at the midpedicular line into the epidural space. Vertebral body osteophytes, perineural, facet joint, and epidural scarring were ablated until the annulus was revealed.

The exiting and transitting nerve roots were mobilized and decompressed medially and laterally until the axilla of the root at the apex of the safe working zone was displayed. The nerve was cleared of perineural fibrosis. Clearance was extended to the bone margin of the superior notch and the superior foraminal ligament. The superior foraminal ligament extends from the ascending facet joint to the transverse process and may become adherent to the exiting nerve root and bind onto the nerve, causing local hyperemia and inflammation. Osteophytes along the ascending facet joint and in the superior notch, dorsum of the vertebral margin, and the vertebral shoulder (shoulder osteophytes) were ablated under endoscopic vision.

In the presence of disc protrusion in the epidural or foraminal zone, the disc was entered and cleared by laser ablation and manual punches. The epidural space was explored with a 2-mm flexible controllable fiberoptic endoscope with a 1-mm working channel through which was passed an end-firing laser fiber for additional clearance of sequestra, osteophytes, and scarring in the epidural space.

Follow-up

Patients were discharged the day after surgery. The muscle balance physiotherapy regime was restarted the first day after surgery and amplified with neural mobilization drills.

A pain diary was maintained by patients to identify the intensity and location of residual pain. Patients were followed-up at 6 and 12 weeks, 6 months, and annually thereafter unless clinical indications required closer supervision. Follow-up questionnaires were obtained at each visit. These questionnaires were bar coded into the Spinal Foundation database and computerized for subsequent analysis. Patients who no longer required support were contacted by postal questionnaire combined with telephone appraisal and confirmation.

RESULTS

The cohort consisted of 101 men and 99 women. The average age of the patients was 56 years (range 22 to 83). The average follow-up period was 34 months. All patients had back, buttock, or leg pain with or without sciatica syndrome. One hundred two patients had predominantly left-sided leg pain and 98 right-sided. All patients stayed in the hospital less than 24 hours.

At 2-year follow-up, 96% cohort integrity was maintained. Calculations were made with Microsoft Access software. Seven patients were lost to follow-up. One patient died of breast metastases 19 months after surgery.

The overall duration of symptoms was 6.1 years (range 5 to 11, standard deviation 2.4). The average duration of the immediate symptom exacerbation prior to surgery was 28 months (range 2 to 96, standard deviation 24.5).

Eighteen patients were involved in litigation or compensation claims.

One hundred six patients had obtained opinions from one or more spinal/orthopedic surgeons or neurosurgeons prior to referral to the Spinal Foundation and had been deemed unsuitable for surgery. These patients included 46 patients with prior failed open conventional lumbar spinal surgery. The Oswestry disability index demonstrated that 48% patients scored a good or excellent index. Ten percent of patients did not show any improvement, 6% were worse, and the remaining 36% of patients improved.

Seventy-four patients had been through *coping courses,* which included pain clinic visits, facet joint injections, epidural injections, extensive physiotherapy with or without the use of morphine sulfate (MST), acupuncture treatment, and transcutaneous electrical nerve stimulation. A preemptive trauma history was obtained from 35 patients; 26 of the traumas were work related and 9 resulted from road traffic accidents.

If all the patients in this study were taken as a group, the Oswestry disability index, on a global scale, demonstrated that 55% had excellent or good results (11% excellent results and 44% good results) for back pain, 52% for buttock pain, and 53% for leg pain. For patients who had no previous operations, the corresponding values were 58%, 53%, and 55%. At 2-year follow-up review, 18 patients (9%) showed continuing degeneration and were worse on their Oswestry disability index, but only 2% patients described their pain as worse than before.

Seventy-nine percent of patients achieved more than 50% of their preoperative rehabilitation objectives selected as their goals prior to surgery within the PTAS; 62% of patients were satisfied with the targets that they had achieved; and 75% of patients were satisfied with their management and the results obtained.

Visual analogue pain scores demonstrated that 12% of patients were pain free, 44% had a visual analogue pain index greater than 50%, and only 2% were worse at the 2-year review.

Prior Open Operations

Forty-six patients had between one and four conventional open operations on the spine. Perineural fibrosis with or without epidural fibrosis was identified in all patients. This was confirmed with MR scanning in those cases without instrumented fusion and by the operative endoscopic findings. In the 37 patients who had undergone one previous operation, endoscopic laser foraminoplasty resulted in an excellent or good Oswestry disability index of 51% for back pain, 33% for buttock pain, and 29% for leg pain. However, when overall results are assessed for all the patients who had previous open operations, 49% improved to the good and excellent category, and an additional 35% patients were improved.

Rheumatoid and Seronegative Spondyarthritis

One patient was being treated for rheumatoid arthritis at the time of operation. She was seropositive for rheumatoid arthritis. On the Oswestry disability score, she scored an index of 80%, 84%, and 76% for back, buttock, and leg pain, respectively. She achieved 94% of her proposed achievement targets before the end of 2 years and an 86% improvement on the visual analogue pain index.

There were three patients with seronegative arthritis. One of these three patients had an excellent result, another achieved an improved level, and the third was unchanged.

Spondylolytic Spondylolisthesis

There were 11 patients with grade I spondylolytic spondylolisthesis. The listhesis occurred at L4–5 in five patients and at L5–S1 in six patients. Ten patients achieved excellent or good results using the Oswestry disability index. Only one patient had a poor outcome because of bilateral perineural and epidural scarring from previous open surgery and fusion. One of the patients had two levels involved (L4–5 and L5–S1). This patient had full recovery from back, buttock, and leg pain and all neurologic symptoms.

There were five patients with grade II spondylolytic spondylolisthesis. Three patients achieved excellent or good results using the Oswestry disability index. One of these five patients was worse at review. This patient was the only patient who had dynamic listhesis that demonstrated slipping into anterior listhesis in flexion and retrolisthesis in extension on the dynamic lateral weight-bearing x-ray films.

Coronary and Vascular Disease

Eight patients had severe coronary and peripheral or cerebral vascular disease. Six of these eight patients were considered inoperable by open surgery because of significant anesthetic risk. Five of the eight patients had excellent-to-good outcome, two improved, and one did not have any change.

Preoperative Foot Drop

There were seven patients who had foot drop grade 1 to 2 prior to surgery. All these patients had the foot drop for more than 3 years and demonstrated improvement in dorsiflexion power at the ankle at the end of 2 years (grade 4/5), although none reached normal power.

MST Usage

Fourteen patients were on MST prior to surgery. Only one patient was still taking MST and one patient was continuing with strong analgesics at the end of 2 years. Eight of these 14 patients had excellent-to-good results, whereas the other six achieved an improved Oswestry disability index.

Multiple Sclerosis

Two patients had multiple sclerosis diagnosed prior to surgery and were wheelchair bound. In these two patients, the visual analogue pain index improved by more than 80%. The Oswestry disability index fell in the poor category because of the underlying pathology, but both could move about using crutches without much difficulty at review. One other patient was diagnosed as having multiple sclerosis a few months after endoscopic laser foraminoplasty. This patient's Oswestry disability index was worse at review, although the pain symptoms remained improved.

DISCUSSION

Many sources have been attributed as causes of sciatica and back and buttock pain, but they have not been examined using aware state patient feedback combined with posterolateral endoscopy as a means of true verification (27).

Viviprudence System

Spinal probing and discography followed by endoscopic laser foraminoplasty represents part of a treatment algorithm termed viviprudence. The viviprudence system is based on detailed analysis of the clinical presentation, clinical and postural examination, and dynamic weight-bearing x-ray films, followed by advanced spinal physiotherapy using the muscle balance approach. Failure of the symptoms to respond sufficiently to specific dynamic postural restabilization and correction of segmental loading leads to MRI scanning.

Experience with spinal endoscopy reveals that the MRI scan is a planning tool rather than a definitive diagnostic tool. The essential and distinctive step in viviprudence is spinal probing. This dictates the direction of further treatment and the choice between intervention and further investigation. Combined with the preparatory examinations and investigations, it indicates those levels that may be treated by laser disc decompression and those requiring endoscopic laser foraminoplasty. Spinal probing allows multiple sites in and around the foramen, epidural space, and disc to be probed with the patient in the aware state. The evoked response is compared to the presenting symptoms and is matched for distribution and severity. At each probing, the anatomic position of the probe is determined by biplanar x-ray evaluation.

Discography is performed as an adjunct to determine the site of degeneration within the disc, the presence of annular collections, and the site of annular leaks. The amount of dye readily accepted by the intradiscal space provides an indication of the amount of intradiscal degeneration and is recorded as the acceptance volume. If discography on a contained disc produces radicular pain, then this further endorses that disc as the index level for the pain. Similarly, if a leak reproduces the patient's pain, then this identifies the targeted disc as a contributor to that evoked pain.

Several reports have questioned the reliability of discography when used alone (10,47). At the Spinal Foundation, discography by itself is not deemed a reliable locator of back pain or peripheral compressive neuropathy.

If symptom reproduction is equivocal or symptoms arise in similar fashion at more than one level, then a therapeutic discogram of 80 mg depomedrone is inserted at the most sensitive level. Adjacent levels can be treated with instilled radiopaque dye (hydraulic discogram) or with bupivacaine (Marcaine) local anesthetic (bupivacaine discogram). This provides the basis for a differential discogram. If the symptoms are ameliorated for more than 10 days, then those symptoms that were relieved may be presumed to arise from the level treated with the therapeutic discogram. If relief lasts for only 5 hours, then the site of relieved symptoms may be presumed to arise from the bupivacaine discogram level; but if relief is for about 18 hours, then the symptoms may be presumed to arise from the hydraulic discogram level. In this process of viviprudence, patients complete a pain diary for 6 weeks. After the outcome has been evaluated, the defined index level is addressed with the appropriate minimalist technique.

If clear symptom reproduction occurs at the time of spinal probing and discography, then endoscopic laser foraminoplasty is effected with direct visualization of the extraforaminal, foraminal, epidural, and intradiscal zones and definition and clearance of the pain sites lying therein.

Magnetic Resonance Imaging Scans and Their Shortcomings

Endoscopy reveals that static MRI fails to demonstrate the tethering and impaction on local structures of the superior facet joint, infolded ligamentum flavum, facet joint capsule, foraminal ligament, and superior foraminal ligament. Endoscopy demonstrates that dorsal and shoulder osteophytes not only encroach on the foramen but tether to the nerves and may impinge on the posterior longitudinal ligament. These features are difficult to detect on the MR scan. Static MRI fails to demonstrate the degree of inflammation and irritation within these structures and within the disc.

In addition, it is unable to determine accurately the longevity of a disc protrusion unless it is acutely edematous. The presence of disc protrusions may be directly misleading when compared to the side and site of the true pathology subsequently located by aware state endoscopy.

A number of patients who were thought to have no compression on the nerves on MR scans because of "fat lucency" around the nerve were found to have significant edema of the nerve sheath causing compression of the nerve within the exit foramen. The latter arose in the presence of a dynamically impacting ascending facet joint.

Endoscopy also reveals that the MR scan underestimates the degree of local scarring, vascular hyperemia, and thrombosis occurring within. The mechanism of defining local and referred pain is further obfuscated by the fact that the local structures, when irritated or sensitized, produce distributions of pain otherwise deemed atypical.

The function of the foramen is a delicate balance between the size of he foraminal boundaries and the status of their contents. This balance is easily compromised by pathology, irritation, or sensitization of tethered tissues and abnormal motion. The latter is currently better determined by weight-bearing standing and sitting x-ray films in flexion and extension.

Questionnaires

The questionnaires in this study used the Oswestry disability questionnaire score as an index, PSS, VAPS, and PTAS. The McNab score was initially tried but was considered to be unsatisfactory in identifying the true disability of the patient. As it is a postoperative score it does not reflect performance gain after treatment. The Oswestry disability questionnaire meets all the validation criteria required to assess the outcome of management of spinal conditions (9,30). We did not observe a direct correlation between the Oswestry disability index, PSS, VAPS, and PTAS. Therefore, each index or score is of value in its own right as a means to highlight variables of benefit or inadequacy of the technique and has been evaluated accordingly.

Outcomes

Current concepts in the management of degenerative disease of the spine are limited in concept and hampered by a construction based on indirect diagnosis that inevitably arises from operating on the unresponsive anesthetized patient.

The foramen as a site for compressive entrapment of the nerve root (23) and the anatomic structures that participate in its formation are established. The effect of structural variations, prior surgery, perineural scarring, facet joint and bone disease, and degenerative conditions on the dynamics of the foramen and on the contrivance of lateral recess stenosis is poorly recognized.

In this prospective study we present the results of management of back pain using the viviprudence system of aware state and endoscopic diagnosis of the causes of pain followed by pain source ablation in the epidural, foraminal, and extraforaminal zones combined with lateral recess and intradiscal decompression by means of endoscopic laser foraminoplasty.

Oswestry Disability Index

Using an Oswestry disability index of 50 or more to determine good and excellent outcomes, 55% of patients exceeded this score for back pain, 52% for buttock pain, and 53% for leg pain. The global improvement was 82%, 79%, and 81%, respectively (fair, good, and excellent). In patients with one prior operation, the corresponding values were 51%, 33%, and 29%. Forty-one (89%) of 46 patients who had one to four open operations improved.

Satisfaction Scores

Seventy-two percent of patients were satisfied with the outcome of the procedure.

We believe the reason for the high satisfaction scores was as follows. Fifty-three percent of patients in this study had been left hopelessly without any choice of treatment and had failed to respond to either conservative management or open surgery. Time spent communicating and establishing a good rapport with the patient and providing full information about the operative procedure helped us to obtain better information about painful sites during operation in the aware state and better perioperative rehabilitation. The excellent satisfaction rating that occasionally was reported despite only partial improvement with the Oswestry disability index was obtained because a large proportion of these patients had existed for several years with severe pain that was ameliorated sufficiently to restore quality of life, if only with partial improvement in function.

Visual Analogue Pain Score

On the visual analogue pain scale, 56% patients had more than a 50% improvement, whereas 2% had deterioration of pain symptoms after surgery.

Patient Target Achievement Score

Sixty-two percent of patients were satisfied with the targets achieved specific to their needs, which were chosen prior to surgery. Patients chose 25 objectives that they aspired to achieve as a result of treatment prior to intervention. They had to achieve a successful result in more than half of these objectives to be deemed satisfied.

Revision Surgery

Five percent of patients required revision surgery. Five patients underwent successful revision endoscopic laser foraminoplasty, and five underwent exploration and fusion at other centers.

Multiple Sclerosis

Multiple sclerosis patients are susceptible to complications, such as altered sensations in the legs, after general anesthesia; therefore, many such patients are managed nonoperatively. The patients in this study had marked improvement in pain levels after endoscopic laser foraminoplasty and some functional improvement despite the underlying irreversible status of the pathology.

Spondylolytic Spondylolisthesis

The pain associated with spondylolytic spondylolisthesis can arise from the degenerate deformed disc, neural compression at the foramen, growth of nerve fibers into the pars interarticularis defect, and scarring and entrapment of nerves at the index level.

In this study, endoscopy demonstrated that all patients operated for spondylolytic spondylolisthesis had bony compression and scarring at the foramen. Scarring and adhesions were observed between the spondylolisthetic defect and the disc, between the nerve and disc, and between the bony prominence and the nerve. That 10 of 11 grade I and 3 of 5 grade II spondylolytic spondylisthesis patients had sustained excellent results indicates that endoscopic laser foraminoplasty provides a minimalist day-case technique for the treatment of this pathology.

Dynamic and Adynamic Lateral Recess Stenosis

Management of lateral stenosis conventionally depends on interpretation of the MR scan and clinical findings and leads to a decision to proceed to conservative management, decompression, or fusion. The extent of bony excision needed to bring about adequate decompression is not defined (14,19,28,29,52). The excision of bone at the time of decompression may cause an increase in motion of the spinal segment that, depending on extent, may or may not amount to ''instability'' (40). Excision of a posterior stabilizing structure, the interspinous and supraspinous ligament, as is done in laminectomy, has been shown to significantly increase spinal motion (15). However, many patients with lateral recess decompression undergo spinal fusion to forestall occurrence of the hypothetical, incompletely understood ''spinal instability.''

Weight-bearing x-ray films obtained with the patient standing and sitting both in flexion and extension serve to demonstrate dynamic and adynamic degenerative spondylolisthesis and retrolisthesis. Endoscopic visualization of the foramen has enabled us to identify impaction of nerves and soft tissues arising from indenting facet joint osteophytes, dorsal or shoulder osteophytes, or overriding hyperflexing or hyperextending hypertrophic facet joints. These effects are aggravated by abnormal movements that can be detected on dynamic flexion and extension weight-bearing x-ray films.

Patients can be substratified into those with anterior spondylolisthesis and those with retrolisthesism, which displace during flexion and extension (dynamic group) that corrects to normal alignment or not. Alternatively there is a group with fixed displacement (adynamic group). In this study, 35% had retrolisthesis and 37% had anterior listhesis.

Particular attention to postoperative muscle balance rehabilitation is required for the dynamic group after endoscopic laser foraminoplasty. Endoscopic laser foraminoplasty appears to be encouragingly effective in all these groups. In all groups the best results are achieved when adequate clearance of shoulder and superior facet osteophytes have been ablated, sufficient undercutting has been achieved to allow endoscopic access beyond the foraminal isthmus, and the push-up test is negative at the end of the procedure.

Impact of Multiple Operations

Forty-six patients in this study had conventional surgical interventions without any improvement in their preoperative conditions. These patients had been treated with extended pain management courses after they had been deemed inoperable. All were taking narcotics or nonnarcotic analgesics.

Careful application of viviprudence and the diagnostic tools of spinal probing and discography, their analysis and interpretation, along with deliberate attempts at identification of the exact source of pain endoscopically have allowed us to assist these patients. Resection of scarring, removal of tethering of the nerve to shoulder, superior notch, and dorsal osteophytes, mobilization of the nerve from adherent disc wall, posterior longitudinal ligament, and superior foraminal ligament, and resection of the ascending facet joint have all contributed variously to the amelioration of symptoms. The inflamed tissues produce unexpected atypical distributions of pain, ablation of which may account for the success of the posterolateral exploration and ablation achieved with the endoscopic laser foraminoplasty.

More than half of the patients had good relief of back pain, but the clearance of buttock and leg pain was less effective. This may be a reflection of limitations in technical ability and experience in the ablation of scar tissue, the clearance of the superior notch, especially at the L5–S1 level and more especially in males with narrow android pelvises, and the undercutting of the foramen in grossly settled segments.

Postoperative Flares

Postoperative flares occurred in 28% of patients and were significant in 12%. The flare represented a recurrence of symptoms usually between 5 and 21 days after surgery. The onset of such symptoms coincides with the inflammatory process and may represent revascularization and remodeling of the laser-ablated bone, healing and removal of intradiscal ablated contents, and accumulation of breakdown products in the small operative space caused by the intervention. Timely caudal epidural steroid infiltration with manipulation under anesthesia has helped to relieve symptoms, maintain neural mobility, and restore patients to their appropriate physiotherapy regime with satisfactory outcome.

That these patients responded to steroid infiltration supports the inflammatory hypothesis of the cause of the flare. The flare occasionally has lasted up to 12 weeks. Inappropriate or untimely physiotherapy allowing neural mobilization may promote bleeding and the formation of adhesions between the foraminal margins and epidural surfaces and inflamed neural sheath causing recurrence of scarring and poor outcome. This may explain the recurrence of pain in patients who initially had relief from pain for failed conventional surgery.

Complications

One patient suffered neurologic deficit after surgery. Despite the use of light aware state analgesia and sedation, we failed to establish good communication with this woman of non-

English origin. Prior to this procedure she had extensive foraminal scarring in the absence of prior surgery. She suffered severe dysesthesia postoperatively with ipsilateral (grade 2) foot drop. Nerve conduction studies suggested diminished nerve conduction velocity at the foramen. However, 2 years later her power has recovered considerably (grade 4), but she still has some dysesthesia in the L5 dermatome. It is unlikely that direct nerve damage occurred, but residual swelling of the nerve with proximal nerve root entrapment in the residual scar may account for this unsatisfactory postoperative outcome. The patient refused a postoperative MRI scan.

One patient had an aseptic discitis. He had symptoms of severe painful discitis, but he was afebrile and had normal blood test results. Because of persistent back pain and spasm, he was treated empirically with antibiotics. His symptoms resolved progressively over a 3-month period, and the patient refused biopsy.

Neurologic Recovery

All patients presenting with foot drop arising after prior conventional operations underwent endoscopic laser foraminoplasty. Visualization of the foramen under endoscopy demonstrated combinations of severe foraminal and epidural scarring, osteophytic encroachment into the foramina, and extraforaminal bone ingrowth from prior paravertebral bone graft compressing the exiting nerve at the index level. Conventional midline exploration would have allowed limited access to these pathologic entities; hence, the prevalent concept of reexploration for the relief of long-standing compressive neuropathy is unrewarding. However, encouraging results were obtained after endoscopic laser foraminoplasty, and had this intervention occurred earlier then the results might have been better.

Postfusion Performance Outcomes

Among the six patients who had a spinal fusion, the four patients who had an anterior lumbar spinal fusion obtained the best results with endoscopic laser foraminoplasty. The two patients with a posterior lumbar intervertebral fusion had poor or worse outcomes. A patient who had a noninstrumented posterolateral fusion and a patient with a GRAF ligament stabilization demonstrated satisfactory outcomes. The patients with anterior fusion achieved better results compared to those with posterior fusion. We believe the posterior fusion has a direct correlation with extensive scar formation in these cases and poor outcome.

Blood Loss

Blood loss was limited to short episodes of bleeding until the bleeding source was sealed with the holmium:YAG laser.

Scarring

Scarring was far more prevalent and dense than preoperative MR scanning would suggest. Mature scarring arising from operations more than 3 years prior was significantly underestimated. Postoperative scarring associated with significant early postoperative symptoms possibly associated with postoperative bleeding demonstrated hemosiderin pigmentation. Patients who had prior postoperative infection demonstrated tenacious and dense scarring.

Scarring almost always was associated with vascular bands. The exiting or traversing nerve often was hyperemic and particularly tender at discrete points along its course. A cause was sought for wherever the nerve was inflamed or irritated. This discrete length would be either tethered to inflamed perineural scarring, adjacent impacting ascending facet joint, superior foraminal osteophytes, superior foraminal ligament, foraminal ligament, and facet joint capsule, or adherent to the disc wall or shoulder or dorsal osteophytes. Conversely, scarring could be found at areas of quiescent nerve. Therefore, scarring can coexist with asymptomatic nerves. This bears out clinical and MR scan experience. However, once inflammation or irritation occurs in the perineural scarring and tethering just described and is associated with abnormal movement patterns and impaction and traction on the foraminal and epidural structures, then this is associated with pain that can resist conservative measures and is ably treated by endoscopic laser foraminoplasty without the need for fusion.

Swelling and engorgement of veins and thrombosis therein have been noted endoscopically in the perineural region. These features have been suggested as a cause of lateral recess stenotic symptoms by compromising the space in the spinal exit foramen or compromising neural drainage (10,38,39).

It is likely that chemical irritants cause edema of the nerve and irritation of adjacent tissues and scar (18). Dynamic stenosis arising from either lateral recess encroachment or disc settlement combined with abnormal movements, such as listhesis or facet joint overriding, could lead to further irritation and compression of the nerve causing a vicious cycle of compression, irritation, edema, and further compression. Endoscopic visualization of the edematous inflamed sheath has been observed in the patients in this study, particularly in those with listhesis and settlement or flexion or extension overstrain.

Many theories abound concerning the role of mediators both in the dorsal ganglion and centrally evoked. These theories have been constructed based on the perception that no nociceptive organic structural cause exists to account for the pain. The central and dorsal root ganglion findings may merely reflect the mediator response to enduring and genuine painful stimulation.

Sequestration

Eight of 12 patients with a sequestrated disc had localized back pain as well as buttock and leg pain. Pain arose from the sequestrated disc and the foramen. Two failed to sustain their improvement after six months and were operated elsewhere for sequestrectomy and fusion. On retrospective analysis we recognized that the cause of pain in the leg and buttock was alleviated by the foraminal surgery, but the persistent back pain was due to the intraspinal component, which had been inadequately cleared. Ten of 12 patients had good-to-excellent results and were treated later in the series. This reflects improved technique, experience, and equipment and indicates that this technique can be used for sequestrectomy at this juncture.

Untreatable Patients

One hundred six of these patients were considered untreatable by surgeons elsewhere because either they had been operated before with conventional surgery or no treatable pathology was identifiable on the MR scan. Additional patients were advised against surgery, but surgery had been offered on a deferred basis pending the outcome of pain management therapy. This indicates that there is a well-found reticence to offer conventional surgery except to the most classic of-presenting pathology. This results in a large number of patients being consigned to coping courses and psychological counseling. Many of the patients presenting to the Spinal Foundation had participated in coping courses or pain management programs for extended periods of time until frustration at the enduring symptoms and degraded lifestyle led them to cease attendance with preexisting levels of pain. Viviprudence and keyhole day-case surgery offers a promising opportunity to ameliorate patients' symptoms with sustained results and benefit to the healthcare provider budget.

MST

Fourteen patients in this series were on constant MST therapy. To many spinal surgeons this is a caveat to surgical intervention, yet with endoscopic laser foraminoplasty, this group of patients fared well, with only two requiring medication 2 years later. One patient had taking 300 mg of MST twice a day prior to surgery and at review was on a maintenance dose of 10 mg. The other patient had taking a similar dosage but at review required modest doses of dihydrocodeine. These findings call into question the appropriateness of the prescription of long-term high doses of MST and raises the thesis that these patients need further investigation with viviprudence to locate the source of their pain and endoscopic laser foraminoplasty as an appropriate treatment.

Learning Curve Effect

It should be stressed that this report represents our preliminary surgical experience with this technique, which has been evolving during the treatment of this cohort. The first 98 patients were treated with a fiberoptic endoscope and the remainder with a solid, round, rod lens endoscope developed with Richard Wolf endoscopes. The initial learning curve encompassed several features, including the technique of developing access, definition of structures, appreciation of new unknown pain sources, and ablation of same as we developed the technique. Our report reflects the compass of all the patients treated with this technique without preferential exclusion of the early group.

As our experience grew, the process of extended endoscopic exploration of the foramen, extraforaminal zone, and epidural space and more extensive tissue ablation gradually increased with commensurately higher dosages of laser energy utilization. This was accompanied by more extensive undercutting, scar ablation, and osteophyte resection and more extensive accelerated surgery.

Shortcomings of Endoscopic Laser Foraminoplasty

Endoscopic laser foraminoplasty ideally is used to treat unilateral unisegmental pathology; however, in many cases of bilateral pain, both symptomatic sides improve with endoscopic laser foraminoplasty performed unilaterally. We presume this is because the removal of breakdown products from the index level effects amelioration of irritation on the contralateral side.

For multiple-level pathology, endoscopic laser foraminoplasty at the index level may be supplemented with a minimalist intervention at the adjacent level with benefit. This was not attempted in this reported series.

Endoscopic laser foraminoplasty is a technically demanding procedure that usually requires 90 to 120 minutes to accomplish once the learning curve has been overcome. More technically challenging cases may be undertaken, but this will result in larger amounts of ablation being required with elongated operating times; however, this is being offset by more modern and versatile resection endoscopic mechanical instrumentation.

Equipment Development

The initial endoscope was fiber optic, with a short depth of field and poor lighting and image resolution. The introduction of the rod lens system presented a quantum leap in visualization. Currently there exists a comprehensive system of endoscopic spinal endoscopes, manual tools, side ports, side arms, power burrs, power osteotomes, and side-firing laser probes. The current endoscopic systems are elliptical in shape and facilitate foraminal access, but they were not available for use in this study.

Recurrent Pathology

There has been no symptomatic or MRI evidence of recurrent perineural fibrosis. The results are sufficiently encouraging for us to extend the application of this new endoscopic laser-assisted procedure to replace the need for minimal intervention fenestrectomy, conventional undercutting and fusion in patients with large protrusions, sequestra, settlement, predominantly unisegmental unilateral scarring, or lateral recess stenosis.

Future Application

That so little tissue handling could benefit so many patients who had no available alternatives emphasizes our lack of understanding of back pain and our persistent overreliance on major, potentially damaging surgical procedures such as instrumented or noninstrumented fusions to treat such symptoms.

Endoscopic laser foraminoplasty offers a minimalist procedure that may have increasingly wider application in the future as an alternative to conventional discectomy, decompression, and soft and solid fusion. It also may be used increasingly to treat patients currently denied surgery and who are destined for pain clinic and coping courses until frustration causes them to cease seeking further support from such sources.

The results of endoscopic laser foraminoplasty reported in this study represent the initial attempts to address degenerative disc disease of the spine, lateral recess syndrome, and failed back surgery as a complex of multiple sources of pain production. The principal cause of the ''failure'' of conventional spinal surgery is attributed to ''operating on the wrong level'' (33). Viviprudence and endoscopy indicate that the cause of failure is not only a failure to identify the level but also the pain site therein.

SUMMARY

Endoscopic laser foraminoplasty provides a minimalist means of determining the source of back, buttock, or leg pain either individually or in combination. It allows specific ablation of these pain sources and offers perineural neurolysis and root mobilization, osteophytectomy, and discectomy combined with facet joint resection and prophylactic foraminal undercutting. The process of aware state spinal probing and discography followed by endoscopic laser foraminoplasty is a promising means of identifying and treating the source of the pain of failed back surgery, treating back pain and sciatica of indeterminate origin, and treating lateral recess stenosis and spondylolytic spondylolisthesis. It serves as a useful means of keyhole perineural neurolysis without extensive exploration and fusion and has particular value in the treatment of the elderly or infirm. Endoscopic laser foraminoplasty avoids the morbidity associated with open spinal surgery. Because it identifies and localizes the source of pain before intervention is attempted, it can be offered as a means of treating chronic degenerative disc disease, especially in those in whom conventional treatment is deemed inadvisable. This technique evaluated in its developmental phase offers wider application in the future.

REFERENCES

1. Almay BGL, Johansson F, Von Knorring L, et al. Substance P in CSF of patients with chronic pain syndromes. *Pain* 1988;33:3–9.
2. Anand P, Gibson SJ, Yiangou Y, et al. Phi-like immunoreactive co-locates with the VIP-containing in human lumbosacral spinal cord. *Neurosci Lett* 1984;46:191–196.
3. Andersson SA, Carlsson CA, Eriksson M. *Akupunktur: fran to till vetenskap.* Malmo: Liber, Forlog, 1984.
4. Angtuaco EJC, Holder JC, Boop WC, et al. Computed tomographic discography in the evaluation of extreme lateral disc herniation. *Neurosurgery* 1984;14:350–351.
5. Caspar W, Campbell B, Barbier D, Kretschmmer R, Gotfried Y. The Caspar microsurgical discectomy and comparison with a conventional standard lumbar disc procedure. *Neurosurgery* 1991;28.78–87.
6. Casper GD, Hartman VL, Mullins LL. Results of a clinical trial of the holmium : YAG laser in disc decompression utilizing a side-firing fiber: a two-year follow-up. *Lasers Surg Med* 1996;19:90–96.
7. Casper GD, Mullins LL, Hartman VL. Laser assisted disc decompression: an alternative treatment modality in Medicare population. *J Oklahoma State Med Assoc* 1996;89:11–15.
8. Choy DS, Michelsen J, Getrajdman G, Diwan S. Percutaneous laser disc decompression: an update—spring 1992. *J Clin Laser Med Surg* 1992;10:177–184.
9. Deyo RA, Battie M, Beurskens, et al. Outcome measures for low back pain research: a proposal for standardised use. *Spine* 1998;23:2003–2013.
10. Evans JG. Neurogenic intermittent claudication. *Br Med J* 1964;2:985–987.
11. Fairbank JCT. The incidence of back pain in Britain. In: Hukins DWL, Mulholland RC, eds. *Back pain. Methods for clinical investigation and assessment.* Manchester: Manchester University Press, 1986.
12. Gerber BE, al Khodairy AT, Morscher E, Hefti F. Offene laserchirurgie am bewegungsapparat [Open laser surgery on the locomotor apparatus]. *Orthopade* 1996;25:56–63.
13. Gerber BE, Siebert WE, Morscher E. Chirurgische laseranwendung am bewegungsapparat [Surgical use of laser on the locomotor apparatus] [Editorial]. *Orthopade* 1996;25:1–2.
14. Goel VK, Goyal S, Clark C, Nishiyama K, Nye T. Kinematics of the whole lumbar spine: effects of discectomy. *Spine* 1985;10:543–554.
15. Goswami AKD. *Laminotomy versus laminectomy: is there a difference in stability? A biomechanical study on cadaveric spines.* Thesis submitted for MCh(Orth). Liverpool: University of Liverpool, 1994.
16. Henry JL. Effects of substance P on functionally identified units in cat spinal cord. *Brain Res* 1976;114:439–451.
17. Hijikata S, Yamagishi M, Nakayama T, et al. Percutaneous discectomy: a new treatment method for lumbar disc herniation. *J Toden Hosp* 1975;5:5–13.
18. Hoyland JA, Freemont JA, Jayson MIV. Intervertebral foramen venous obstruction—a cause of perineural fibrosis. *Spine* 1989;14:558–568.
19. Johnsson K, Willner S. Postoperative instability after decompression of lumbar spinal stenosis. *Spine* 1986;11:107–110.
20. Kambin P. Arthroscopic microdiscectomy of the lumbar spine. *Clin Sports Med* 1993;12:143–150.
21. Kambin P. Diagnostic and therapeutic spinal arthroscopy. *Neurosurg Clin North Am* 1996;7:65–76.
22. Kambin P, Casey K, O'Brien E, Zhou L. Transforaminal arthroscopic foraminal decompression of lateral recess stenosis. *J Neurosurg* 1996;84:462–467.
23. Kirkaldy Willis WH. The relationship of the structural pathology to the nerve root. *Spine* 1984;9:49–52.
24. Knight MTN. Laser assisted percutaneous and endoscopic lumbar discectomy. In: Ramani PS. ed. *Textbook of spinal surgery.* Mumbai, India: Department of Neuro and Spinal Surgery, C.T.M. Medical College and Hospital 1996:449–454.
25. Knight MTN, Pantoja S. KTP/532 Percutaneous laser disc decompression for lumbar disc prolapse. *Clin Neurosci* 1996;49:330–336.
26. Knight KTN, Vajda A, Jakab GV, Awan S. Endoscopic laser foraminoplasty on the lumbar spine—early experience. *J Minimally Invas Neurosurg* 1998;41:5–9.
27. Kushlick SD, Ulstrom CL, Michael CJ. The tissue origin of low back pain: a report of pain response to tissue stimulation during operations on lumbar spine using local anaesthesia. *Orthop Clin North Am* 1991;22:181–187.
28. Lee CK. Lumbar spinal instability (olisthesis) after extensive spinal decompression. *Spine* 1983;8:429–433.
29. Lehmann TR, Wilson MA, Crowninshield RD. Load response characteristics of lumbar spine following surgical destabilisation. Presented at 28th Annual Orthopaedic Research Society meeting, paper no. 240, Los Angeles, January 19–21, 1981.
30. Little DG, MacDonbald D. The use of percentage change of Oswestry disability index score as an outcome measure in lumbar spinal surgery. *Spine* 1994;19:2139–2143.
31. Mathews HH. Transforaminal endoscopic microdiscectomy. *Neurosurg Clin North Am* 1996;7:59–63.
32. Mayer HM. Spine update. Percutaneous lumbar disc surgery. *Spine* 1994;19:2719–2723.
33. McCulloch J. Complications of lumbar microdiscectomy. *Acta Orthop Belg* 1987;53:272–275.

34. Mooney V. The failed back: an orthopaedic view. *Int Disabil Stud* 1988;10:32–36.
35. Nachemson A. Recent advances in the treatment of low back pain. *Int Orthop* 1985;9:1–10.
36. Nettelbladt E. Antalet reumatikerinvalder I Sverige under en 30–arsperiod. *OPMEAR* 1985;30:54–56.
37. Onik G, Mooney V, Maroon, JC, et al. Automated percutaneous discectomy: a prospective multi-institutional study. *Neurosurgery* 1990;26:228–232.
38. Parke WW, Gammell K, Rothman RH. Arterial vascularisation of the lumbosacral spinal nerve roots. *J Bone Joint Surg* 1981;63A:53–62.
39. Parke WW, Watnabe R. The intrinsic vasculature of the lumbosacral nerve roots. *Spine* 1985;10:508–515.
40. Posner I, White AA, Edwards T, et al. A biomechanical analysis of the clinical stability of lumbar and the lumbosacral spine. *Spine* 1982;7:374–389.
41. Quigley MR. Percutaneous laser discectomy. *Neurosurg Clin North Am* 1996;7:37–42.
42. Quigley MR, Maroon JC. Laser discectomy: a review. *Spine* 1994;19:53–56.
43. Regan JJ, McAfee PC, Mack MJ. *Atlas of endoscopic spine surgery.* St. Louis, MI: Quality Medical Publishing, 1995.
44. Report of the Commission on the Evaluation of Pain. *Soc Security Bull* 1987;50:13–44.
45. Rydevik B, Brown MD, Lundborg G. Pathoanatomy and pathophysiology of nerve root compression. *Spine* 1984;9:7–15.
46. Scholz M, Deli M, Wildforster U, et al. MRI-guided endoscopy in the brain: a feasibility study. *J Minimally Invas Neurosurg* 1996;39:33–37.
47. Shapiro R. Lumbar discography: an outdated procedure [Letter]. *J Neurosurg* 1986;64:686.
48. Sherk HH. The use of lasers in orthopaedic procedures. *J Bone Joint Surg* 1993;75A:768–776.
49. Simpson JM. Indications for laser surgery in the treatment of degenerative disk disease of the lumbar spine. *J South Orthop Assoc* 1996;5:174–180.
50. Spitzer WO, LeBlank FE, Dupuis M, et al. Scientific approach to the assessment and management of activity related disorders: a monograph for clinicians. Report of the Quebec task force on spinal disorders. *Spine* 1987;12[Suppl]:S1–S59.
51. Terenius L. Endorphins and pain. *Frontiers Hormone Res* 1981;8:162–167.
52. Tibrewal SB, Pearcy MJ, Portek I, et al. A prospective study of lumbar spinal movements before and after discectomy. Proceedings of the International Society for the Study of Lumbar Spine, Montreal, Canada, June 3–7, 1984.
53. Varga PP, ed. *Lumbalis spinalis stenosis.* New York: Springer, 1995.
54. Von Knorring L, Almay BGL, Johansson F, et al. Pain perceptions and endorphin levels in cerebrospinal fluid. *Pain* 1978;5:359–365.
55. Weber H. Lumbar disc herniation: a prospective study of prognostic factors including a controlled trial. Part I. *J Oslo City Hosp* 1978;28:33–40.
56. Weber H. Lumbar disc herniation: a prospective study of prognostic factors including a controlled trial. Part II. *J Oslo City Hosp* 1978;28:89–95.
57. Weisenfield-Hallin Z, Hokfelt T, Lundberg JM, et al. Immunoreactive calcitonin gene-related peptide and substance-P coexist in sensory neurons to the spinal cord and interact in spinal behavioral responses of the rat. *Neurosci Lett* 1984;52:199–204.

Lumbar Spinal Stenosis
edited by Robert Gunzburg and Marek Szpalski
Lippincott Williams & Wilkins, Philadelphia, © 2000.

27

Current Trends in Surgery for Patients with Lumbar Spinal Stenosis of the Degenerative Variety

Dan M. Spengler

Department of Orthopaedics and Rehabilitation, Vanderbilt University Medical Center, Nashville, Tennessee 37232

Patients older than 65 years of age who have lumbar spinal stenosis comprise one of the most common cohort groups to undergo surgical intervention (9), and the number of elderly patients in this group is projected to increase over the next several decades in the United States. This review of the current trends with regard to surgical intervention for patients with lumbar spinal stenosis seems appropriate as well as timely.

Although the biochemical and biomechanical properties of the intervertebral disc change significantly with age, the reported incidence of low back pain does not necessarily increase in the elderly. Valkenburg and co-workers (11) reported that low back pain complaints diminish for both men and women beginning at age 55. This observation is important for orthopedists to recognize, because elderly patients who present with low back pain complaints must be assessed thoroughly to ensure that their complaints are related to the musculoskeletal system as opposed to other disorders that may result in similar complaints (e.g., neoplasm, infection, aneurysm). Patients who present with lumbar spinal stenosis also may suffer from cervical spinal stenosis. Patients with cervical stenosis may develop signs and symptoms of cervical myelopathy, a condition that often requires more immediate surgical intervention. Because cervical myelopathy can result in lower extremity complaints, a careful consideration of this entity must be included in the overall differential diagnosis for elderly patients with spinal stenosis.

CLINICAL EVALUATION

Patient history and physical examination remain most important in the clinical assessment of patients who present for evaluation of low back pain and/or sciatica. The history may alert the clinician to pursue a more exhaustive diagnostic assessment if various red flags are elicited during the interview. The more important questions that should be discussed include a history of trauma, weight loss, fever, infection, night pain, bladder dysfunction, weakness, cancer, and osteoporosis. In addition, patient older than 60 years or younger than 20 years may suggest a more thorough review. Patients with symptoms from lumbar spinal stenosis usually have vague complaints of low back pain with or without radiation to the lower extremities. Pain may increase with walking or, in some patients, the pain may actually be more of an issue at night. The literature suggests that those patients who complain of an increase in pain

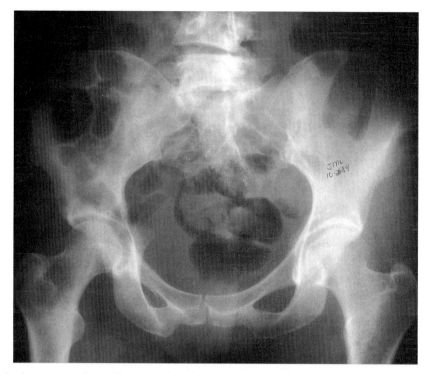

FIG. 1. Anteroposterior radiograph of the pelvis in a 60-year-woman who presented with low back pain and right thigh pain. The lesion in the right greater trochanter was missed initially. The metastatic adenocarcinoma was recognized after the patient underwent an unsuccessful decompression for what was thought to be lumbar stenosis.

complaints with a change in posture or position more likely will improve after appropriate surgical intervention (4). Likewise, patients who have diabetes, previous surgery, psychological issues, back pain worse than leg pain, and no history of claudication type pain likely will not do as well as other patients (4).

The physical examination of patients with lumbar spinal stenosis generally does not reveal major neurologic deficits (8). Patients typically have a flattened lumbar lordosis with increased pain on lumbar extension. Sciatic tension signs are seldom present (8). Minor neurologic findings are common and include weakness of the extensor hallucis longus and various sensory changes. Red flags on physical examination would include a lax anal sphincter, perineal numbness, and/or major neurologic deficits. Plain radiographs of the lumbar spine and pelvis in patients with lumbar stenosis reveal the expected changes typical in an elderly group of patients. Plain radiographs are important, however, to exclude other significant bony changes, such as neoplasia, infection, and spinal deformity (Fig. 1). After the history and physical examination, the clinician must carefully reflect on a thorough differential diagnosis to minimize the chance for an errant diagnosis (Fig. 2).

IMAGING STUDIES

To objectively finalize the diagnosis of lumbar spinal stenosis, advanced imaging studies are necessary. High-resolution magnetic resonance imaging and/or a lumbar myelogram with postmyelogram computed tomography can be recommended. If an associated spinal deformity

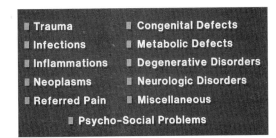

■ Trauma	■ Congenital Defects
■ Infections	■ Metabolic Defects
■ Inflammations	■ Degenerative Disorders
■ Neoplasms	■ Neurologic Disorders
■ Referred Pain	■ Miscellaneous
	■ Psycho–Social Problems

FIG. 2. Differential diagnosis table for low back pain.

or metal surgical implants are present, the myelogram is preferred. How then does one formulate the diagnosis of spinal stenosis? Previous authors have shown that bony measurements alone do not reliably identify patients with degenerative spinal stenosis (2). In most patients, both the degenerative changes that occur in the zygapophyseal joints as well as the soft tissue narrowing associated with the ligamentum flavum create the narrowed spinal canal with a compressed dural sac (2). The diagnosis of lumbar spinal stenosis in the degenerative spine is warranted when the anteroposterior diameter of the dural sac is 10 mm or less (Fig. 3) (2,8). In normal subjects, the anteroposterior diameter of the dural sac is approximately 15 mm. Lateral recess stenosis is somewhat more difficult to diagnose, but a recess smaller than 2 mm suggests stenosis laterally.

NONOPERATIVE TREATMENT

Once the diagnosis of lumbar stenosis is confirmed, the patient has an option of treatments that may circumvent or delay the need for surgical intervention. However, if significant

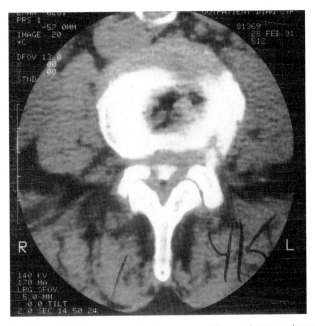

FIG. 3. Axial section from a lumbar computed tomographic myelogram demonstrates marked lumbar spinal stenosis, primarily from the ligamentum flavum and the enlarged zygapophyseal joints.

neurologic deficits are present, I recommend prompt surgical decompression. Nonoperative approaches include symptomatic treatment and activation. Patients may notice a decrease in symptoms with salicylates or nonsteroidal antiinflammatory drugs. Both types of medications can be associated with complications, especially in an elderly population. Most commonly gastrointestinal distress and/or gastrointestinal bleeding may occur. Patients need to be followed carefully so that these complications can be appropriately recognized and managed. Epidural steroid injections are useful to consider before recommending surgical intervention. Epidural steroid injections may be associated with a range of complications but, in general, such an approach is less invasive than surgery. If patients notice significant symptomatic relief with one of the approaches described, a physical therapy program can be initiated to enhance aerobic conditioning and trunk strengthening, depending on the goals and objectives of the individual patient. Selected patients may notice some improvement with an abdominal binder. If this symptomatic treatment is ineffective, surgical intervention may be recommended, assuming the patient's quality of life is adversely impacted to the point where an elective surgical procedure is warranted. This decision is reached interactively by the patient and surgeon. The surgeon must emphasize that no result can be guaranteed, and approximately 15% of patients will not improve or actually will experience worsened symptoms after surgery (8).

SURGICAL INTERVENTION

A number of factors are considered in the surgical decision analysis. The surgical indications for most patients include the fact that nonoperative treatment did not provide relief. In addition, the patient must view his or her quality of life as unacceptable. Certainly, progressive neurologic deficits or a cauda equina syndrome would justify prompt surgery, but such presentations are most uncommon in elderly patients with lumbar stenosis.

Other surgical considerations include age, health, comorbidities, and associated spinal conditions. Two main issues need to be addressed in any patient who is a candidate for surgical intervention. First, the type of decompression most likely to result in adequate neural relief should be recommended. Second, the issue of surgical stabilization should be discussed. Is fusion necessary and, if so, what type?

Surgical decompression can be achieved successfully through a variety of approaches, which include multiple laminotomies, wide laminectomies, and laminoplasty. Postacchini et al. (6) compared patients with lumbar stenosis who underwent multiple laminotomies versus those who underwent wide laminectomy. They reported no significant differences in clinical outcome at 4-year follow-up. They observed that multiple laminotomies took longer to perform and that patients who underwent multiple laminotomies had a 12% (3 of 26) chance for nerve root injury. In addition, 9 (26%) of 35 patients who underwent multiple laminotomies had to be converted to wide laminectomy later. The clinical outcomes for patients with lumbar spinal stenosis who undergo surgical decompression without fusion varies from 59% to 85% good-to-excellent results (1,5,7,8,10).

DEGENERATIVE SPONDYLOLISTHESIS WITH LUMBAR STENOSIS

Most authors agree that patients who have degenerative spondylolisthesis and lumbar stenosis should undergo both surgical decompression and surgical stabilization. The one remaining controversial issue is whether spinal instrumentation should be used. Fischgrund and co-workers (3) performed a prospective study on patients with degenerative spondylolisthesis.

In addition to decompression, one group was fused by the traditional *in situ* posterolateral approach. The other group of patients underwent spinal instrumentation in addition to the posterolateral fusion. At 2-year follow-up, no significant changes in outcomes were observed between the two groups of patients (3). With respect to fusion, however, the instrumented patients had a much higher fusion rate. My indications for instrumentation in these patients would include a dynamic instability greater than 5 mm, evidence of progression of the spondylolisthesis over time, history of smoking, and a patient who requires a more extensive decompression to sufficiently compromise spinal stability. Outcome expectations in patients who undergo decompression and fusion for degenerative spondylolisthesis range from 80% to 90% good results.

LUMBAR STENOSIS ASSOCIATED WITH SPINAL DEFORMITY

Patients who have lumbar stenosis associated with a spinal deformity present a challenge for optimal management. Although only a paucity of objective data exists with respect to these patients, certain principles remain useful. If a patient with a spinal deformity has a focal or single-level spinal compression with radicular complaints that are consistent with the imaging finding, the best approach may be a "keyhole" decompression without fusion (Fig. 4). This approach can be affirmed further by performing a single nerve root injection preoperatively to see if symptomatic relief is obtained. The patient must be informed that curve progression is a possibility after decompression. If progression occurs, a more extensive spinal fusion will be necessary. Patients who have significant rotatory deformities and/or lateral lithesis at the site of neural compression should, in my opinion, have both decompression and an instrumented fusion (Figs. 5 and 6). Although the outcome for patients who have scoliosis and stenosis is less favorable than for patients with spinal stenosis who have no deformity, the surgeon should likely note good outcomes in 70% to 75% of patients.

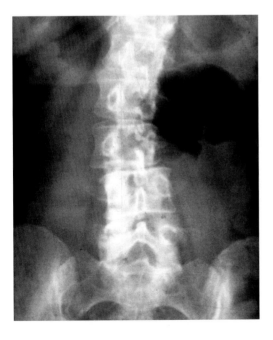

FIG. 4. Anteroposterior radiograph of the lumbar spine reveals the type of spinal deformity in which a "keyhole" decompression would be warranted if the imaging studies revealed a single-level problem that is affirmed by a selective nerve root injection.

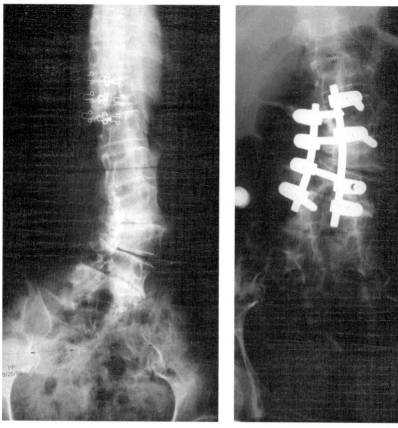

A   B

FIG. 5. Anteroposterior radiographs taken preoperatively **(A)** and postoperatively **(B)** in a 53-year-old woman with a significant rotatory deformity in the midlumbar area. Computed tomographic myelogram confirmed marked spinal stenosis. Spinal instrumentation and fusion were performed in addition to lumbar decompression to prevent curve progression.

WHEN TO FUSE PATIENTS WITH LUMBAR SPINAL STENOSIS

I recommend that all patients with degenerative or isthmic spondylolisthesis have spinal fusion in addition to an appropriate decompression. I instrument approximately 70% of these patients. I also recommend spinal fusion for any patient who has evidence of segmental hypermobility or instability on dynamic motion radiographs. Those patients with multiple previous spinal surgeries who present with another symptomatic stenotic level also are candidates for surgical fusion in addition to decompression. I also recommend surgical fusion for any patient who needs to have spinal stability compromised to adequately decompress the neural elements (e.g., resection of the facet joint). Finally, those patients with spinal deformity who require decompression and who are not candidates for "keyhole" decompression should undergo fusion.

COMPLICATIONS

Although the focus of this review is not on surgical complications, mention of complications must be made to put the risk-to-benefit ratio in perspective. In general, the rate of complica-

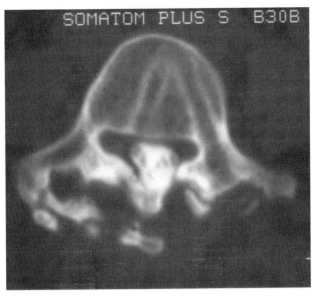

FIG. 7. Axial computed tomographic scan of a patient who presented with no function in the right L5 nerve root secondary to improper surgical placement of a lumbar pedicle screw.

tions will rise in proportion to the length of the procedure and the associated medical/surgical conditions exhibited by the patient. In a healthy elderly patient who undergoes only a single-level decompression for stenosis, the most likely complication would be a dural tear. Repair usually is uncomplicated, with no long-term consequence. In patients who undergo extensive decompression and fusion for stenosis, complications are more likely. In my 5-year experience with 148 patients who underwent lumbar fusion, I noted complications in 15% of the primary cases (no prior surgery) and 24% of the revision cases. In addition, the complication rate was 21% for patients who underwent an instrumented spinal fusion versus 16% for those who underwent *in situ* fusion without instrumentation. Thus, complications certainly occur in these patients. A realistic review of the common problems likely to be encountered (5% or greater) should be undertaken with the patient to ensure that the patient understands the potential risks that may occur when a spinal surgeon attempts to provide the benefits of surgery. Complications related to technical mishaps can be minimized by careful surgical technique and by thoughtful preoperative planning (Fig. 7).

SUMMARY

Patients commonly present for evaluation and management of their lumbar stenosis. I believe that the surgical outcomes for these patients remains good. To optimize outcome, proper surgical selection must be combined with a proper surgical procedure. The techniques and perioperative management must be excellent. To combine all of these parameters with good postoperative rehabilitation will lead to an improved quality of life for our patients and a keen sense of accomplishment for the surgeon.

REFERENCES

1. Anahsinen O, Herro A, Turunen V, et al. Surgical outcome of 438 patients treated surgically for lumbar spinal stenosis. *Spine* 1997;22:2278–2282.

2. Bolender N, Schonstrom N, Spengler D. Role of computed tomography and myelography in the diagnosis of central spinal stenosis. *J Bone Joint Surg* 1985;67A:240–246.

3. Fischgrund J, MacKay M, Herkowitz H, et al. Degenerative lumbar spondylolisthesis with spinal stenosis: a prospective randomized study comparing decompressive laminectomy and arthrodesis with and without spinal instrumentation. *Spine* 1997;22:2807–2812.

4. Gary J. Lumbar spinal stenosis: postoperative results in terms of posture related pain. *J Neurosurg* 1990;72: 71–74.

5. Mardjetko S, Connolly P, Shott S. Degenerative lumbar spondylolisthesis, a meta-analysis of literature 1970–1993. *Spine* 1994;19:22565–22655.

6. Postacchini F, Cinotti G, Perugia D, Gumina S. The surgical treatment of central lumbar stenosis. Multiple laminotomy compared with total laminectomy. *J Bone Joint Surg* 1993;75B:386–392.

7. Sivlers H, Lewis P, Usch H. Decompressive lumbar laminectomy for spinal stenosis. *J Neurosurg* 1993;78: 695–701.

8. Spengler D. Current concepts review. Degenerative stenosis of the lumbar spine. *J Bone Joint Surg* 1987;69A: 305–308.

9. Spivak J. Current concepts review: degenerative lumbar spinal stenosis. *J Bone Joint Surg* 1998;80A:1053–1066.

10. Tuite G, Stern J, Doran S. Outcome after laminectomy for lumbar spinal stenosis, part I: clinical correlations. *J Neurosurg* 1994;81:699–706.

11. Valkenburg H, Huanen H. Epidemiology of low back pain. NIAMMD Workshop of Idiopathic Low Back Pain, Miami, Florida, 1980.

Lumbar Spinal Stenosis
edited by Robert Gunzburg and Marek Szpalski
Lippincott Williams & Wilkins, Philadelphia, © 2000.

28

Pedicular Fixation in Lumbar Stenosis

Bruce E. Fredrickson

*Department of Orthopedic Surgery, SUNY Health Science Center—Syracuse,
Syracuse, New York 13202*

Lumbar spinal stenosis has multiple causes; however, the most frequent cause is degenerative. Less frequent causes include congenital stenosis in otherwise normal people and stenosis related to various genetic abnormalities, such as dwarfism. Conservative measures to relieve the discomfort caused by neural compression include various antiinflammatory agents, rest, exercises, and various forms of epidural injections. Surgical treatment of these problems always incorporates some form of spinal canal decompression. This can be accomplished in multiple ways, but generally it involves removal of the lamina, a portion of the facet complexes, and redundant ligaments.

The presurgical anatomy generally includes some combination of disc space settling with secondary annular bulging, facet overgrowth, subluxation of the facets with migration of the superior facet proximally, and infolding of the redundant capsular and ligamentous structures. The disc collapse may be associated with either a coronal or sagittal plane deformity, depending on the degree and location of disc loss. Subluxation of the vertebras likewise may be seen as disc height is lost and the annular structures become redundant. The degree of subluxation appears to be dependent first on the amount of disc collapse, second on the orientation of the disc to the horizontal plane, and third on the orientation of the facet joints.

The postoperative anatomy is different from the preoperative anatomy in that there is always some resection of the bony and ligamentous structures. Resection of these structures may predispose the spine to further deformity. Neither the preoperative imbalances nor the postoperative potential instability can be addressed adequately with conservative measures. Serious consideration must be given to stabilization (arthrodesis) of the spine if either significant preoperative imbalance exists or potential postoperative instability is created.

The use of internal fixation in conjunction with a spinal arthrodesis for this problem has been attempted for a number of years The goals of such instrumentation are first to reduce any coronal or sagittal plane imbalance and second to maintain these positions while the arthrodesis heals. It was only with the development of pedicular fixation that these two goals could be met satisfactorily. Earlier forms of fixation, including facet screws and various hook/rod combinations, proved to be inadequate or potentially even to increase spinal deformities.

Several studies have tried to determine if arthrodesis in conjunction with stabilization is superior to decompression alone and whether instrumentation provides any further benefit. The majority of these studies have looked at degenerative spondylolisthesis; there are no good comparative studies for other forms of imbalance. Herkowitz and Kurz (2) in 1991 reported a prospective comparative study between decompression and decompression and fusion. Their results favored decompression and fusion over decompression alone. Zdeblick

(4) in 1993 attempted to determine whether instrumentation added further improvement over fusion alone. He demonstrated an improved fusion rate with the use of pedicular instrumentation. Bridwell et al. (1) in 1993 also reported on the use of instrumented versus noninstrumented fusions for degenerative spondylolisthesis. They found improved functional outcome in patients with instrumentation in addition to improved spinal balance and fusion rates. Fishgrund et al. (3) in 1997 reported on a study similar to that of Bridwell et al. They reported an improved fusion rate with the use of instrumentation as did Zdeblick and Bridwell et al.; however, their clinical outcomes were statistically similar. It appears from review of the literature that fusion combined with instrumentation is beneficial in a select group of patients. Those with degenerative spondylolisthesis appear to have a higher fusion rate and improved clinical result with instrumentation (Fig. 1). Instrumentation for other lumbar deformities has not been shown to date to be beneficial in a prospective randomized trial; however, numerous case studies have documented its effectiveness in reducing and holding deformities while the arthrodesis is consolidating (Fig. 2).

Selection of the appropriate pedicle screw system must consider the following issues: (i) the biocompatibility and mechanics of the specific device; (ii) the ease of insertion from the surgeon's standpoint; (iii) the flexibility of the system to adapt to multiple changes in local anatomy; and (iv) the profile of the system as it affects the ability of local musculature to provide adequate vascularization to the bone graft site. Not every system is appropriate for every case; however, certain generalities can be stated about each of the four points.

Two materials currently are in use for spinal fixation systems. The first is 316 L stainless steel and the second is titanium and titanium alloys. The two materials differ in their mechanical properties; stainless steel is approximately twice as stiff as the titanium implant and approximately 28% stronger in ultimate strength if it has the same geometry. However, the corrosion and abrasion properties of titanium are superior to those of stainless steel. Histologic

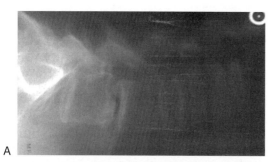

A

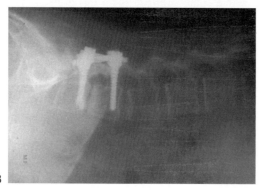

B

FIG. 1. Preoperative anteroposterior **(A)** and lateral **(B)** x-ray films of the lumbar spine in a patient with typical symptoms of pseudoclaudication and findings of degenerative spondylolisthesis.

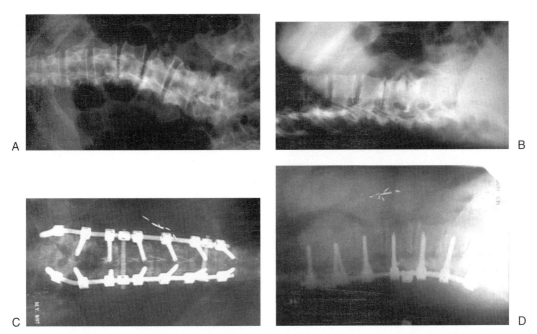

FIG. 2. Preoperative anteroposterior **(A)** and lateral **(B)** x-ray films of a patient with collapsing lumbar scoliosis secondary to degenerative changes. Postoperative anteroposterior **(C)** and lateral **(D)** x-ray films show reduction of the deformity, recreation of normal lumbar lordosis, and the low profile of the SDRS system.

studies suggest that titanium implants are better tolerated than stainless steel implants. Imaging of the two materials shows a significant improvement in the computed tomographic and magnetic resonance images with titanium (Fig. 3).

The locking mechanism between the rod and pedicle screw has proved to be one of the more critical areas in selection of the system for individual physicians. The locking mechanism not only determines the stability of the device in terms of slipping of the screw on the rod, but it also is extremely important in terms of ease of insertion and overall profile of the device. The wedgelock system is unique in that it does not rely on a thread/nut connection. This eliminates the difficulty of cross threading and at the same time significantly reduces wear debris. Figure 4 illustrates the axial stability of various systems, and Fig. 5 shows the torsional stability of the same systems. The ideal locking mechanism would have a very low profile that allows maximum contact of the surrounding musculature with the bone graft and yet provides the most rigid fixation between the rod and the screw. Table 1 shows the comparative data between various systems on the market.

Screw design is extremely important in terms of the ultimate and fatigue strength of the screw and its pullout resistance. The majority of pedicle screws today have a thicker proximal inner diameter and a thinner distal one. This optimizes strength in the area of the pedicle where fatigue fracture has proved to be most common and optimizes pullout strength within the cancellous bone by the larger distal thread. Figure 6 shows comparative pullout strength between some of the screws currently on the market.

The ideal stiffness of a specific implant construct is not known. We know that increasing stiffness in a system can lead to improved fusion rates; however, as the system becomes too

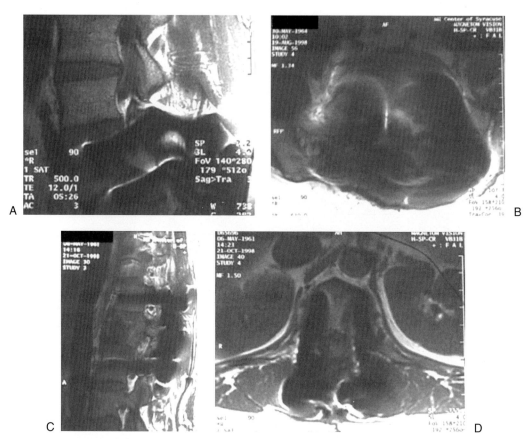

FIG. 3. Sagittal **(A)** and axial **(B)** magnetic resonance images of the stainless steel implant with significant artifact precluding any useful interpretation. Sagittal **(C)** and axial **(D)** magnetic resonance images of a titanium segmental implant. Interpretation is possible even with the artifact created.

TABLE 1. *Mechanical properties*

Material	Young's modulus (GPa)	Ultimate strength[a] (MPa)	Yield strength[a] (MPa)	Abrasion (μm)	Corrosion $1/R_p(M\Omega^{-1}\ cm^{-2})$
316L stainless steel	193	965	690	—	1.52 ± .52
High-strength 316L stainless steel	193	1,105	860	33 ± 6	—
C.P. titanium (grade IV)	104	550	485	—	—
Ti 6Al-4V (ELI)	114	860	795	21 ± 9	0.66 ± .42
Anodized Ti 6Al-4V (ELI)	—	—	—	7.9 ± 1.5	—

[a] Minimum acceptable strength
From refs. 1–4.

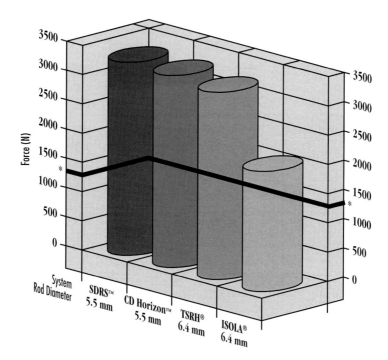

FIG. 4. Component axial slip strength results. Forces from flexion or extension are simulated. Axial pushdown load was recorded at 1.5 mm of slip. (Courtesy of Surgical Dynamics, a subsidiary of Tyco Healthcare Group, Norwalk, Connecticut.)

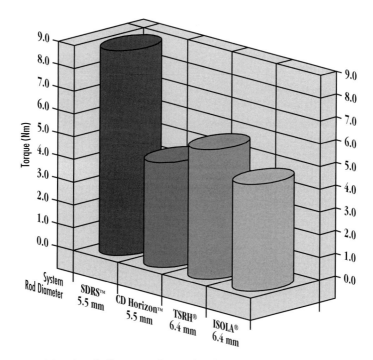

FIG. 5. Component torsional slip strength results. Torsional loads simulate rotational forces tested. Recorded at 5 degrees of slip. (Courtesy of Surgical Dynamics, a subsidiary of Tyco Healthcare Group, Norwalk, Connecticut.)

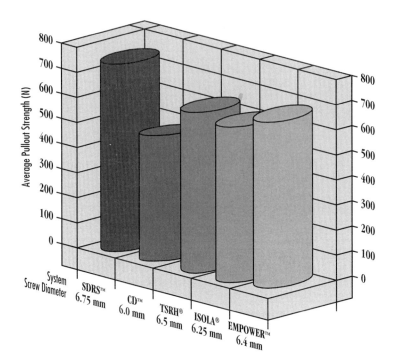

FIG. 6. Screw pullout strength. (Courtesy of Surgical Dynamics, a subsidiary of Tyco Healthcare Group, Norwalk, Connecticut.)

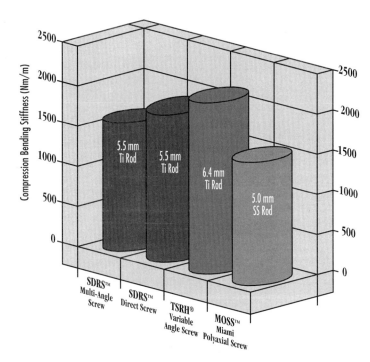

FIG. 7. Construct compression bending stiffness. Excessive flexibility may lead to pseudoarthritis. (Courtesy of Surgical Dynamics, a subsidiary of Tyco Healthcare Group, Norwalk, Connecticut.)

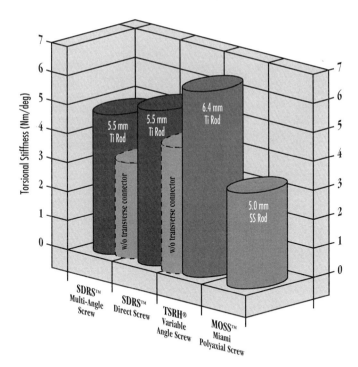

FIG. 8. Construct torsional stiffness. (Courtesy of Surgical Dynamics, a subsidiary of Tyco Healthcare Group, Norwalk, Connecticut.)

stiff some degree of stress shielding of the underlying bone occurs. Until further information is available about the dichotomy between stiffness and stress shielding, clinical experience indicates that the currently available systems all provide reasonable degrees of stiffness with only a few exceptions (Figs. 7 and 8).

Fatigue strength is the last important parameter that must be assessed. There currently exist ASTM standards that allow comparison among the various systems. Any system eventually will fail if the fusion does not consolidate; therefore, a minimum resistance of the system to fatigue is necessary. Figures 9 and 10 show typical fatigue strengths of systems currently on the market.

The three system characteristics other than biocompatibility and mechanics include the ease of insertion, flexibility, and profile of device. These three characteristics all interrelate and can only be assessed fully in the operating room. Many systems that appear to be easy to insert in cadavers become extremely difficult with the added soft tissues. Additionally, it is only as one attempts to use systems for increasingly complex cases that one can better appreciate the true flexibility and adaptability of a system.

SURGICAL SECTION

The following surgical technique is for a single-level instrumentation and fusion at L5–S1 using the SDRS (Surgical Dynamics, Norwalk, Connecticut) spinal fixation system.

Burr the initial cortex at the entry point for your screw. Use the detachable bone probes for your initial pedicle preparation. There are two types of probe shafts: grooved and solid.

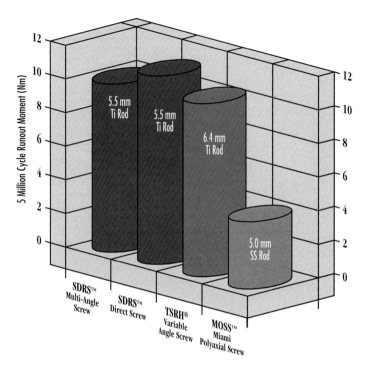

FIG. 9. Construct fatigue gauged by the number of repetitive loadings a spinal construct can withstand at a specific stress level. (Courtesy of Surgical Dynamics, a subsidiary of Tyco Healthcare Group, Norwalk, Connecticut.)

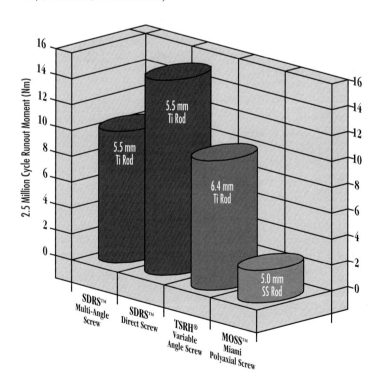

FIG. 10. Interconnection fatigue isolates the fatigue strength of one component, such as a screw or hook, and its connection to the spinal rod. (Courtesy of Surgical Dynamics, a subsidiary of Tyco Healthcare Group, Norwalk, Connecticut.)

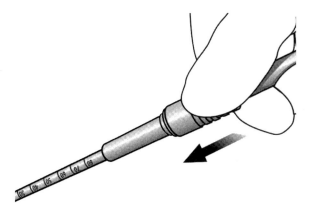

FIG. 11. Push the collet on the T-handle forward to connect and disconnect probe shafts. (Courtesy of Surgical Dynamics, a subsidiary of Tyco Healthcare Group, Norwalk, Connecticut.)

Push the T-handle forward (Fig. 11) to connect or disconnect probe shafts. Insert the probe (Fig. 12) and detach the handle. Continue until all four probes are placed. Use grooved probes for the patient's left side and solid probes for patient's right side (Fig. 13).

SRDS screws are self-tapping, but the author chooses to use the tap provided. Tap each screw site using the ratcheting T-handle, tap, and drill sleeve that also serves as a soft tissue protector. Tap to the preferred depth using the calibrated markings from the shaft of the tap (Fig. 14).

Assemble selected screws onto screw inserter using the arrows for alignment and entering from the gold side of the screw. Tighten the knob to hold the screw (Fig. 15). Insert screws into each pedicle. The inserter is removed by turning the knob counterclockwise and sliding the inserter in the opposite direction of the arrows on the screws and inserter (Fig. 16).

Rods are available precut in 10-mm increments for lumbar surgeries. You can cut to length as desired. Use the rod bender to contour the rod as needed. Hold the bent rod with the rod holder and drop into head of screws.

Assemble the locking cap with the cap holder. Squeeze the initial squeezer to start the

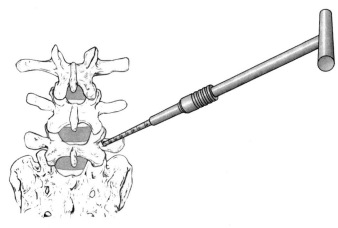

FIG. 12. Insert probe into the pedicle to the appropriate depth mark. (Courtesy of Surgical Dynamics, a subsidiary of Tyco Healthcare Group, Norwalk, Connecticut.)

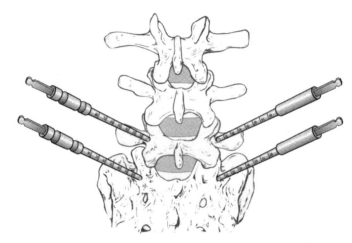

FIG. 13. Insert probes on each side. Use grooved probes on one side to determine probe orientation on sagittal x-ray film. (Courtesy of Surgical Dynamics, a subsidiary of Tyco Healthcare Group, Norwalk, Connecticut.)

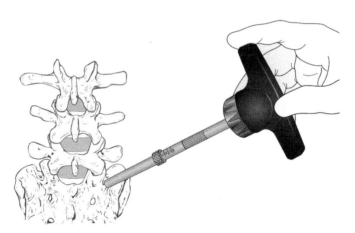

FIG. 14. Tap appropriate depth through the drill sleeve that serves as a soft tissue protector. Screws are self-tapping; thus, surgeons may choose not to tap. (Courtesy of Surgical Dynamics, a subsidiary of Tyco Healthcare Group, Norwalk, Connecticut.)

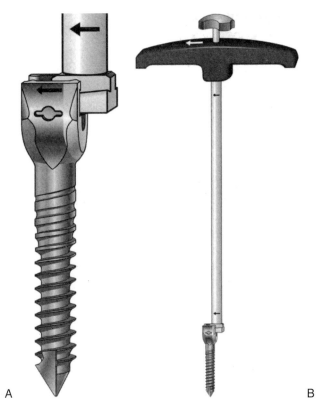

A   B

FIG. 15. A: Assemble selected screw onto screw inserter using the arrows for alignment. **B:** Tighten the knob to hold the screw. (Courtesy of Surgical Dynamics, a subsidiary of Tyco Healthcare Group, Norwalk, Connecticut.)

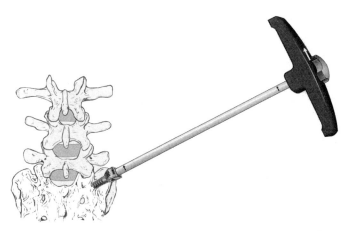

FIG. 16. Insert screw to the proper depth. Remove inserter by twisting knob counterclockwise and sliding the inserter in the opposite direction of the arrows on the screw and inserter. Repeat steps for remaining screws. (Courtesy of Surgical Dynamics, a subsidiary of Tyco Healthcare Group, Norwalk, Connecticut.)

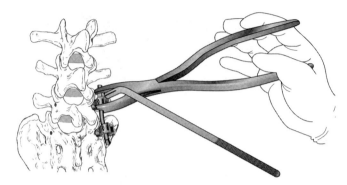

FIG. 17. Assemble cap with cap holder. Squeeze with the initial squeezer to start the cap. (Courtesy of Surgical Dynamics, a subsidiary of Tyco Healthcare Group, Norwalk, Connecticut.)

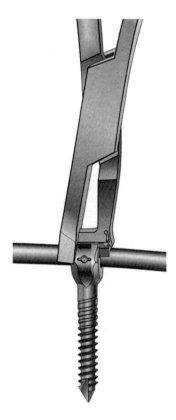

FIG. 18. Use the cap inserter/removal tool to start locking cap. With arm down, the cap will stop halfway across, allowing the screw to slide freely but blocking the rod from springing free. With arm up, the cap will go 80% across, which holds distraction/compression in most cases. (Courtesy of Surgical Dynamics, a subsidiary of Tyco Healthcare Group, Norwalk, Connecticut.)

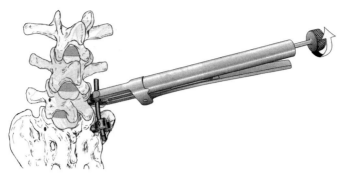

FIG. 19. Rod reduction. Place rod persuader on screw head and turn knob clockwise until rod is fully seated into the head of the screw. (Courtesy of Surgical Dynamics, a subsidiary of Tyco Healthcare Group, Norwalk, Connecticut.)

locking cap (Fig. 17). Alternatively you can use the single-hand method by using the cap inserter/removal tool to start the locking cap (Fig. 18).

Rod reduction or persuasion may be necessary to accomplish certain surgical goals, such as reduction of spondylolisthesis. To accomplish this maneuver, SDRS has an inline reduction tool that aligns directly with the screw shaft. This avoids taking up additional room on the rod or rocking the rod, which can occur with reduction systems designed to operate offset from the screw shaft. Place the rod persuader on the screw head and turn the knob clockwise until the rod is fully seated into the head of the screw (Fig. 19). Use an appropriate angled cap squeezer to start the locking cap (Fig. 20). Remove the rod persuader once the cap is started.

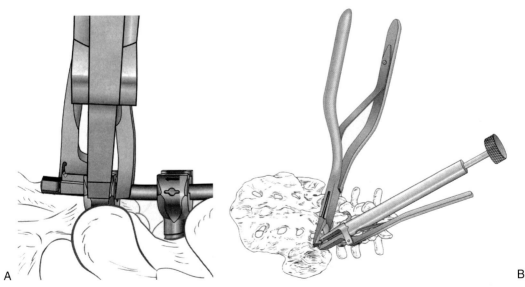

A

B

FIG. 20. A: Use appropriate angled cap inserter with locking cap. Click into first tab using the cap squeezer. **B:** Remove rod persuader once the locking cap engages in the first tab. (Courtesy of Surgical Dynamics, a subsidiary of Tyco Healthcare Group, Norwalk, Connecticut.)

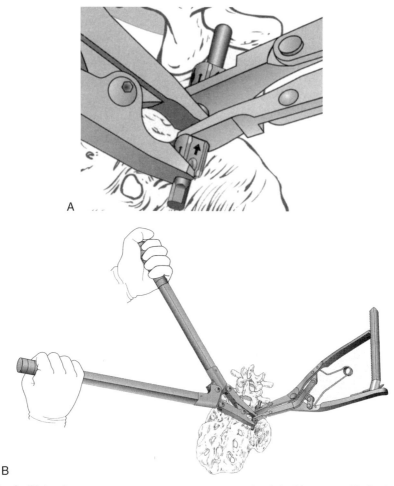

FIG. 21. **A:** Distract or compress screws as necessary. Lock locking cap with final squeezing tool. **B:** Repeat procedure on the other side. A rod gripper can be placed behind the screw being locked to prevent rod migration. (Courtesy of Surgical Dynamics, a subsidiary of Tyco Healthcare Group, Norwalk, Connecticut.)

Distract or compress screws as necessary. Lock the locking cap with the final squeezing tool and repeat until all caps are locked (Fig. 21). For *in situ* fixation, use a rod gripper behind the screw being locked during the final locking.

The cross connector consists of cross-bar clamps, a half rod, and locking caps. Cut and bend the half rod as required. Assemble the cross-bar clamp by sliding onto the screw inserter and aligning the arrows on the implant and inserter. Twist the clamp on the rod and slide the inserter out opposite of the arrows. Repeat on the opposite side (Fig. 22).

Drop the transverse road into clamp heads. Insert the locking cap using the cap holder and initial squeezer (Fig. 23). Use the final squeezer to lock the locking caps (Fig. 24).

If locking cap removal is desired, you have two options. If the cap is not completely locked you can use the cap inserter/removal tool. Place the front peg into the hole on the locking cap, then squeeze and remove cap (Fig. 25). If the cap is completely locked, use the ratcheting removal tool. Always remove the cap by pushing it opposite the arrow (Fig. 26).

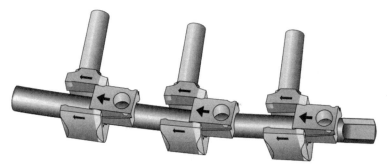

FIG. 22. Preassemble offset connectors on rod. (Courtesy of Surgical Dynamics, a subsidiary of Tyco Healthcare Group, Norwalk, Connecticut.)

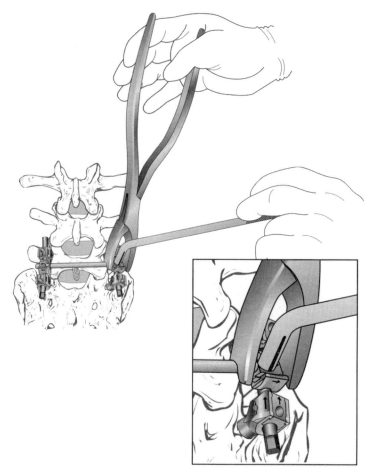

FIG. 23. Cut transverse rod connector as desired and drop into clamp heads. Using cap holder, place the cap on the transverse rod connector. Tighten and lock with the initial cap squeezer. (Courtesy of Surgical Dynamics, a subsidiary of Tyco Healthcare Group, Norwalk, Connecticut.)

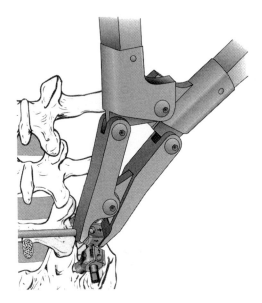

FIG. 24. Use final squeezer if necessary to lock cap. (Courtesy of Surgical Dynamics, a subsidiary of Tyco Healthcare Group, Norwalk, Connecticut.)

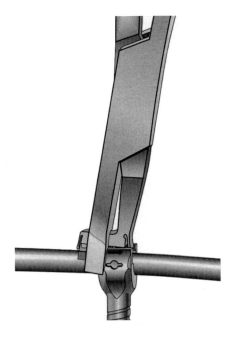

FIG. 25. Prior to complete locking, use cap inserter/removal tool. Place front peg into hole on locking cap. Squeeze tool and remove cap. (Courtesy of Surgical Dynamics, a subsidiary of Tyco Healthcare Group, Norwalk, Connecticut.)

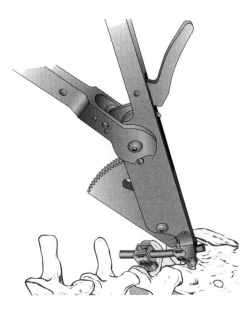

FIG. 26. After complete locking, use ratcheting removal tool. Push cap in the opposite direction of the locking cap. (Courtesy of Surgical Dynamics, a subsidiary of Tyco Healthcare Group, Norwalk, Connecticut.)

CONCLUSIONS

Pedicular fixation is the preferred method of internal fixation in cases of lumbar spinal stenosis that requires fusion. Selection of the appropriate system depends on (i) biocompatibility and mechanics of the device, (ii) ease of insertion, (iii) flexibility of the system, and (iv) profile of the device. Appropriate selection of the system used definitely can enhance the surgeon's ability to reduce and maintain proper spinal balance, fusion rates, and clinical outcomes.

REFERENCES

1. Bridwell KH, Sedgewick TA, O'Brien MF, Lenke LG, Baldus C. The role of fusion and instrumentation in the treatment of degenerative spondylolisthesis with spinal stenosis. *J Spinal Disord* 1993;6:461–472.
2. Herkowitz HN, Kurz LT. Degenerative lumbar spondylolisthesis with spinal stenosis. A prospective study comparing decompression with decompression and intertransverse process arthrodesis. *J Bone Joint Surg Am* 1991;73: 802–808.
3. Fishgrund JS, Mackay M, Herkowitz HN, Brower R, Montgomery DM, Kurz LT. 1997 Volvo Award winner in clinical studies. Degenerative lumbar spondylolisthesis with spinal stenosis: a prospective, randomized study comparing decompressive laminectomy and arthrodesis with and without spinal instrumentation. *Spine* 1997;22: 2807–2812.
4. Zdeblick TA. A prospective, randomized study of lumbar fusion. Preliminary results. *Spine* 1993;18:982–991.

Lumbar Spinal Stenosis
edited by Robert Gunzburg and Marek Szpalski
Lippincott Williams & Wilkins, Philadelphia, © 2000.

29

Instrumented Posterolateral Interbody Fusion

Patrick J. Depraetere

Heilig-Hartziekenhuis, 8800 Roeselare, Belgium

This chapter presents our experience from 1997 and 1998 with the application of instrumented posterolateral interbody fusion (PLIF), its fusion rate, and clinical outcome. Our results are compared with data reported in the literature.

The rationale of fusion is simple: Eliminate pathologic motion to relieve pain. Bluntly stated: "If it doesn't move, it doesn't hurt." However, anyone acquainted with spinal fusion might be aware that the pursuit of full fusion perhaps is not so important in terms of clinical outcome, as we probably all have encountered patients without union or with partial union who do well after surgery. Yet the need for full fusion is generally accepted. As 80% of the load on the spine is carried by the anterior column, it seems logical and biomechanically correct to fuse the anterior column, a procedure that is preferred in our hospital, but which apparently does not prevail in the literature (3). The controversies are aimed more at the need for additional posterior instrumentation.

Some studies, such as the clinical study of Thomson et al. (7) from Aarhus, concluded that in 130 patients with bilateral intertransverse process arthrodesis (BIPA) with and without instrumentation, fusion rate and clinical results were statistically equal. However, more retrospective and prospective studies, such as the randomized study of Zdeblick (8), show a higher fusion rate of 80% to 90% with instrumentation in contrast to the noninstrumented cases with a fusion rate of approximately 65%. Fischgrund et al. (4) reported a prospective analysis of 67 patients and stated that successful arthrodesis was obtained in 83% of the instrumented cases and only 45% of the noninstrumented ones. However, in this study, clinical outcome was not clearly correlated with higher fusion rate.

A recent meta-analysis (6) of four prospective studies indicated a better outcome (with pain as the main parameter) and concluded slightly in favor of fusion with posterior instrumentation.

Additional spinal instrumentation is expected to increase fusion rate, shorten rehabilitation time, and probably improve clinical results or patient satisfaction. However, we also must bear in mind the inherent disadvantages of this procedure: increased surgical trauma with greater blood loss, longer operation time, and risk of screw misplacement, which are factors that might have a negative influence on outcome.

MATERIALS AND METHODS

From January 1997 to August 1998, 94 patients underwent spinal instrumentation for various disorders: severe degenerated disc syndrome, spinal stenosis, degenerative facet syndrome with lateral recess stenosis and narrowing of the neural foramen, postlaminectomy instability (failed back syndrome), and spondylolisthesis.

The most important determination is the most appropriate surgical procedure, not only in terms of fusion rate but also in terms of clinical outcome. The operative options in lumbar spinal stenosis are decompressive laminectomy; decompression with arthrodesis; and decompression, arthrodesis, and spinal instrumentation (2).

The predominant preoperative symptoms were radicular pain or paresis, including neurogenic claudication in 73.5% of patients, low back pain only in 2%, and mixed radicular and vertebral symptoms without predominance in 24.5%.

Eight patients underwent instrumented PLIF and 14 had BIPA. Patient distribution, average age, and levels of implant were as follows: 38 women (33 PLIF and 5 BIPA) and 56 men (47 PLIF and 9), giving a ratio of 40% women and 60% men who were included in this study.

Ages ranged from 24 to 76 years for women (average 51 years 6 months) and 25 to 77 years for men (average 53 years 5 months).

The most frequently involved level was L4–5 with 83 cages inserted, followed by L5–S1 with 52 cages, and, in decreasing order, L3–4 with 34, L2–1 with 20, and L1–2 with 4. A total of 193 cages were used. Three patients had a single cage placed at the midline because the configuration of the cage and the available intersomatic space did not match. Of the 80 PLIF cases, 25 patients received 54 PEEK (polyether-ether-ketone) cages, 54 patients received 139 titanium cages, and 1 patient had autologous bone grafts harvested from the iliac crest.

RESULTS

Follow-up duration varied from 3 months to 1 year 10 months. Sixteen of 25 patients with PEEK cages had follow-up of more than 1 year. All the patients with PEEK cages were evaluated at 1, 3, 6, and 12 months, according to their functional and economic status, daily-life activities, and clinical signs. Improvement rate evolved steadily to 81% after 1 year. We also measured the bone density in the cages and the adjacent endplates to assess the speed and extent of fusion.

Of the 80 instrumented PLIF patients we reviewed, four dropped out for various reasons. One patient died of unrelated causes, two patients did not comply with the follow-up protocol, and one alcoholic woman showed up once, approximately 1 year after surgery.

Of the remaining 76 patients, 9 had a fair-to-poor outcome and 67 had excellent-to-good results (12% and 88%, respectively). As these values do not distinguish between patients on prolonged sick leave before surgery and other patients, the excellent-to-good result may be underestimated. Furthermore, in Belgium the tradition of granting generous sick leave benefits does not encourage employees to return to work. A Finnish report of 438 patients illustrates this point. An important retrospective study by Airaksinen et al. (1) reported that 60% of preoperatively (self) employed patients returned to work versus only 31% of patients on sick leave.

Complications were minor and included two superficial infections, one delayed fusion of the 25 PEEK cage patients (operated August 28, 1998), and five nonunion of the 51 titanium cases. Fusion was obtained in 93% of the titanium cages and 96% of the PEEK cages. The overall fusion rate in our series was 92%. No instrumentation had to be removed, and there was no material fracture or displacement.

Fusion was assessed on plain dynamic x-ray images with the following criteria for titanium cages: no angulation of more than 5 degrees while bending and the absence of a black line between cage and adjacent endplates. For PEEK cages, the evaluation was much easier and unambiguous. Radiologically confirmed fusion of the latter occurred within 2 to 6 months; rod/screw (18 patients) or plate/screw (7 patients) combinations did not influence the speed of fusion.

CONCLUSION

It is important for spinal surgeons to define some standard treatment of well-defined conditions, such as spinal stenosis and spondylolisthesis. This is especially true in a health care system where third party insurance companies attempt to impose their treatment algorithms.

Key questions are as follows: "Is fusion rate really higher in combination with posterior instrumentation?" and "Is clinical outcome better in patients with a higher fusion rate?" The answer to the first question, in our opinion and that of others (5), certainly is "affirmative." The answer to the second question is "probably yes."

Despite the skepticism of the last 10 years, a growing number of experienced spine surgeons are in favor of the combination of arthrodesis and posterior instrumentation as state-of-the-art treatment of any spinal disorder that requires fusion, including many cases of lumbar stenosis.

REFERENCES

1. Airaksinen O, Herno A, Turunen V, Saari T, Suomlinen O. Surgical outcome of 438 patients treated surgically for lumbar spine stenosis. *Spine* 1996;22:2278–2282
2. Bridwell KH, Sedgewick TA, O'Brien MF, Lenke LG, Baldus C. The role of fusion and instrumentation in the treatment of degenerative spondylolisthesis with spinal stenosis. *J Spinal Disord* 1993;6:461–472.
3. Caputy A, Luessenhop A. Long-term evaluation of decompressive surgery for degenerative lumbar stenosis. *J Neurosurg* 1992,77:669–676.
4. Fischgrund J, MacKay M, Herkowitz H, et al. Degenerative lumbar spondylolisthesis with spinal stenosis: a prospective randomized study comparing decompressive laminectomy and arthrodesis with and without spinal instrumentation. *Spine* 1997;22:2807–2812.
5. Herkowitz HN. Degenerative lumbar spondylolisthesis. *Spine* 1996;20:1084–1090.
6. Mélot C. Clinical trials in surgery: methodologic and statistical criteria of validity, with example of meta-analysis of randomized trials in spine surgery. In: *Instrumented Fusion of the Degenerative Lumbar Spine*. Philadelphia: Lippincott-Raven, 1996, 281–289.
7. Thomsen K, Christensen F, Eiskjaer S, Hansen E, Fruensgaard S, Bünger C. The effect of pedicle screw instrumentation on functional outcome and fusion rates in posterolateral lumbar spinal fusion: a prospective, randomized clinical study. *Spine* 1997;24:281–322.
8. Zdeblick TA. A prospective, randomized study of lumbar fusion. Preliminary results. *Spine* 1993;18:982–991.

Lumbar Spinal Stenosis
edited by Robert Gunzburg and Marek Szpalski
Lippincott Williams & Wilkins, Philadelphia, © 2000.

30

Posterior Lumbar Interbody Fusion Using an Original Screwed Titanium Device: LIFEC Expandable Cages

A Retrospective Study of 48 Patients with a Minimal Follow-up of 1 Year

David Attia

Département de Chirurgie du Rachis, Clinique Kennedy, Montelimar 26200, France

Posterior lumbar interbody fusion (PLIF) is the most satisfying technique used for lumbar arthrodesis (9–11,17). The graft is set between two large and flat cancellous bony surfaces, in compression, just in the mechanical axis of charge of the lumbar column.

Nevertheless, since its description by Cloward (3–5) in 1943, after many modifications, this technique did not achieve the success expected. Most spine surgeons preferred posterolateral athrodesis (PLA), despite its inherent risk of pedicular screwing, difficulties with bone fusion (6), which requires large muscle release and a large volume of graft harvesting and is performed at a less favorable site, histologically and biomechanically.

The poor results attributed to PLIF are due to technical difficulties and the morbidity, and particularly graft instability, source of migration, and pseudoarthrodesis.

Since the advent of intersomatic cages (2,14), the use of PLIF has been revived. These new devices have several benefits:

- Simplification of the technique
- Immediate stability by preventing collapse of the graft and its migration. However, other problems can occur, such as impaction on vertebral plates, graft resorption, nonfusion, and cage migration.

For this new concept, we considered the following requirements:

- Lordosing action, to maintain the physiologic aspect of the lumbar spine
- Large contact surface between graft and vertebral plates, as in titanium screwed cages
- Good stability, to avoid the risk of migration
- Smaller overall dimensions for easier setting, being as conservative as possible with the posterior elements, facets, interspinal ligament, and, above all, muscle vascularization, and avoiding excessive stretching of neural structures.

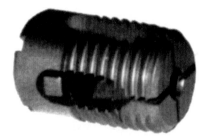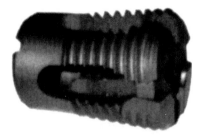

FIG. 1. The LIFEC cage. Note the the 6-degree lordosis while the cage is expanded, flattening of its contact faces, and wide windows.

DESCRIPTION OF THE LIFEC CAGES

Made of TA6V titanium, the LIFEC cage (Advanced Spine, Irvine, CA) has a cylindrical/ovoid shape, which is adapted to the vertebral plate shape. It is threaded, so it is easily set in the disc space by screwing, which provides the first element of stability (Fig. 1). It is hollow and widely fenestrated. After expansion, it has a large internal volume that allows bone graft filling and has large windows that expose the vertebral plates, promoting intersomatic fusion.

The most interesting characteristic is the possibility of expansion *in situ*, as the cage:

• Provides strong bone moorage, which increases its stability
• Is easy to implant because of its smaller overall dimensions when it is not expanded
• Restores disc space height and widens the foramen
• Restores discal lordosis, providing about 6 degrees of anterior sinus.

After expansion and bone filling, the cages are sealed by a titanium screwed cap.

The cage is shaped like a cylinder, is separated into four branches in its anterior part, and is threaded on the outside so that it can be implanted by screwing. Inside, a washer can be pushed from posterior to anterior, which spreads the four branches and expands the cage. This washer is made with two lateral wings that slide through the lateral windows between the branches so as to avoid their sinking in compression. The expansion is achieved, after insertion of the cage inside the disc space, using a specific ancillary device. The cage can be easily unexpanded and removed, if necessary, using a special tool.

Another interesting aspect is that the cage, which initially is cylindrical, turns into a parallelepiped shape. Its upper and lower sides are flattened after expansion, which improves its contact with the endplates.

BIOMECHANICAL STUDIES

Titanium complies with technical requirements of elasticity and high-level mechanical resistance, which allow expansion without breakage. The limit of elasticity was tested in the laboratory to determine the optimal degree of expansion before plasticity, without risk of weakening.

The resistance of the cages also was tested on an INSTRON 8540 machine, at a capacity of 40 kN and a precision of 25 N.

Compression was achieved between two PTFE plates, one fixed and one on a pivot, to adapt the pressure to the obliquity of the cage. This extra-high-density polyethylene has a tensile modulus of 120 to 150 MPa, which is close to that of vertebral plate bone.

Measurements were taken by extensometry gauges (KYOWA 120) in the constraint concentration zones, on the proximal body, and in the transition radius of the side windows. Measurement of distortion was made by blade displacement sensors that were put through the lateral windows of the cage.

Results were as follows:

- Static compression resistance: 11-mm diameter: 11,000 N, 13 mm: 15,000 N, 15 mm: 25,000 N, supported without breakage.
- Dynamic tests: under a charge of triangular cycles of 200 to 3,000 N at a frequency of 8 Hz, each cage underwent 5,000,000 cycles without any deformation, controlled by an optic microscope on the fragility zones.

Efforts were stopped when these values were obtained, because they correspond to loads that are much superior to the physiologic norm of spine loads (1,7,8,12). Shirazi (16) noted that the maximal charge on lumbar vertebrae while bearing 4,000 N was 900 N. Biomechanical studies showed the rebalancing forces on 45-degree kyphosis measured 4,670 N, shared among several vertebrae. Schultz (15) evaluated the lumbar charge with the patient in sitting position at 380 N and in the standing position carrying 8 kg at 2,350 N. Moreover, 1,000,000 cycles correspond to about 4 months of normal activity.

MATERIALS AND METHODS

Materials

Forty-eight consecutive patients (26 men and 22 women; ages 24 to 72 years, average 43.4) with degenerative disc diseases (n = 27), with or without disc herniation (4 cases), failed back surgery syndrome (n = 14), isthmic spondylolisthesis grades I to III (n = 6), and degenerative pseudospondylolisthesis (n = 1) were operated on using a minimally invasive technique and LIFEC expandable cages.

The target level was L4–5 in 14 patients, L5–S1 in 25 patients, and both levels in 9 patients.

Twelve patients had previous surgery: 1 spondylolisthesis with pseudoarthrodesis after posterior instrumented two-level fusion, 11 surgical discectomies (one of which was operated twice before), 1 multioperated with posterior arthrodesis failure, and 2 had previous chemonucleolysis.

Indications for treatment were intractable low back pain in all patients, which was associated with consequent sciatica in 42 cases, sensory deficit in 15, and severe motor deficit in 4. All patients underwent preoperative radiography, computed tomography, and/or magnetic resonance imaging of the lumbar spine (myelography). History of complaints was more than 6 months. Fourteen patients were heavy smokers (more than ten cigarettes per day). Nine patients were on long-term disability preoperatively. The average follow-up was 19 months (range 12 to 27).

Postoperative Evaluation

Patients were seen postoperatively at 6 weeks, 3, 6, 12, and 24 months, and at term.

Anteroposterior, lateral, and Ferguson x-rays views were taken at 3, 12, and 24 months. In cases of doubt about fusion, flexion/extension radiographs were taken at the last visit.

The last term clinical status was evaluated by a score calculated on the following scale (points in parentheses):

- Low back pain and radicular pain: permanent (0); severe, at rest (1); on effort (2); moderate (3); none (4)

- Neurogenic claudication: less than 100 m (0); 100 to 500 m (1); more than 500 m (2); none (3)
- Neurologic deficit: severe (0); moderate (1); none (2)
- Drugs absorption: major, using morphine (0); daily (1); frequent (2); occasional (3); none (4)
- Daily life: impossible (0); impeded (1); slightly limited (2); normal (3).

This score, derived from a Stauffer and Coventry modified score based on 20 points, gives us the relative gain calculated using the formula: (final score − initial score)/(20 − initial score), which is an evaluation of the percentage of recovery.

Fusion success was determined by:

- Absence of any dark halo around a cage on the anteroposterior, lateral, and Ferguson radiographic views
- Continued presence of visible bone within the cages, seen on the lateral view, well observed through the wide lateral windows
- Absence of motion on flexion/extension radiographic views, using a radiographic overlay method to assess angular change at the segment(s).

Surgical Technique

At induction of anesthesia, all patients received an intravenous dose of a third-generation cephalosporin continued every 8 hours for 24 hours postoperatively.

Patients were operated on while in the prone position on iliac crests supports, with the abdomen free of compression. It is essential to obtain a maximal flat back during the installation so as to open maximally the posterior spaces. Reduce the lordosis, but the expansion will give it back by itself.

A small incision is made, with minimal soft and hard tissue dissection when compared to bilateral laminotomy for discectomy at the target level. Most of the articular facets are preserved (always more than half) and the conservation of the interspinous ligament is usually possible. The space need only fit the diameter of the chosen cages. Epidural venous bleeding is controlled by bipolar coagulation with perioperatively controlled hypertension. After neural release and maximal discectomy, prepare the cage location with the specific ancillary, delicately drilling into the space with canulled drills through a guidewire and avoiding an incorrect path in the vertebral plates (Fig. 2).

In contrast to most other cylindrical screwed cages, it is important to achieve minimal refreshment of the vertebral plates, to avoid as much as possible cage sinking into the vertebral plates.

The size of cages to be set is evaluated by taking measurements from preoperative imaging studies, but the final element of choice is the stability of the drill in the space, considering that the drill diameter is 1.5 mm smaller than the corresponding cage before expansion.

While setting the cage and expanding it *in situ,* obtain widening of the disc space, reopening of the foramen, and restoration of lordosis. Then complete the bone refreshing through the windows, using a 3-mm angulated curette inside the cage after expansion, without any risk of removing the cortical bone on charge in contact with the cage.

Well-cleaned and morselized bone from the initial release can be used as graft for fusion. The graft can be completed if necessary by using bone harvested from the posterior iliac crest. The disc space can be filled with graft between and lateral to the cages.

Expansion increases the anterior diameter by 2 to 2.5 mm. This expansion, with subchondral support (without going to cancellous endplate bone), allows minimal bone resection and

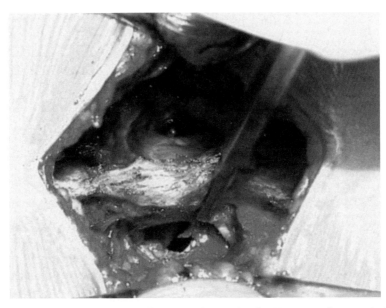

FIG. 2. The surgical approach. L5–S1 level. Cage size is 13 mm and expanded. There is conservation of the interspinous ligament and two thirds of the facets (in this case). There is no excessive lateral muscle release.

avoids root stretch injury, which is in contrast to most other cylindrical screwed titanium cages available. Under these conditions, we consider this technique to be minimally invasive surgery.

Generally, ambulation began on the first postoperative day; hospitalization averaged 5 postoperative days. Patients wore a lumbar belt all the time for 1.5 months and decreasingly during the following month.

Results

Complications included one case of foot drop, after delirium tremens, without compression at surgical revision, on postoperative day 1. An ischemic aspect of the L5 root was noted. This patient showed complete recovery after 3 months.

No cage breakage or migration occurred at any time after implantation in any patient. No LIFEC cages needed to be removed, and there were no other complications (Fig. 3).

The results were statistically the same for smokers and nonsmokers, and for obese people (6 cases) and nonobese, whatever the level or number of levels.

Forty percent (19 or 47) of the patients had a pathologic junction level seen on magnetic resonance imaging as a black disc on T2 without herniation. There was a minor difference in the result, which consisted of residual mild low back pain that was moderate and not disabling and did not require medication.

There was also a minor difference, although not statistically significant, among patients with previous surgery, with mild residual radicular pain in some cases.

There was one failure that was an error of indication in a 52-year-old obese woman who had severe osteoporosis and degenerative instability at the upper level. Early impingement of the cages in the vertebral endplates occurred; the patient was reoperated after 5 months by two-level posterior arthrodesis, with a medium final result (score increase from 13 to 14).

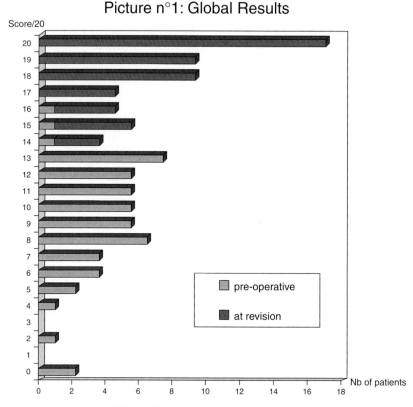

FIG. 3. Overall results of LIFEC use.

There were three mediocre results (but all improved their scores, with a gain of 40% to 44%):

- One patient had atypical positional low back pain and a psychiatric hysterical profile. His sciatica improved.
- One patient improved his score from 11 to 15, for a relative gain of 44%. This patient was 53-year-old man, disabled by schizophrenia, who was operated on because of L5–S1 major collapsed degenerative disc disease, with pathologic unstable junction.
- One 52-year-old patient, with chronic degenerative severe L5–S1 and moderate L4–L5 discopathy, suffered bilateral sciatica for many years with sensory deficit and distal S1 radicular pain by disafferentation. His pain decreased by using daily low doses of neuroleptics.

There were 44 satisfying results (91.4%): 16 patients (36%) had an excellent result (with a final score of 20 of 20, gain 100%), and 28 patients (58.3%) had good results (gain more than 60%).

Radiologic fusion seems complete on x-ray films in all patients but one, who has a halo around the cages noted on the anteroposterior view and no motion on dynamic x-ray films. This patient had complete improvement of his radicular pain, but still had residual low back pain from stage V to III; he is satisfied with the result.

Analysis of the results shows a large decrease in cases of sciatica. Sciatica disappeared in

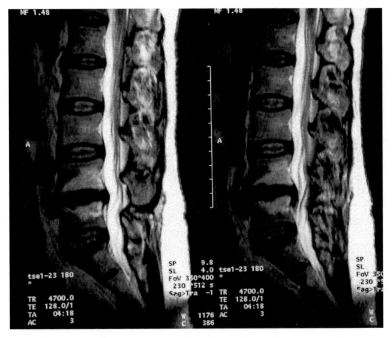

FIG. 4. Magnetic resonance image shows disc herniation with degenerative severe aspect, type Modic I, in a 36-year-old woman with chronic low back pain and bilateral sciatica.

31 patients; decreased to moderate and not limiting in 14 patients, most after previous surgery due to fibrosis; 3 patients suffer on effort, and no patient suffers at rest.

Low back pain disappeared in 26 patients; decreased to moderate in 17 patients; 5 patients suffer on effort, most due to the existence of degenerative adjacent level; and no patient suffers at rest.

Results on neurogenic limping and neurologic deficit are excellent. It disappeared in all but one patient, who was the failure subject.

Daily life improved significantly as follows:

- Initially, 9 patients were disabled and 16 considered their lives to be impeded postoperatively.
- Finally, 37 patients have a normal life, 10 patients feel "slightly limited" because they had to change work or stop participating in a sport, and 1 feels impeded (the failure subject) (Figs. 4 and 5).

DISCUSSION

The benefits of interbody fusion increasingly are being recognized. Biomechanically it is the ideal place for spinal fusion; it is the best way to widen back the disc space; it is less aggressive than posterior fusion for the paravertebral muscles; and it requires less volume of graft, which limits the morbidity associated with iliac crest harvesting. Other elements to consider are the dangers of pedicular screwing (6) and the instability at the junction level, because of possible damage to the lower part of the facet and the high lever arm of posterior fixation.

Even though there is no consensus on how to perform interbody fusion, the literature seems

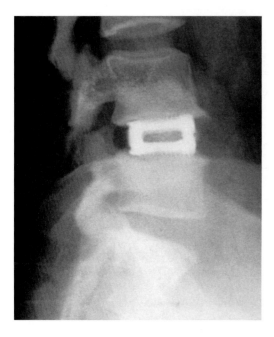

FIG. 5. Complete clinical recovery at 9-month follow-up. Radiologic aspect of the fusion shows good restoration of the lordosis and no impingement on the vertebral plates.

to favor cylindrical titanium screwed cages. The disadvantages of these devices are their excessive exterior size, which involves risk of stretching on neural structures, and the need for subsequent bone and facet removal if the chosen procedure is a PLIF. Anterior lumbar interbody fusion has its own difficulties and complications (10), so we do not routinely use this technique.

The LIFEC device for PLIF reduces the overall dimensions, such that:

- Expansion increases the anterior diameter by 2 to 2.5 mm, after the cage is implanted in the disc space,
- The goal is to refresh the bone of vertebral plates to the subchondral level, but not cancellous bone, to achieve strong support for expansion. Then the endplates can be deeper refreshed through the windows on the surface that is not under charge, but which is in contact with the graft.

Especially in cases of recurrent surgery, expansion provides a real advantage in reducing the traction on such retracted and fibrous roots and avoiding extensive neural release.

Other advantages of expansion include:

- Procuring strong bone anchorage and avoiding any risk of migration. However, the right size to completely fill the space must be chosen (do not underestimate the size).
- Restoring physiologic lordosis. A study comparing two series of 20 patients, presented by Noriega Trueba and Noriega Gonzalez (13) at the Spanish Spine Society Congress, recently demonstrated the superiority of this device to restore lordosis in contrast to other cylindrical titanium screwed cages.
- Improving surface contact with the endplates when the upper and lower faces of the cage are flattened.
- Bringing immediate stability, which results in quick recovery. In our patients, most of the time posterior synthesis was not required (Fig. 6).

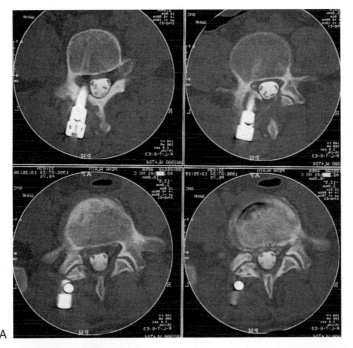

A

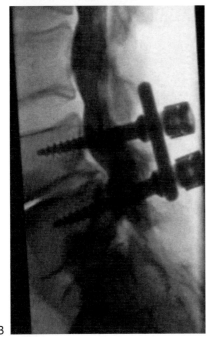

B

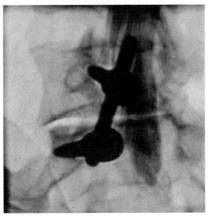

C

FIG. 6. A 33-year-old man, who was a work accident victim, underwent nine surgeries from 1989 to 1995 and was disabled for 3 years. He had permanent low back pain, left sciatica, and foot drop. He was treated with lumbar brace, morphine, and neuroleptics. Walfing perimeter: 100 m. Note disc collapse, persistent disc herniation, L5 left root injury caused by the intercanalar screw, and absence of posterior fusion. Despite fibrosis, there was no problem with surgical technique. Fusion was achieved after 3 months. At 17-month follow-up there was no lumbar or radicular pain. There was neurologic recovery of foot and toe extensors from 2 to 4 + normal lumbar active motion, and he was not wearing a lumbar belt. He was back to work after 6 months. **A:** Computed tomographic scan showing the direct L5 left root injury caused by the intracanalar screw and the absence of fusion. **B:** Lateral view myelogram showing disc collapse and persistent disc herniation. **C:** Oblique view myelogram showing malposition of the screw injuring the root. *(Figure continues.)*

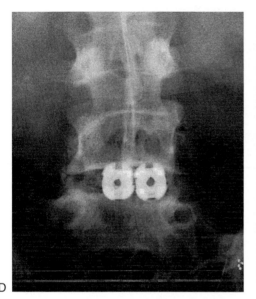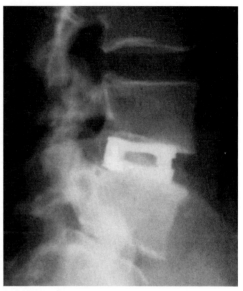

D   E

FIG. 6. *Continued.* **D:** Anteroposterior view postoperative x-ray film. **E:** Lateral view postoperative x-ray film showing fusion in good position and correction of lordosis and disc height.

CONCLUSION

Posterior lumbar interbody fusion remains a palliative surgery for degenerative disc diseases by suppressing natural disc motion. Clinically it results in near complete recovery. Anatomically it is associated with a good rate of fusion, restored physiologic lordosis, good disc opening, and foramen widening. It results in minimal complications, is a safe and conservative procedure, with an ancillary simplified to its minimum, is a technique that is not difficult for surgeons once they become accustomed to it, and is easy to teach to other spine surgeons.

At follow-up of 12 to 27 months, LIFEC expandable cages gave 91.7% satisfactory functional and radiologic results. No patient became worse.

This new device is stand-alone stable, maintains disc height and lumbar physiologic lordosis, favors interbody fusion, provides good pain relief, and leads to early recovery.

REFERENCES

1. Blaimont P, Alamel M. Biomécanique de l'arthrodèse lombaire. *Acta Orthop Belg* 1981;47:605–618.
2. Brantigan JW, Steffee AD. A carbon fiber implant to aid interbody fusion: two-year clinical results in the first 26 patients. *Spine* 1993;18:2106–2107.
3. Cloward RB. The treatment of ruptured lumbar intervertebral discs by vertebral fusion. Indications, operative technique. After care. *J Neurosurg* 1953;10:154–158.
4. Cloward RB. Lesions of intervertebral discs and their treatment by interbody fusion methods. *Clin Orthop* 1963; 4:27–32.
5. Cloward RB. Posterior lumbar interbody fusion updated. *Clin Orthop* 1985;193:16–19.
6. Davne SH, Myers DL. Complications of lumbar spinal fusion with transpedicular instrumentation. *Spine* 1992; 17:S184–S189.
7. Diop A, Skalli W, Lavaste F. Tests et épreuves biomécaniques incontournables pour le développement d'une nouvelle instrumentation rachidienne. *Cah Enseign SOFCOT* 1995;53:20–27.
8. Evans JM. Biomechanics of lumbar fusion. *Clin Orthop* 1983;193:38–46.
9. Hutter CG. Posterior intervertebral body fusion, a 25 year study. *Clin Orthop* 1983;179:86–96.
10. Lerat JL, Basso MP, Moyen B. Arthrodèse lombaire intersomatique postérieure—comparaison avec les autres méthodes d'arthrodèse. Technique—indications-résultats. *Cah Enseign SOFCOT* 198728:275–280.

11. Lin PM. Posterior lumbar interbody fusion technique. Complications and pitfalls. *Clin Orthop* 1985;193:90–102.
12. Nachemson A. The loads of lumbar discs in different positions of the body. *Clin Orthop* 1965;45:107–122.
13. Noriega Trueba JJ, Noriega Gonzalez D. Analisis comparativo de la angulacion sagital lumbar despues de la realizacion de un PLIF con implantes metalicos cilindricos y expansivos. Proceedings of the Annual Meeting of the Spanish Spine Society (GEER), Murcia, 1998.
14. Ray CD. Threaded titanium cages for lumbar interbody fusion. *Spine* 1997;22:667–679.
15. Schultz C. Andersson GB. Analysis of loads on the lumbar spine. *Spine* 1981;6:76–82.
16. Shirazi A. Finite element evaluation of contact loads on facets of L2-L3 segments in complex loads. *Spine* 1991;16:494–502.
17. Wiltberger BL. Intervertebral body fusion by the use of posterior bone dowel. *Clin Orthop* 1964;35:69–79.

Lumbar Spinal Stenosis
edited by Robert Gunzburg and Marek Szpalski
Lippincott Williams & Wilkins, Philadelphia, © 2000.

31

Dynamic versus Rigid Spinal Implants

Archibald von Strempel, Andreas Neekritz, *Phillip de Muelenaere, and
†Guillaume du Toit

*Annastift, Department III, 30625 Hannover, Germany; *Muelmed Hospital, Arcadia,
South Africa 0083; and †Constantiaberg Medi-Clinic, Cape Town, South Africa 7800*

The last decade has seen a rapid increase in the use of implants in spinal surgery, not only for deformity surgery but also for degenerative disorders, particularly of the lumbosacral spine. Utilization of implants for this latter surgery has been controversial. Critics maintain that an equal rate of success can be achieved without implants (where fusion is performed with decompression) while at the same time avoiding implant complications (33). In contrast, the use of implants for correction of spinal deformities and stabilization of unstable fractures and tumorous vertebral destruction is generally accepted.

In a review of the literature, Boos and Webb (4) determined that the use of stable internal fixation with pedicle screws to achieve fusion in the degenerative spine has a higher fusion rate than without instrumentation.

A further advantage of the stable implants is the ability to influence alignment of the spine, especially in multisegmental fusions. Decompression can be achieved without the risk of destabilizing the motion segment.

Development of modern internal fixation systems utilizing pedicle screws that were applied to spinal fractures were more stable than the old hook-based systems and had several advantages (7,10,24): (i) shorter instrumentation and fusion, (ii) improved ability to correct deformities, and (iii) shorter period of immobilization.

Increasing experience and longer follow-up periods have resulted in numerous reports about implant breakages and dislocations (1,3,16,22,27).

Other reports indicated a possible stress-shielding effect leading to decrease in bone density in the instrumented segment of the fusion (17).

This chapter reports the results of a prospective multicenter study on use of the segmental spinal correction system (SSCS). This system provides a choice between conventional rigid pedicle screws that create a constrained linkage and a screw with a head that articulates in one plane. All other components in the system are similar and interchangeable.

This study attempted to determine (i) the differential fusion rates in rigid and dynamic instrumentation and (ii) the difference in implant failure rates between the two systems.

MATERIALS AND METHODS

Initial results are presented of a prospective multicenter study of patients undergoing spinal fusion for degenerative low back disorders (degenerative disc disease) using the SSCS system. The initial 218 patients have been followed-up for 2 years and were operated between 1993 and 1995.

The SSCS implants used in this study were stainless steel (they now are available in titanium) and had the following specifications:

Screws

- Rigid-head screw with a cylindrical thread, outside thread diameter of 6.0 mm, and inside shank diameter of 4.0 mm with a self-cutting thread and a blunt tip.
- Dynamic screw with an uniaxial articulated head in the sagittal plane and identical thread specifications.
- Screws are fixed onto the rod by a sharp-tipped grub screw.

Rods

- Varying lengths with an outside diameter of 6.25 mm and a circumferential grooved nonprogressive thread surface to improve fixation.

Cross connectors

- Identical specifications to the rods and mounted on the rods with clamps of similar construction to the screw heads.

Figure 1

- Hinged screw, rigid screw, and circumferentially grooved rod.

A posterolateral fusion was performed in all patients. Autogenous iliac bone was used throughout.

At follow-up, the state of the fusion and implant integrity were assessed by independent examiners using anteroposterior and lateral x-ray films.

The state of the fusion was graded as follows (12):

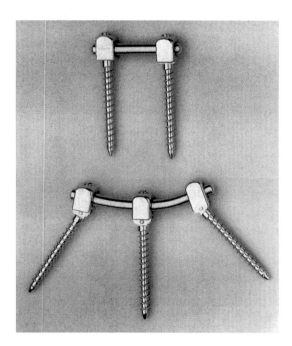

FIG. 1. Rigid screws, hinged screws, and profiled rod.

1. Solid fusion: continuous trabecular pattern of bone formation
2. Not sure: continuous bone formation but amorphous and not clearly trabecular
3. Not solid: amorphous and noncontinuous bone formation.

Implant failures were divided into the following categories:

1. Screw breakage
2. Rod breakage
3. Screw-rod interface loosening
4. Rod-transverse stabilizer interface loosening
5. Screw-bone interface loosening.

In the study group the following complications were specifically recorded:

1. Wound infection
2. Neurological deterioration
3. Implant dislodgment
4. Necessity for revision operation.

All patients were mobilized within the first 5 days of operation. Neither casts nor rigid braces were used.

Rigid screws were only used in single-level fusions, and a direct comparison could be made with dynamic monosegmental instrumentation. At the beginning of the study, rigid screws only were used for single-level instrumentation. After the first follow-up examinations, hinged screws also were used in single-level instrumentations because of some implant breakages of the rigid screws.

In multisegmental fusions, some surgeons preferred nonsequential instrumentation. The results of these patients could be compared with those in whom every segment was instrumented. In both groups with multilevel instrumentation only hinged screws were used.

Statistical analysis of the results was performed using the p exact test for unmatched pairs. Significance was $\alpha = 0.05$. The difference was considered significant for $p < 0.05$ ($p < \alpha$). The following groups were matched: (i) rigid versus hinged screws in single-level instrumentations, and (ii) each segment screwed versus nonsequential instrumentation in multilevel instrumentation (only hinged screws).

RESULTS

Originally 222 patients were followed-up for a minimum of 24 months. Four patients were excluded because of incorrect instrumentation wherein a combination of rigid and hinged screws were used in multisegmental instrumentation.

Among the 218 patients included in this study, there were 102 women (average age 46.8 years, range 19 to 79) and 116 men (average age 46.0 years, range 16 to 74). The age distribution is shown in Fig. 2. The patients were divided into the following groups:

1. Monosegmental instrumentation: 57 patients with rigid and 44 patients with hinged screws.
2. Multisegmental instrumentation: 99 patients with sequential fixation of each level and 18 in whom levels were skipped.

There was no significant difference in age or gender between the two groups. This study was confined to patients with degenerative disorders of the lumbar spine.

Table 1 shows the segments that were instrumented. For the monosegmental rigid instrumentation, 114 rods, 228 screws, and 1 cross connector were used. For the monosegmental dynamic instrumentation, 88 rods, 176 screws, and 13 cross connectors were implanted. For

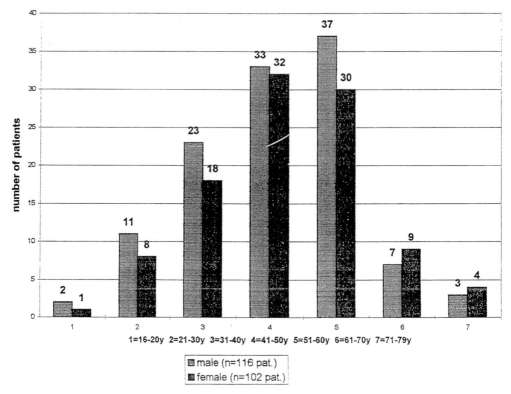

FIG. 2. Age and gender of the patients.

TABLE 1. *Kind of instrumentation*

Segments	Monosegmental instrumentation with rigid or hinged screws (n = 101 patients)	
	Rigid screws	Hinged screws
L2/L3	0	3
L3/L4	2	3
L4/L5	13	4
L5/S1	42	34
Total	57	44

Segments	Multisegmental instrumentation with hinged screws (n = 117 patients)	
	Each segment screwed	Skipping a segment
T12–L3	1	0
L2–L4	1	0
L3–L5	1	0
L2–S1	2	3[a]
L3–S1	23	1[b]
L4–S1	71	14
Total	99	18

[a] 1 × L2,L4,S1;1 × L2,L3,L4,S1;1 × L2,L3,S1.
[b] 1 × L3,S2.

the multisegmental instrumentations, 234 rods, 809 screws, and 10 cross connectors were used.

The mean operating time for the monosegmental instrumentation was 205.9 ± 64.3 minutes and for the multisegmental instrumentation was 229.0 ± 69.7 minutes. The mean blood loss was 836.7 ± 807.4 mL and 961.7 ± 816.0 mL, respectively.

Fusion Rate

Fusion rates are shown in Figs. 3–7. The fusion rate at 24 months among the group with monosegmental instrumentation was 93.2% for hinged screws and 91.2% for rigid screws. The difference was not statistically significant.

Among the group with multisegmental instrumentation in which each segment was fixed, the fusion rate was 95.0%. In the group in which segments were skipped there was a statistically significant lower fusion rate of 83.3% ($p = 0.045$).

Within the first follow-up after 3 months. 61.1% of the single-level instrumentations with hinged screws showed a solid fusion but only 24.5% of the patients with rigid instrumentation were solidly fused. This difference was statistically significant ($p = 0.003$).

In total, the fusion rate for patients instrumented with hinged screws (Fig. 7) was 48.1% after 3 months and 93.2% after 24 months.

Implant-related Complications

In the group with single-level fusions, more implant-related complications occurred among the fusions with rigid instrumentation than with dynamic instrumentation. The difference is

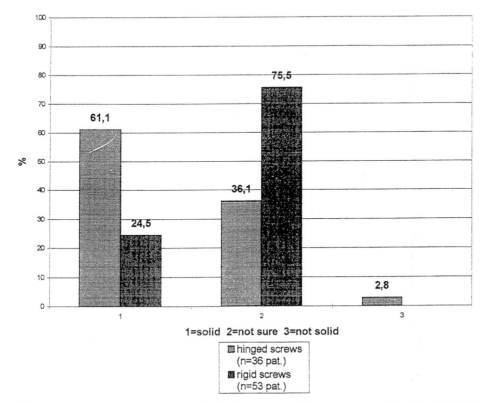

FIG. 3. Bone formation after 3 months for the group with monosegmental instrumentation.

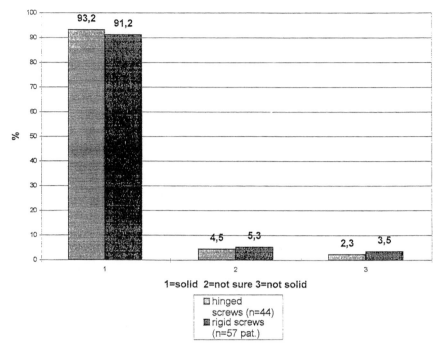

FIG. 4. Bone formation after 24 months for the group with monosegmental instrumentation.

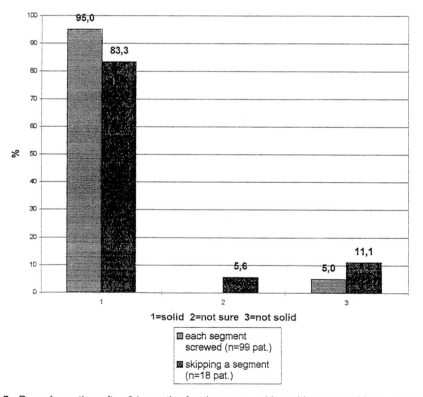

FIG. 5. Bone formation after 24 months for the group with multisegmental instrumentation.

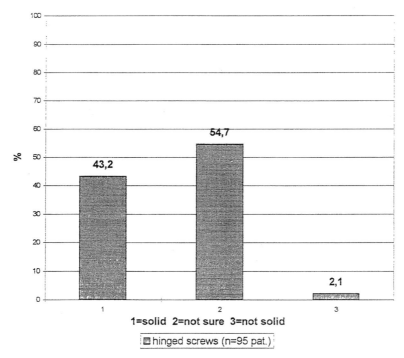

FIG. 6. Bone formation after 3 months for the group with multisegmental instrumentation (each segment screwed and skipping a level).

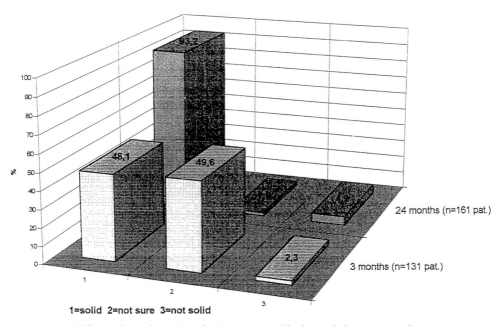

FIG. 7. Bone formation for the group with dynamic instrumentation.

TABLE 2. *Implant-related complications*

Monosegmental instrumentation (n = 101 patients)		
	Hinged screws	Rigid screws
Screw breakage	—	5/228 (2.2%)
Rod breakage	—	—
Screw dislocation	—	—
Screw-rod interface loosening	1/176 (0.6%)	—
Rod-transverse stabilizer interface loosening	—	—
Multisegmental instrumentation with hinged screws (n = 117 patients)		
	Each segment screwed	Skipping a segment
Screw breakage	4/728 (0.5%)	1/80 (1.3%)
Rod breakage	4/198 (2.0%)	1/36 (2.8%)
Screw dislocation	—	—
Screw-rod interface loosening	1/728 (0.1%)	—
Rod-transverse stabilizer interface loosening	—	—
Dynamic monosegmental and multisegmental instrumentation with hinged screws (n = 161 patients)		
Screw breakage	5/984 (0.5%)	
Rod breakage	5/322 (1.5%)	
Screw dislocation	—	
Screw-rod interface loosening	2/984 (0.2%)	
Rod-transverse stabilizer interface loosening	—	

statistically significant (p = 0.00005). The individual complications are listed in Table 2. Loosening of the screw-rod interface occurred in one patient and probably was due to inadequate tightening of the grub screw during surgery. Implant-related complications in the groups with multisegmental instrumentations (as shown in Table 2) are not statistically significant.

In all the dynamic breakages (monosegmental and multisegmental) there were 0.5% screw breakages and 1.5% rod breakages.

Failure of the hinge mechanism in the dynamic screws was not noted.

Complications

Seven patients (3.2%) developed deep wound infections. Postoperative malposition of screws was found in eight cases (3.7%).

There was an improvement in motor deficit in six patients postoperatively, but in three patients (1.44%) permanent motor and sensory deficit occurred as a result of the surgery.

A total of 28 revison operations were performed on 26 patients (12%), in 7 because of wound infections, in 2 because of malposition of the screws, in 1 because of neurological deficit due to the operation, and in 18 to remove implants and repair a painful pseudarthrosis in five patients.

DISCUSSION

This study proves that there is a statistically significant higher rate of screw breakage using rigid SSCS screws in single-level fusion compared to mechanically identical hinged SSCS screws.

A similar comparison was not possible in multilevel fusions because the use of rigid SSCS screws is contraindicated in such fusions.

When compared with other reports in the literature, there was a significantly lower rate of screw and rod breakages using the dynamic SSCS system.

A total of 984 hinged screws were implanted. There were only 5 breakages (0.5%) and 5 broken rods (1.5%) of 322 rods implanted with the hinged screws. Dynamic instrumentation was utilized in 161 patients in whom there were a total of 9 implant failures (5.6%).

McAfee et al. (18) reported 4.2% screw breakages affecting 10% of their patients. Bailey et al. (3) reported 2.6% screw breakages among their patients. Yuan (31) also reported a 2.6% screw breakage rate and a 0.7% rod or plate breakage rate. In addition to other implant-related complications, Ohlin et al. (22) reported a 6.0% screw breakage rate. Temple et al. (27) reported 6.6% screw breakage affecting 17% of patients. Similar values were reported by Anand and Tanna (1), who reported 6.6% screw failures in 17.8% of affected patients. Marchesi et al. (16) reported a very high 15% screw breakage rate in nontraumatic patients. At a 6- to 24-month follow-up, West et al. (29) reviewed 124 patients and found 2.3% broken screws affecting 9.6% of patients. Steffee and Brantigan (26) had 33 broken screws of 1,314 (2.5%) affecting 13.9% of patients.

In a 12-month retrospective follow-up of 617 patients, Esses et al. (9) reported a 4.4% implant complication rate. At 5 years Davne and Myers (6) found 1.1% broken screws in 496 (4.3%) patients.

When comparing the results of the present study with those utilizing rigid rod-screw or plate-screw combinations, there is a lower failure rate of implants in our study.

This is attributed to the articulated connection between the head (which is fixed to the rod) and the shaft of the screw. In contrast to implants used in long bones, spinal implants cannot be protected by adequate external immobilization when the patient is allowed to get of bed.

Spinal implants are enormously stressed during walking, standing, and sitting. Constrained linkages, especially in multisegmented instrumentation fusions, are overstrained, which may result in fatigue failure.

In the spinal implant system under review, there is perpetual potential sagittal mobility at the hinge site between the screw head and the shank of the screw (i.e., mechanically between the longitudinally orientated rod and the sagittally placed screw shank). This is a uniaxial semiconstrained linkage that reduces flexion strain on the implant. This facilitates insertion of a dynamic implant versus a rigid implant where the rod has to be absolutely accurately contoured or else it preloads the implant. One of the requirements for proper bone union is immobilization, and appropriate implants should produce this effect. An obvious source of concern with a dynamic implant is its ability to adequately immobilize the instrumented segment. In an *in vitro* biomechanical study of this device, it was shown that hinged screws afford an equal degree of stability to the tested construct as a rigid system (28).

Some authors are of the opinion that noninstrumented fusions produce a better quality fusion than instrumented fusions (19). Most authors report a clear superiority of instrumented fusions over noninstrumented fusions (2,15,20,25,31,32). In our study, the fusion rate with dynamic instrumentation was in the upper range of those reported by other investigators utilizing internal fixation. We compared our results with those using rigid or semirigid instrument systems (8,23,25,31,32) because a comparable study with a dynamic implant system (with a permanently articulating rod-screw connection) did not exist.

Assessment of the state of fusion and detection of a pseudarthrosis in a posterolateral spinal fusion are difficult. An anteroposterior x-ray film is probably the most appropriate investigation to assess a continuum of bony trabeculae between the transverse processes. If the bone in this region is in continuity but not clearly trabecular in nature, the fusion status must be regarded as uncertain. A deficiency of bony continuity is regarded as a definite nonunion of the graft (5,12,21).

The stress-shielding effect of rigid implants on long bones is well known; therefore, it is recommended that such rigid devices be removed to prevent formation of cancelli of the long bone (11,13,14).

In the field of spinal surgery, the effects of rigid implants on bone quality are largely unknown. McAfee et al. (18) using a canine model demonstrated a correlation between the rigidity of the spinal implant and loss of bone density.

It is probable that the reduced stress on the implant with a dynamic fixation system not only reduces the risk of the implant breaking but also reduces the stress-shielding effect on bone, thereby enhancing the quality of the bone fusion.

CONCLUSION

Implant-related problems reduce the benefit of instrumented fusions for degenerative spinal disorders, although a higher fusion rate probably can be achieved than with noninstrumented fusions. Through the use of dynamic instrumentation (semiconstrained linkage between rod and screw with a hinged screw), the rate of screw and rod breakage was reduced compared to rigid instrumentation. The bone fusion rate attained is comparable to the best results obtained by other investigators. The articulated connection between the rod and the screw in the sagittal plane is considered the reason for the lower rate of implant failure because of a reduction of flexion strain. Part of the load sharing is transferred from the implant to the spine. IN addition to the positive effect on the implant, further studies are required to assess the extent of reduction of the stress-shielding effect on bone.

To date, rigidity has been regarded as paramount in achieving adequate spine fusion, but the present study suggests that dynamic instrumentation achieves the same degree of stability and fusion in the degenerate spine but with a lesser risk of implant failure and possibly less stress shielding of bone.

REFERENCES

1. Anand N, Tanna DD. Unconventional pedicle spinal instrumentation. *Spine* 1994;19:2150–2158.
2. Axelsson P, Johnsson R, Strömqvist B, Arvidsson M, Herrlin K. Posterolateral lumbar fusion. *Acta Orthop Scand* 1994;65:309–314.
3. Bailey SI, Bartolozzi P, Bertagnoli R, et al. The BWM spinal fixator system. A preliminary report of a 2-year prospective, international multicenter study in a range of indications requiring surgical intervention for bone grafting and pedicle screw fixation. *Spine* 1996;21:2006–2015.
4. Boos N, Webb JK. Pedicle screw fixation in spinal disorders: a European view. *Eur Spine J* 1997;8:2–18.
5. Brantigan JW. Pseudarthrosis rate after allograft posterior lumbar interbody fusion with pedicle screw and plate fixation. *Spine* 1994;19:1271–1280.
6. Davne SH, Myers DL. Complications of lumbar spinal fusion with transpedicular instrumentation. *Spine* 1992; 17[Suppl]:185–189.
7. Dick W. The ''fixateur interne'' as a versatile implant for spine surgery. *Spine* 1987;12:882–900.
8. Enker P, Steffee AD. Interbody fusion and instrumentation. *Clin Orthop* 1994;300:90–101.
9. Esses SI, Sachs BL, Dreyzin V. Complications associated with the technique of pedicle screw fixation. A selected survey of ABS members. *Spine* 1993;18:2231–2239.
10. Gurr KR, McAfee PC, Shih C-M. Biomechanical analysis of posterior instrumentation systems after decompressive laminectomy. An unstable calf spine model. *J Bone Joint Surg* 1988;70A:680–691.
11. Jasmine MS, Dahners LE, Gilbert JA. Reduction of stress shielding beneath a boneplate by use of polymeric underplate. An experimental study in dogs. *Clin Orthop* 1989;246:293–299.
12. Jorgenson SS, Lowe TG, France J, Sabin J. A prospective analysis of autograft versus allograft in posterolateral lumbar fusion in the same patient. A minimum of 1-year follow-up in 144 patients. *Spine* 1994;19:2048–2053.
13. Korvick DL, Newbrey JW, Bagby GW. Stress shielding reduced by a silicon plate-bone interface. A canine experiment. *Acta Orthop Scand* 1989;60:611–616.

14. Låftman P, Nilsson OS, Brosjö O. Stress shielding by rigid fixation studied in osteomized rabbit tibiae. *Acta Orthop Scand* 1989;60:718–722.
15. Lorenz M, Zindrick M, Schwaegler P, et al. A comparison of single-level fusions with and without hardware. *Spine* 1991;16[Suppl]:455–458.
16. Marchesi DG, Thalgott JS, Aebi M. Application and results of the AO internal fixation system in nontraumatic indications. *Spine* 1991;16[Suppl]:162–169.
17. McAfee PC, Farey ID, Sutterlin CE, Gurr KR, Warden KE, Cunningham BW. The effect of spinal implant rigidity on vertebral bone density. A canine model. *Spine* 1991;16[Suppl]:190–197.
18. McAfee PC, Weiland DJ, Carlow JJ. Survivorship analysis of pedicle spinal instrumentation. *Spine* 1991; 16[Suppl]:422–427.
19. McGuire RA, Amundson GM. The use of primary internal fixation in spondylolisthesis. *Spine* 1993;18: 1662–1671.
20. Meril AJ. Direct current stimulation of allograft in anterior and posterior lumbar interbody fusions. *Spine* 1994; 19:2393–2398.
21. Millan MM, Cooper R, Haid R. Lumbar and lumbosacral fusions using Cotrel-Dubousset pedicle screws and rods. *Spine* 1994;19:430–434.
22. Ohlin A, Karlsson M, Düppe H, Hasserius R, Redlund-Johnell I. Complications after transpedicular stabilization of the spine. A survivorship analysis of 163 cases. *Spine* 1994;19:2774–2779.
23. Ricciardi JE, Pflueger PC, Isaza JE, Whitecloud TS III. Transpedicular fixation for the treatment of isthmic spondylolisthesis in adults. *Spine* 1995;20:1917–1922.
24. Roy-Camille R, Saillant G, Berteaux D, Salgado V. Osteosynthesis of thoraco-lumbar spine fractures with metal plates screwed through the vertebral pedicles. *Reconstr Surg Traumatol* 1976;15:2–16.
25. Schwab FJ, Nazarian DG, Mahmud F, Michelsen CB. Effects of spinal instrumentation on fusion of the lumbosacral spine. *Spine* 1995;20:2023–2028.
26. Steffee AD, Brantigan JW. The variable screw placement spinal fixation system. Report of a prospective study of 250 patients enrolled in food and drug administration clinical trials. *Spine* 1993;18:1160–1172.
27. Temple HT, Kruse RW, van Dam BE. Lumbar and lumbosacral fusion using Steffee instrumentation. *Spine* 1994;19:537–541.
28. von Strempel AH, Krönauer I, Morlock M, Schneider E. Stability of the instrumented spine: dynamic versus rigid instrumentation. In: Haher TR, Merola AA, eds. *Spine: State of the Art Reviews.* Hanley and Belfus: Philadelphia, 1996;10:397–408.
29. West JL III, Ogilvie JW, Bradford DS. Complications of the variable screw plate pedicle screw fixation. *Spine* 1991;16:576–579.
30. Wood GW II, Boyd RJ, Carothers TA, et al. The effect of pedicle screw/plate fixation on lumbar/lumbosacral autogenous bone graft fusions in patients with degenerative disc disease. *Spine* 1995;20:819–830.
31. Yuan HA, Garfin SR, Dickman CA, Mardjetko SM. A historical cohort study of pedicle screw fixation in thoracic, lumbar, and sacral spinal fusions. *Spine* 1994;19[Suppl]:2279–2296.
32. Zdeblick TA. A prospective, randomized study of lumbar fusion. *Spine* 1993;18:983–991.
33. Zucherman J, Hsu K, Picetti G III, White A, Wynne G, Taylor L. Clinical efficacy of spinal instrumentation in lumbar degenerative disc disease. *Spine* 1992;17:835–836.

Lumbar Spinal Stenosis
edited by Robert Gunzburg and Marek Szpalski
Lippincott Williams & Wilkins, Philadelphia, © 2000.

32

The Utility of Interbody Arthrodesis Using BAK Cages in Treatment

Stephen D. Kuslich

Spinology, Inc., Stillwater, Minnesota 55082

Lumbar spinal stenosis is a pathologic state wherein the internal dimensions of the spinal canal are reduced to such an extent that neurologic symptoms occur. Symptoms might include paresthesias and dysesthesias in the lower extremities and, in more severe cases, neurologic deficits. It is generally agreed that surgical nerve root decompression is the appropriate treatment when neurologic symptoms are disabling and prolonged (3,9). Fusion may be added to the decompression in an effort to treat any instability that might be aggravating the stenosis or to treat the low back pain component.

Following the pivotal equine work of Bagby (1) demonstrating the usefulness of hollow metal cages in spinal fusion, cages have become popular for fusion of the lower lumbar spine in humans. Some were designed for use with pedicle fixation systems (e.g., Brantigan and Harms cages), whereas others were designed to be stand-alone systems (e.g., BAK and Ray cages). As one of the inventors and designers of the BAK system, I am most familiar with that product. The utility of cages for the treatment of spinal stenosis has not been clearly defined. To the best of my knowledge, there are no scientific studies that rigorously establish the utility of cages in this condition. All other forms of instrumentation share this lack of convincing scientific evidence for safety and effectiveness. But, on the basis of theoretical considerations and early experience, cage fusion is feasible and may soon become a preferred method in certain forms of spinal stenosis.

• For example, the United States multicenter BAK Food and Drug Administration trial (1,200+ cases, 19 medical centers, 1992 to 1996) proved that back and leg pain could be significantly improved by the performance of an interbody fusion using a hollow, threaded titanium cage filled with bone graft. That study included many cases of spinal stenosis (8). Based on the findings of that study and on my own experience, I will attempt to provide some information about indications and contraindications for the use of cages in spinal stenosis.

The ideal treatment of spinal stenosis requires a detailed knowledge of the pathoanatomy involved in the individual patient, because each case is unique. Following that, an appropriate conservative or surgical intervention is undertaken in an effort to relieve the symptoms. Ideally, patients and surgeons will choose the least dangerous, simplest, most durable, and most cost-effective means of treatment. Obviously, this ideal may be difficult or impossible to achieve in every patient.

To obtain satisfactory results, the physician must be skilled in the evaluation of symptoms and signs, and proficient in the interpretation of radiographic and physiologic tests. Also, the physician must be able to understand the risks and benefits of several therapeutic interventions and be able to provide the appropriate intervention at the correct time and with a high level of technical competence. Not uncommonly, additional difficulties arise when the patient presents with other significant disease conditions, e.g., cardiovascular disease, arthritis, obesity, central nervous system dysfunction, diabetes, or osteoporosis. As often as not, the physician must choose between doing what may be done technically and doing what can be done safely. Because of the inherent complexity and difficulty of this mandate, the evaluation and treatment of spinal stenosis represents one of the most challenging clinical conditions that any spinal practitioner is required to manage.

SYMPTOMS

Stenosis involving compression of a single nerve root in the subarticular or foraminal zones produce symptoms that are indistinguishable from disc herniation, except that the symptoms are usually long standing in cases of stenosis. In most cases, the symptoms occur gradually, over a period of years, as patients progress into the later decades of life. Usually these symptoms take the form of numbness and tingling in the legs and feet when the patient walks long distances. Later on, pain in the buttock and legs develops, and the distance walked before symptom onset begins to shorten. Eventually, the simple act of standing may generate symptoms. A particular type of pain in the legs, sometimes called "pseudoclaudication," occurs with standing and walking. It is similar but not identical to muscle ischemic pain. Weakness or muscle paralysis may be present. Cauda equina syndrome with sphincter paralysis is rare, unless there is an acute decrease in canal size, as might occur when a patient with severe, preexisting stenosis develops a large central disc hernia.

Low back pain is a common concomitant symptom, but the pathology causing low back pain is different than the pathology causing nerve compression (7). Unfortunately, simple nerve element decompression cannot be expected to alleviate the back pain component.

PATHOLOGY

A variety of pathologic states can produce spinal stenosis. Congenital narrowing predisposes the nerve elements to impingement by any other mechanism. In rough order of frequency, the following pathologic states can generate the stenosis:

- Degenerative remodeling of the architecture of the vertebral bodies, including the formation of "spurs" on the facets and vertebral endplates
- Intervertebral disc bulging, protrusion, or herniation
- Thickening, swelling, or cyst formation in the facet joints
- Thickening, swelling, or cyst formation in the ligamentum flavum
- Caudal descent of the pedicle resulting from narrowing of the intervertebral disc or due to compression fracture of the vertebral bodies
- Spodylolisthesis, degenerative or isthmic
- Interspinal canal mass formation, resulting from infection, hematoma, tumor, or even synovial and fibrotic reaction to a foreign body such as a spinal implant, suture, or medicinal agent.

PATHOPHYSIOLOGY

The pathophysiology of spinal stenosis is not entirely understood, but research studies suggest that symptoms are related to blood flow problems in the spinal nerve elements. Blood flow may be compromised by direct compression at high pressures or by venous pooling in low-pressure compression. Preexisting atherosclerosis will exacerbate the problem (8).

If the ischemia is mild, sensory symptoms predominate. If the compression is more severe, radicular pain is generated and motor conduction is affected. The compression may be intermittent or sustained. Symptoms are usually body-position dependent. The nerves recover well from intermittent compression, but prolonged ischemia may lead to permanent deficits.

AUTHOR'S RESEARCH INTO THE ORIGIN OF SPINAL AND RADICULAR PAIN

I have reported the methods, results, and conclusions drawn from more than 20 years of observations made during the performance of decompression operations on disc hernia and spinal stenosis cases using local anesthesia while patients were awake and responsive during the procedure. These unique experiments allowed me to determine the tissue origin of spinal pain in the individual patient and to generate hypotheses regarding the pathophysiology of spinal and sciatic pain conditions (8).

My experiments determined the following:

- Most tissues of the spine are insensitive to mechanical stimulation.
- The outer annulus of the disc is the primary tissue responsible for mechanical low back pain.
- The posterior longitudinal ligament is the most sensitive portion of the degenerating disc.
- The facet capsule can and does produce mechanical low back pain when it is inflamed or mechanically traumatized (especially in older individuals).
- Some individuals can ''feel'' their degenerating discs (about two thirds of humans), whereas others cannot (about one third).
- In some individuals, in certain stages of degeneration, the inferior facet may abut against the back of the disc (especially during extension of the spine) causing low back pain, with or without nerve compression and leg pain.
- Nerve root ischemia secondary to compression is the main cause of radicular pain.
- Epidural scar tissue is not itself painful, but fibrosis may tether nerves and make them more susceptible to tension or compression.
- Despite all that has been written about the ''chemical theory'' of radicular pain, I remain convinced that the primary pathology is mechanical, i.e., tension and/or compression of the nerve elements. The rapid relief of radicular pain immediately following decompression of even long-standing sciatica argues strongly against the chemical hypothesis.

SURGICAL PLANNING

When conservative treatments are ineffective, the physician may be forced to consider a surgical solution. The following issues need to be addressed:

- What is the proportion of lumbar to radicular symptoms? In other words, is the patient suffering from back pain, leg pain, or both?
- What is the extent, nature, and location of nerve element compression, e.g., is the compression central, subarticular, foraminal, extraforaminal, or a combination?

- How many levels and sites are involved, and to what degree?
- Is the compression static or dynamic?
- Is the compressing tissue hard or soft?
- What is the stability status of the involved motion segments, and what will they be after decompression?

Unfortunately, answers to these questions may be difficult or impossible to determine preoperatively or even intraoperatively. Sometimes the surgeon must simply make a judgment call before or during surgery and hope for the best. Surgery for spinal stenosis is not an exact science. No amount of case studies, meta-analyses, or Monday morning, *ex post facto* pontificating by academic professors will ever reduce this field to a simple cookbook or algorithmic formula.

The role of arthrodesis in the management of spinal stenosis is uncertain and controversial. My experience and reading of the literature lead me to believe, that under certain circumstances, arthrodesis is not only preferable, it is positively indicated if good results are to be assured. I agree with Wiltse et al. (11), Herkowitz and Kurz (5), and others that certain forms of stenosis are best treated by arthrodesis, in addition to, or in some cases, instead of decompression. These situations are as follows:

- Significant spondylolisthesis
- Significant scoliosis or kyphosis
- Second surgery for stenosis at the same segment
- Iatrogenic instability caused by generous laminectomy, facetectomy, or foraminotomy
- When radical discectomy is performed.

The type of fusion remains a matter of individual choice, because few controlled studies have been done to define this decision. Good-to-excellent results have been reported when surgeons used the following techniques:

- Posterolateral fusion without fixation
- Posterolateral fusion with fixation
- Anterior and posterolateral fusion with fixation
- Anterior fusion with posterior fixation
- Posterior lumbar interbody fusion (PLIF) without fixation (2)
- Posterior lumbar interbody fusion with fixation
- Anterior lumbar interbody fusion (ALIF) alone.

Fischgrund et al. (4) presented a prospective randomized study comparing posterolateral arthrodesis with and without instrumentation in cases of degenerative spondylolisthesis and spinal stenosis. They concluded that although instrumentation may lead to a higher fusion rate, the clinical outcome, in terms of back and leg pain relief, is not positively affected by the addition of instrumentation.

Two recent studies indicate that anterior interbody fusion alone, without decompression, is more effective than decompression alone for the surgical treatment of degenerative spondylolisthesis with associated stenosis (6,10).

Based on my experience and knowledge of the literature, I suggest the following course of action.

WHEN, WHERE, AND HOW TO OPERATE FOR LUMBAR STENOSIS

When to Operate?

- When the symptoms are at least moderately severe and/or disabling.
- When symptoms do not respond to a reasonable period of time and conservative treatment;

usually 3–6 months of activity modification, bracing, exercises, oral medications, and injections.
- When the patient is physically, emotionally and mentally capable to withstanding the operation, i.e., when the risks and benefits analysis dictates a surgical solution.
- When the surgeon is convinced that he or she clearly understands the pathoanatomy, pathophysiology, and stability status of the motion segments involved.
- When the surgeon is convinced that the planned operation will adequately decompress the involved areas, without causing later instability and/or restenosis.
- When the surgeon is convinced that the planned operation will correct the preexisting instability or will compensate for the decompression-induced instability.
- When the surgeon is convinced that he or she is technically capable of performing the indicated operation.

Where to Operate?

- At all levels and sites where significant, symptom-producing nerve tension or compression is present; based on a careful analysis of the symptoms, physical signs, and preoperative radiographic and physiologic studies of the patient.
- At other areas and sites where it is reasonable to assume that stenosis problems might occur in the near future, e.g., moderately stenotic lesions at adjacent levels.

How to Operate?

The exact choice of operation will always remain a judgment call, based on the experience and training of the surgeon and guided by the state of the science at the time. The past 2 decades have produced a great deal of scientific information about the subject of spinal stenosis. Our understanding of the pathoanatomy and pathophysiology of the condition has improved. Computed tomographic and magnetic resonance imaging technologies have greatly enhanced our diagnostic abilities. Surgical technologies are rapidly evolving, but the choice of procedure for each form of the disease is still controversial and unclear.

I consider the following rules to be prudent:

- When the symptoms are mainly radicular, and
- When the stenosis is static and isolated to one or two segments, and
- When the compression is mainly subarticular or foraminal, and
- When a simple posterior or lateral decompression can be accomplished with little threat of iatrogenic instability,

I recommend central, and/or subarticular and/or foraminal microsurgical decompressions, alone, using local and regional anesthesia, without any attempt at fusion.

- When the symptoms are a balanced combination of back and leg symptoms, and
- When the segment is only mildly unstable (e.g., grade I degenerative spodylolisthesis), and
- When the stenosis is only mild to moderate, and subarticular, or ''up-down'' due to decent of the pedicle, and
- When the stenosis involves only one or two motion segments, and
- When the anterior approach is feasible (i.e., the great vessels can be mobilized without fear of laceration or embolization)

I recommend anterior interbody fusion with interbody implants, without concomitant decompression. I say this because the cage procedure can distract the disc sufficiently to open the foramen and reduce and/or eliminate the subarticular compression by preventing sagittal plane instability. If the stenotic symptoms are not relieved, a simple but complete posterior decompression can be done later without concerns about iatrogenic instability.

If the anterior approach is not feasible, I recommend posterior decompression and PLIF with cages, or posterolateral fusion without instrumentation.

• When the stenosis is severe, but all other factors in the previous paragraph are true,

I recommend posterior decompression followed by PLIF or ALIF using interbody implants, as long as the field of surgery is limited to no more than two motion segments.

• When more than two segments are involved,

I believe that some other form of segmental fixation, e.g., pedicle systems, should be used.

• If there is a radiologic diagnosis of stenosis, but the symptoms are mainly low back pain, and the preoperative instability is not severe,

The surgeon should disregard the stenosis and proceed to an interbody fusion (anterior if possible) of the involved motion segments using interbody implants, without decompression.

• If there is preoperative evidence of deformity or significant segmental instability (unbalanced scoliosis, lateral displacement, or grade II or greater spondylolisthesis),

The surgeon should perform a posterior decompression followed by pedicle-based stabilization and posterolateral fusion, with or without correction of the deformity, depending on circumstances. Cages or bone graft can be used in the anterior column, if needed.

CASE EXAMPLES

The following illustrative cases demonstrate some of the lessons we have learned about the use and misuse of interbody cages in the treatment of spinal stenosis.

Case 1

A 40-year-old manual laborer with a 6-year history of back and leg pains since falling from a scaffold.

Sagittal magnetic resonance imaging demonstrates severe disc damage with dehydration of the disc and retrolisthesis (Fig. 1). Moderately severe subarticular stenosis was present.

Treatment consisted of posterior decompression by partial facetectomy followed by PLIF with BAK cages using ''progressive local anesthesia'' (Fig. 2).

The result is complete relief of back and leg pains over 6 years of follow-up.

Case 2

A 50-year-old man with many years of leg and back pains not responding to conservative treatments.

Lateral x-ray film demonstrates grade I degenerative spondylolisthesis with marked loss of disc height (Fig. 3).

Magnetic resonance imaging reveals subarticular stenosis and degenerative changes at L4–5 and relatively normal middle-aged discs above and below (Fig. 4).

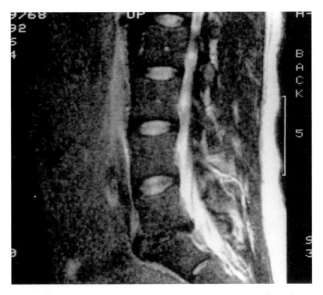

FIG. 1. Sagittal magnetic resonance image demonstrates severe disc damage with dehydration of the disc and retrolisthesis. Moderately severe subarticular stenosis was present.

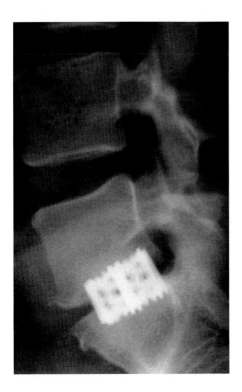

FIG. 2. Treatment consisted of posterior decompression by partial facetectomy followed by posterior lumbar interbody fusion with BAK cages using "progressive local anesthesia."

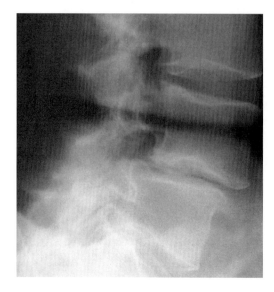

FIG. 3. Lateral x-ray film demonstrates grade I degenerative spondylolisthesis with marked loss of disc height.

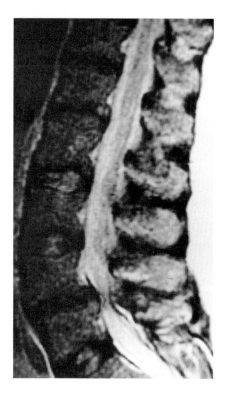

FIG. 4. Magnetic resonance imaging reveals subarticular stenosis and degenerative changes at L4–5 and reveals relatively normal middle-aged discs above and below.

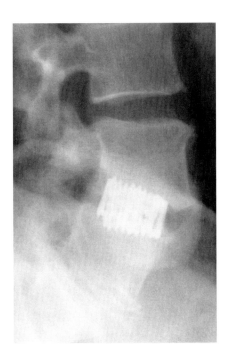

FIG. 5. X-ray film taken 36 months after posterior lumbar interbody fusion with BAK cages shows solid fusion and maintenance of partial reduction.

X-ray film taken at 36 months after PLIF with BAK cages shows solid fusion and maintenance of partial reduction (Fig. 5). Pain is relieved and the patient is fully employed.

Case 3

A 44-year-old woman who had three previous decompressions for herniated nucleus pulposus and recurrences presents with a 6-year history of back and leg pain, is taking codeine daily, and is finding it difficult to perform gainful employment.

Lateral x-ray film shows severe loss of disc height and slight retrolisthesis at L4–5 (Fig. 6).

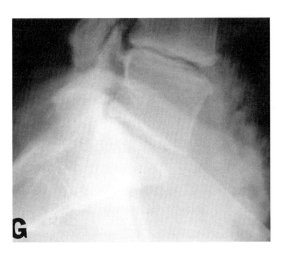

FIG. 6. Lateral x-ray film shows severe loss of disc height and slight retrolisthesis at L4–5.

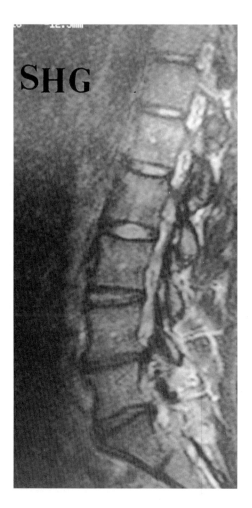

FIG. 7. Magnetic resonance imaging shows subarticular stenosis due to disc bulge and retrolisthesis and facet hypertrophy.

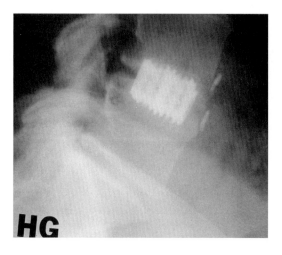

FIG. 8. Treatment by anterior lumbar interbody fusion with BAK cages at L4–5, without a fourth attempt at decompression.

Magnetic resonance imaging shows subarticular stenosis due to disc bulge and retrolisthesis and facet hypertrophy (Fig. 7).

The patient underwent treatment by ALIF with BAK cages at L4–5, without a fourth attempt at decompression (Fig. 8).

The result is nearly complete relief of back pain and elimination of leg pain, although some sensory paresthesias remain. She is fully employed and no longer taking medications more that 3 years after the fusion operation.

Case 4

A 44-year-old woman presents with many years of back and leg pain without history of injury.

Lateral x-ray film show grade I degenerative spondylolisthesis at L4–5 (Fig. 9).

Magnetic resonance imaging shows degenerative disc disease (DDD) at L4–5 and L5–S1, with slip at L4–5 and subarticular stenosis (Fig. 10). Discography is positive at L4–5 and L5–S1.

Posterior decompression at L4–5 is immediately followed by ALIF at L4–5 and L5–S1 using BAK instrumentation (Fig. 11). At 1 year, pain is improved but the superior endplate at L4–5 appears to be un-united. Nothing is done other than providing comfort measures.

At 2 years, the back pain is mostly relieved and the lateral x-ray film shows solid incorporation of bone into the implant (Fig. 12).

This case demonstrates an important principle. If the pain is improving and the implants are not migrating, simply continue observation. In almost all instances, the segment eventually will fuse, especially if the patient remains active!

Case 5

A 41-year-old male presents with long-standing low back pain and sciatica.

Lateral x-ray film shows grade II isthmic spondylolisthesis and DDD at L5–S1 (Fig. 13).

Magnetic resonance imaging reveals the same plus foraminal stenosis of the L5 root (Fig. 14). A posterior decompression, including partial removal of the right pedicle, is followed by PLIF with BAK cages. Reduction is not achieved. Postoperatively, the patient requires a long time to achieve any reduction in pain.

During the first few weeks following surgery, one implant displaced posteriorly about 8 mm (Fig. 15). At 2 years, he has improved enough to work at light-duty occupations, but

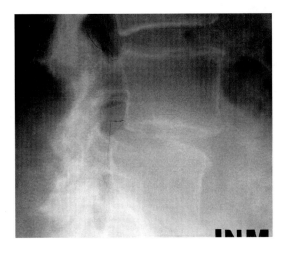

FIG. 9. Lateral x-ray film shows grade I degenerative spondylolisthesis at L4–5.

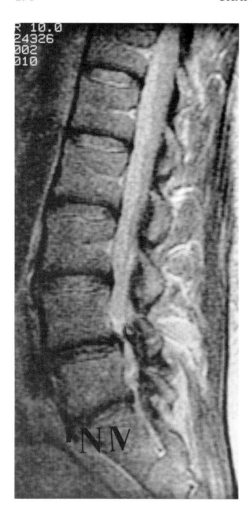

FIG. 10. Magnetic resonance imaging shows DDD at L4–5 and L5–S1, with slip at L4–5 and subarticular stenosis. Discography is positive at L4–5 and L5–S1.

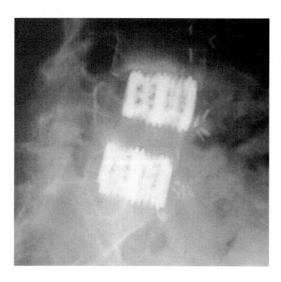

FIG. 11. Posterior decompression at L4–5 is immediately followed by anterior lumbar interbody fusion at L4–5 and L5–S1 using BAK instrumentation.

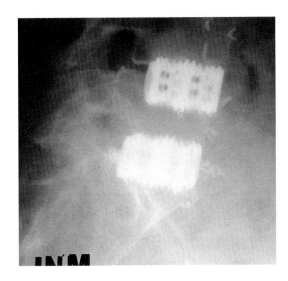

FIG. 12. At 2 years the back pain is mostly relieved and the lateral x-ray film shows solid incorporation of bone into the implant.

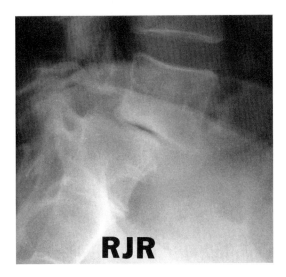

FIG. 13. Lateral x-ray film shows grade II isthmic spondylolisthesis and DDD at L5–S1.

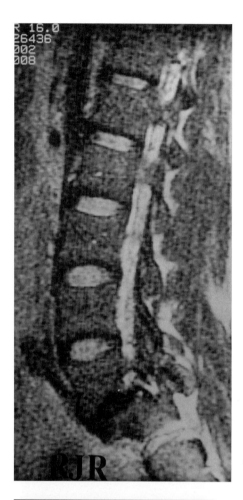

FIG. 14. Magnetic resonance imaging reveals the same plus foraminal stenosis of the L5 root. A posterior decompression, including partial removal of the right pedicle, is followed by posterior lumbar interbody fusion with BAK cages.

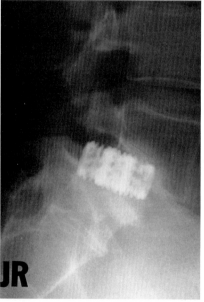

FIG. 15. During the first few weeks following surgery, one implant displaced posteriorly about 8 mm.

some leg pains remain. He is offered a revision, but decides against it. He is better than he was preoperatively, but not good. We consider his case a failure that might need a difficult revision at some time in the future. The lesson: Stand-alone cages are not indicated in grade II or greater slips.

CONCLUSION

Spinal arthrodesis with interbody cages is a useful and successful method for treating certain forms of spinal stenosis with back pain and/or minor forms of instability.

REFERENCES

1. Bagby GW. Arthrodesis by the distraction-compression using a stainless steel implant. *Orthopaedics* 1988;11: 931–934.
2. Cloward RB. Long-term result of PLIF. In: Lin PM, ed. *Posterior lumbar interbody fusion.* Springfield, IL: Charles C. Thomas, 1982.
3. Epstein NE, Epstein EE. Surgery for spinal stenosis. In: Weisel WW, Weinstein JN, Herkowitz HN, Dvorak J, Bell GR, eds. *The lumbar spine,* 2nd ed. Philadelphia: WB Saunders, 1996:737–765.
4. Fischgrund J, MacKay M, Herkowitz H, et al. Degenerative lumbar spondylolisthesis with spinal stenosis: a prospective, randomized study, comparing arthrodesis with and without instrumentation. North American Spine Society Annual Meeting, October 1996.
5. Herkowitz HN, Kurz LT. Degenerative lumbar spondylolisthesis with spinal stenosis. A prospective study comparing decompression with decompression and intertransverse process arthrodesis. *J Bone Joint Surg* 1991; 73A:802–808.
6. Kim NH, Kim DJ. Anterior interbody fusion for spondylolisthesis. *Orthopedics* 1991;14:1069–1076.
7. Kuslich SD, Ulstrom CL. The tissue origin of low back pain and sciatica: a report of pain response to tissue stimulation during operations on the lumbar spine using local anesthesia. *Orthop Clin North Am* 1991;22: 181–187.
8. Kuslich SD, Ulstrom CL, Griffin SL, Ahern JW, Dowdle JD. The Bagby and Kuslich method of lumbar interbody fusion. *Spine* 1998;23:1267–1278.
9. Porter R. Pathophysiology of neurogenic claudication. In: Weisel WW, Weinstein JN, Herkowitz HN, Dvorak J, Bell GR, eds. *The lumbar spine,* 2nd ed. Philadelphia: WB Saunders, 1996:717–722.
10. Satomi K, Hirabayahi K, Toyama Y, Fujimura U. A clinical study of degenerative spondylolisthesis. *Spine* 1992;17:1329–1336.
11. Wiltse LL, Kirkaldy-Willis WH, McIvor GW. The treatment of spinal stenosis. *Clin Orthop* 1976;115:83–91.

Lumbar Spinal Stenosis
edited by Robert Gunzburg and Marek Szpalski
Lippincott Williams & Wilkins, Philadelphia, © 2000.

33

Etiology, Evaluation, and Treatment of Patients Who Underwent Failed Lumbar Spine Surgery

Robert S. Biscup

Department of Orthopaedic Surgery, Cleveland Clinic Foundation, Cleveland, Ohio 44195

It is estimated that approximately 350,000 or more spine operations are performed annually, with patients undergoing a variety of surgeries designed to remove pressure off spinal nerves, correct a deformity, and/or fuse painful or unstable spine segments together. New and innovative surgical procedures developed recently offer excellent results that allow most patients to be pain free and lead normal lifestyles in all age groups.

However, approximately 20% of these patients continue to have significant problems after spinal surgery; this represents a large population. These patients, their families, and treating physicians often experience frustration, anger, and sometimes despair over persistent or even worsening symptoms that cannot be explained.

Typically, these individuals had at least one prior back surgery that has failed to effectively treat their problem. They can still have significant pain, difficulty performing their normal daily activities, and neurologic problems, and they often stay out on long-term disability or Worker's Compensation.

Many of these patients are physically challenged and deconditioned. They have a high rate of emotional and psychological problems, including depression, sleep disturbances, narcotic medicine dependence or addiction, marital problems, and generally a poor quality of life. If a work-related injury is present, a high incidence of litigation against employers is common. Ongoing medical care, consultations, and treatment programs often are fragmented, uncoordinated, inconsistent, and somewhat a la carte, with no clear end in sight for this difficult patient population.

However, many of these patients can be helped given recent advances in comprehensive spine care and new surgical techniques, which include minimally invasive and reconstruction surgery. The key is to determine if a potential surgical problem still exists and the chances of success with additional surgery.

PATIENT POPULATION

A patient with failed spine surgery syndrome is someone who had at least one previous surgery (or more) performed longer than 6 months ago. Previous spinal surgeries include:

- Simple laminectomy or microdiscectomy
- Percutaneous disc surgery (including chymopapain)

- Decompression surgery
- Attempted spinal fusion (with or without posterior instrumentation)
- Attempted deformity correction
- Previous surgery involving spine implants
- Previous postoperative wound infections
- Transition syndrome (degeneration above or below previous fusion).

The pathology most frequently encountered in the failed spine surgery patient population can include a variety of conditions that include, but are not limited to:

- Spinal stenosis
- Recurrent disc herniation
- Failed spinal fusion
- Malpositioned spinal hardware
- Failed spinal hardware
- Persistent, recurrent, or new spinal deformity
- Spinal instability
- Postsurgical painful disc degeneration
- Degeneration above or below a fusion
- Recurrent tumor
- Infection.

THE CLEVELAND CLINIC CENTER FOR THE SPINE: PROGRAM FOR FAILED SPINE SURGERY

The Program for Failed Spine Surgery is a comprehensive service provided to Cleveland Clinic Foundation staff doctors, patients, referring physicians, and representatives of managed care organizations. It is one of several coordinated multidisciplinary programs offered under the auspices of the Cleveland Clinic Center for the Spine.

Patients suffering from failed spine surgery syndrome are assessed through a comprehensive multidisciplinary program to effectively evaluate, treat, and study their problem using an innovative approach developed by Cleveland Clinic physicians.

PATIENT ENTRY

The point of entry into the Program for Failed Spine Surgery is through a detailed evaluation by a spine surgeon in the Department of Orthopaedics or Neurosurgery. Patient referrals would be through five avenues:

1. Prior patients treated by Cleveland Clinic Spine Surgeons
2. Patients referred by Cleveland Clinic Staff and network physicians
3. Patients referred by outside orthopedic, neurosurgical, or primary care physicians
4. Direct patient calls
5. Managed care representatives (case managers).

Patient consultations or appointment requests are triaged and arranged through centralized scheduling or through individual physician offices.

INITIAL PATIENT VISIT WITH THE SPINE SURGEON

The unique aspect of this program is that the initial evaluation of the failed spine surgery patient is by an experienced spine surgeon from the Orthopaedic or Neurosurgery Department.

An experienced spine surgeon is the most uniquely qualified physician to determine if the goals of the original surgery were met or if a problem still exists and whether further surgical intervention is indicated.

Prior to the initial visit with the spine surgeon, the patient is told to bring to the scheduled appointment all previous imaging studies, surgery reports, test results, and letters from referring physicians. During the initial visit, a nurse clinician/physician's assistant may see the patient, record patient history on data forms, organize outside films, acquire new imaging films if none are available, organize all information, and "present the case" to the spine surgery staff physician.

After evaluating the failed spine surgery patient, the spine surgery staff physician determines that:

1. A possible surgical problem exists but further imaging or laboratory studies are required (magnetic resonance imaging, myelography/computed tomography, discography, dynamic studies, bone scan, laboratory tests, etc.).
2. A surgical problem exists and schedules surgery if the problem appears straightforward and no risk factors exist.
3. A surgical problem exists with some risk factors. Refer to the multidisciplinary team for a comprehensive evaluation with recommendations for postoperative care.
4. Not a surgical problem. Refer for ongoing conservative management program.
5. Not a surgical problem. Return to referring or primary care physician.

A salient feature of the Program for Failed Spinal Surgery is the collection of outcomes data: both clinical and surgical outcomes. Initial and ongoing collection of outcomes data will assure that meaningful research is conducted to assess accurately the evaluation and management of the patient.

EVALUATION OF SURGICAL OUTCOMES

The technical success of surgery is best measured by radiographic imaging studies. Efforts are being directed to developing an imaging protocol with the Department of Radiology at the Cleveland Clinic Foundation to assess surgical outcomes in spinal surgery. Under this program, the spine radiologist would attempt to answer certain questions posed by the spine surgeon in assessing the results of spinal surgery. A radiology "consult" might attempt to answer questions such as:

1. Is there residual spinal stenosis or nerve compression?
2. Is there a recurrent disc herniation?
3. Is the spine fusion solid or incomplete, or is pseudoarthrosis present?
4. Is there evidence of malpositioning of spinal hardware or implants?
5. Is there evidence of failed or broken spinal hardware?
6. Is there evidence of infection?
7. Is there evidence of spinal instability?
8. Is there a persistent or new spinal deformity?
9. Is there evidence of a new adjacent problem or "transition syndrome" that has developed?
10. Is arachnoiditis or other problems present?

The spine radiologist then would order the most appropriate test(s) to provide objective data that would answer these questions for the spine surgeon. This same protocol would be used in the initial evaluation, when indicated, as well as for ongoing assessment. Data generated would establish the criteria for successful *surgical outcomes.*

Other useful information, such as intraoperative data, laboratory results, complications, length of stay, surgical techniques and constructs, implants, and cost of care, would be collected to round out the complete picture of surgical outcome evaluation. The spine surgeons will meet collectively at regular intervals to review this data, develop new treatment or research protocols, evaluate new and innovative surgical techniques, and perform peer review.

EVALUATION OF CLINICAL OUTCOMES

In contrast to surgical outcomes, *clinical outcomes* measure the functional and behavioral results of the surgical procedure. Activities such as pain relief, medication usage, social activity level, return to work status, sleep status, psychological behavior, physical and functional capacities, and return to sports are a few examples.

To assess the failed spine surgery patient relative to clinical outcomes, a multidisciplinary team has been convened at the Cleveland Clinic Center for the Spine to perform a comprehensive evaluation. When included as part of the initial assessment, this team evaluation helps to determine if the patient is a candidate for additional surgery and the chances of clinical success provided that surgical success is demonstrated.

Patients referred to the multidisciplinary team evaluation for failed spinal surgery is a patient who has already seen a Cleveland Clinic spine surgeon, and the surgeon has determined that the patient *is* a candidate for additional spine surgery. The surgeon at this point is concerned about possible risk factors that might affect the clinical outcome and asks the team for their input into the final decision-making process.

Members of this multidisciplinary team include:

1. Spine surgeon
2. Spine medical specialist
3. Clinical psychologist and pain management specialist
4. Physical and rehabilitation therapist
5. Vocational rehabilitation specialist (if necessary).

Patients are scheduled to see all members of this team consecutively on 1 day, except the spine surgeon (who would have seen the patient previously).

Spine medical specialist. The spine medical specialist interviews and examines the patient, reconstructs the history or care, and determines if all reasonable attempts at ongoing conservative management have been exhausted. During the assessment, the role of the medical spine specialist is the opposite of the surgeon. Comorbidities and/or general health factors such as diabetes, obesity, heart disease, medications, etc., are considered at this point relative to appropriateness and medical risks with further surgery. However, if further surgery is indicated and performed, the medical spine specialist can play an important role in the patient's management to ensure that preoperative rehabilitation goals are being met in the postoperative period.

Clinical psychologist and pain management specialist. The role of the clinical psychologist and pain management specialist is to evaluate the patient's pain behavior, expose psychiatric comorbidity, identify chemical-dependency problems, determine motivation status, explore family relations, and help to identify those risk factors that may contribute to a poor clinical outcome. As with the medical spine specialist, the clinical psychologist can play an important role in postoperative pain management and reregulation of endogenous means of sleep control, mood elevation, family counseling, personal and group therapy, and stress management.

Physical therapy and rehabilitation specialist. The physical therapy specialist evaluates what prior rehabilitation program the patient has participated in and its effectiveness. The therapist also determines which activities aggravate or improves the patient's condition. An assessment is made of general physical health and fitness, physical and functional capacities evaluation, and potential for improvement with or without additional surgery. The emphasis here is on function. The physical therapist will attempt to determine what are realistic physical and functional goals to strive for 1 year after the proposed additional surgery.

Vocational rehabilitation specialist. The vocational rehabilitation specialist interviews the patient regarding employment status and what expectations lie in the future both with and without further surgery. This assessment is extremely important in worker's compensation patients or patients who are seeking disabilities. This may include site visits and a dialog with the patient's employer to assess accurately what opportunities exist for return to work with or without any restrictions.

After these assessments, all members of the team, including the spine surgeon, meet to discuss the case and make appropriate recommendations regarding the ongoing care of the patient, determine if further surgery is indicated, what risk factors are present, and what suggestions are made for postoperative management and rehabilitation. Data are collected establishing baseline clinical parameters that will be used for subsequent evaluations if further surgery is performed. In this context, outcomes criteria are established up front prior to surgery. If possible, clinical case managers are welcomed and encouraged to attend this team meeting and participate in the discussions. At the conclusion of the meeting, the patient is invited to enter the conference room where the recommendations of the team are presented. At the conclusion of this meeting, one of three options is presented:

1. If further surgery is suggested, a follow-up appointment is made with the surgeon to discuss surgery and postoperative treatment protocol.
2. If no surgery, referral for nonsurgical management.
3. Return to the referring physician.

At the conclusion of the assessment, a summary report that outlines the findings of the team along with their recommendations is generated and signed by all participants. Copies are forwarded to referring physicians, case managers, patients, and insurance agencies as necessary and approved.

FOLLOW-UP APPOINTMENT WITH THE SPINE SURGEON

Once it has been determined that the failed spine surgery patient is a good candidate for additional surgery, a follow-up appointment is made to specifically discuss the proposed surgery, risks and complications, and benefits. Realistic outcome expectations are reviewed with the patient and their families, referring physicians, and case managers representing insurance companies. It is important that all participants understand clearly the objectives of surgery and the ultimate clinical and surgical outcome that hopefully will be achieved.

If the patient meets the selection/inclusion criteria for any of a number of clinical research projects that might be ongoing, the opportunity to participate is offered at this time. Preoperative data are collected as indicated to establish further baseline information regarding the proposed surgery, hospital stay, and postoperative rehabilitation program. Patient education activities include the use of videos, patient brochures, and models to assure a complete understanding of the surgical procedure, postoperative pain management, and physical therapy.

POSTOPERATIVE FOLLOW-UP VISITS

After surgery, routine visits are scheduled at 1, 3, 6, 12, and 24 months. At each point, patients are assessed relative to surgical and clinical outcomes criteria determined preoperatively and data recorded. Comanagement including the medical spine specialist, psychology/pain management specialist, physical therapy, and job retraining (if necessary) activities are coordinated with Cleveland Clinic Foundation staff members or outside physicians as indicated for pain management, radiologic assessment, rehabilitation, and ongoing medical care. Referring physicians are informed of patient progress by regular reports and/or letters. Referring physicians are included in the postoperative management of the patient if they request to become a member of the ''team.'' Activity status, return to work, and participation in sports are determined by the patient's spine surgeon, with input from all multidisciplinary team members.

Lumbar Spinal Stenosis
edited by Robert Gunzburg and Marek Szpalski
Lippincott Williams & Wilkins, Philadelphia, © 2000.

34

Lumbar Stenoses and Fusion

Jacques Boulot

Clinique Du Parc, 31400 Toulousse, France

The surgical treatment of lumbar stenoses remains a subject of controversy (1,4,6–8,10–12). The first objective of this surgery is release of the compressed nervous structures. Treatment of degenerative lesions that lead to the stenosis or that are associated with it is not an end goal in itself. What is the exact role of arthrodesis for the treatment of lumbar stenoses?

It can be deduced from the literature (7,11) that isolated decompression can be an adequate and sufficient treatment, with satisfactory results ranging from 64% to 95%.

The most common technique consists of relatively extensive laminectomy possibly combined with arthrectomy, the extent of which varies according to the case. However, this technique can increase preexisting instability and may even, in some case, induce secondary instability (3,6,10). Other authors have reported different rates of preoperative instability, ranging from 2% to 15% when the lumbar spine is initially stable to more than 70% when there is preoperative instability, particularly in the case of degenerative spondylolistheses. For this reason, arthrodesis complementary to decompression often is required. However, few studies with a stringent methodology advocate fusion combined with decompression, except in the case of degenerative spondylolisthesis (1,3,11).

Another issue arises: Does spinal osteosynthesis increase the rate of fusion in the treatment of lumbar stenoses? Here, too, few articles provide a clear-cut view, which makes it difficult to forge a precise opinion on the subject. It seems clear, however, that the use of osteosynthesis in lumbar fusion theoretically offers several advantages: reduced spinal mobility; immediate stabilization of the spine segment(s), thus enabling the fusion to be made with a better mechanical position; possibility to correct an associated deformation; and possible suppression of external compression.

What are the most current indications for arthrodesis for treatment of lumbar stenosis? We believe the following:

- Preoperative instabilities, established and detected
- Potential instabilities, i.e., stenoses that lead the surgeon to consider that a peroperative release will necessitate sacrificing bone to such an extent that it can induce a secondary destabilization
- Degenerative spondylolistheses
- Associated scolioses, rotational dislocation, and stenosis
- Failed back surgery syndrome.

We believe these indications should be compared against the results obtained using fusion and instrumentation for treatment of lumbar stenoses in 46 patients (25 men and 21 women, mean age 63.4 years). Maximum follow-up was 6 years, and minimum follow-up was 2 years (mean 3 years 8 months). All patients were operated by the same surgeon. Thirty-nine percent already had one spine surgery, 19% two, and 6% three and more. All these patients were operated on after failure of conservative treatment or for emergency reasons (equina cauda syndrome, paralyzing sciatica). Seventeen percent of the patients were referred by a pain treatment center.

The fusion was always performed using an autologous graft obtained from bone debris from laminoarthrectomy or harvested from the iliac crest. The graft is posterolateral (in the case of a wide laminoarthrectomy), medial (bridging the fenestration zones), or associated with an interbody graft with Moss-type cages. The instrumentation used was the Cotrel-Bubousset (CD) and Moss-Miami hardware with pedicular screws; the hooks were used in the stenosis deformation association. Usually, there is no postoperative compression. The same examiner reviewed all patients, except two patients who died. Thus, 44 patients were analyzed based on Beaujon's score.

The patients were divided into three groups:

Group I: lumbar stenosis and degenerative spondylolisthesis
Group II: lumbar stenosis and deformation
Group III: isolated stenosis.

GROUP I: ANALYSIS

This group consisted of ten patients (eight women) having lumbar stenoses with degenerative spondylolisthesis. There are 13 spondylolistheses, because three patients exhibited a dual level of slippage. All patients had a slippage at L4–5 and L3–4. The mean preoperative slippage was 6 mm. Only one patient was treated on an emergency basis for equina cauda syndrome. All had a fusion and were instrumented. In principle, the fusion is never extended to L5–S1. The aim of reduction was to restore segmentary lordosis, thus inducing better regional lordosis. The reduction was always quasitotal. The mean postoperative slippage was 2 mm.

Results in group I show that seven patients had excellent results and three had average results. No pseudarthrosis was noticed *a priori*. There was no loss of reduction.

Two questions arise:

1. Is a fusion necessary for degenerative spondylolisthesis?
2. If so, what type of arthrodesis is needed?

Numerous articles have reported on this topic and indicate that laminectomy can be sufficient (4,8,11), but others have shown that a postrelease fixation improves the results (2,6). However, the result can be good even after a loss of correction (2). *In situ*, fixation is possible with a good result, but the local segmentary kyphosis remains identical.

What type of arthrodesis? A posterolateral graft can be sufficient, particularly in patients with a poor medical condition; however, it calls for a large approach that is associated with muscular damage. Isolated, it may deteriorate the correction by plastic deformation of the graft and at a high rate of pseudarthrosis. We would rather add an interbody graft that enables lasting reduction and restoration of disc height.

GROUP II: STENOSES AND DEFORMATION

This group consisted of ten patients (nine females), four of whom had previous surgery. In addition to the classic clinical signs of lumbar stenoses, cruralgia was noted frequently.

The stenosis was associated with either an aged idiopathic scoliosis or a *de novo* degenerative scoliosis, generally postmenopausal. Rotational dislocation was frequent but not always at the compression level. Generally, neurologic compression is on the concave side, although it can be intermittent. In such a case, it is a dynamic stenosis on deformative instability that can be well analyzed with myelography performed with the patient standing up and x-ray films taken in lateral and sagittal bendings. Eight stenoses were released and instrumented, and two others were corrected without intracanal penetration by reduction of the deformation, particularly in instability-induced stenoses.

In all cases, the deformation was fully instrumented with frontal correction and mainly the recovery of a correct sagittal balance. Here again, stage L5–S1 should not, in our opinion, be included in the instrumentation. In the case of patients already operated or with a failed back surgery syndrome, this situation is far more complex and necessitates a specific approach in one or two simultaneous procedures that often include extraction of the hardware and osteotomy of the existing fusion, correction, new instrumentation, and iterative fusion.

In this group of 10 patients, 8 had an excellent result, 1 average, and 1 poor due to pseudarthrosis. In this group it appears essential to treat all the problems within a single procedure, medical condition permitting. However, a simple decompression can be performed on a fragile patient, with limited stenosis and significant stiff and angular curvature.

GROUP III: ISOLATED STENOSES

This group consisted of patients having stenoses without spondylolisthesis and without associated deformation. There were 24 patients (4 females and 20 males). Nine had previous surgery, 2 had congenitally induced stenoses, and 22 had acquired degenerative stenoses, with central intracanalar predominance in 6 cases, lateral (stenosis of the lateral recessus) in 11, or combined central and lateral in 5.

In this group, the fusion was performed because there was:

- One clear preoperative instability shown on the dynamic x-ray films,
- A large peroperative release,
- A destabilizing action had been performed during the surgery, such as cure of a disc herniation,
- An intradiscal space at the stenotic stage,
- One or several preliminary surgeries at the same level, or
- It was a failed back surgery syndrome.

In three cases the fusion was extended to the sacrum.

In this group, there were 68% good or excellent results, 18% average results, and 14% poor results. One patient died of pulmonary embolism.

The results are poorer than in the other groups for several reasons:

1. Arthrodeses were performed only on the most evolved patients or on patients whose stenosis rate was such that alternative solutions to fusion, such as recalibration, could not be performed.
2. In this group, the patients were older, they often already had been operated, and they suffered from one or several associated pathologies (2,3,5,6,11).

Finally, this group contained the maximum number of patients with acute neurologic complications *before* the release surgery (seven patients had equina cauda syndrome).

A survey of the three groups combined shows more than 70% good or excellent results. However, although the analysis shows that the neurogenous claudication and the radiculalgia clearly improved, the lumbago often remained, thus affecting the final result, especially in patients already operated on, who experience the highest number of preoperative and postoperative complications (3,5,10).

COMPLICATIONS

This is an extensive surgery with a high morbidity rate. Two patients died (1 pulmonary embolism, 1 stroke). There were 3 cases of sepsis that resolved after treatment, 1 required extraction of the osteosynthesis material after fusion, 2 postoperative equina cauda syndromes caused by a compressive hematoma, 1 of which regressed completely, 3 dural lesions that occurred in patients who had already been operated on, 1 psychiatric decompensation, and 2 pseudarthroses including 1 symptomatic that was operated with a satisfactory outcome.

CONCLUSION

The arthrodesis should not be systematic.

In our opinion, this surgery should be reserved for the following cases:

• Degenerative spondylolistheses and confirmed preoperative instabilities
• Foreseeable instabilities
• Highly evolved stenosed lumbar canals
• Associated deformations
• Failure of preliminary surgery.

For other cases, techniques such as recalibration (9) or backup ligamentoplasty are preferable.

REFERENCES

1. Deyo RA, Ciol MA, Cherkin DC, Loeser JD, Bigos SJ. Lumbar spinal fusion: a cohort study of complications, reoperations and resource use in the Medicare population. *Spine* 1993;18:1463–1470.
2. Frazier DD, Lipson SJ, Fossel AH, Katz JN. Associations between spinal deformity and outcomes after decompression for spinal stenosis. *Spine* 1997;22:2025–2029.
3. Guigui P, Ulivieri JM, Lassale B, Deburge A. Les réinterventions après chirurgie de la sténose lombaire dégénérative. *Rev Chir Orthop* 1995;81:663–671.
4. Hanley EN. The indications for lumbar spinal fusion with and without instrumentation. *Spine* 1995;20:1435–1535.
5. Herno A, Airaksien O, Saari T, Sihvonen T. Surgical results of lumbar spinal stenosis. A comparison of patients with or without previous back surgery. *Spine* 1995;20:964–969.
6. Katz JN, Lipson SJ, Larson MG, et al. The outcome of decompressive laminectomy for degenerative lumbar stenosis. *J Bone Joint Surg Am* 1991;73A:809–816.
7. Katz JN, Lipson SJ, Lew RA, et al. Lumbar laminectomy alone or with instrumented or non-instrumented arthrodesis in degenerative lumbar spinal stenosis: patient selection, costs and surgical outcomes. *Spine* 1997;22:1123–1131.
8. Sonntag VK, Marciano FF. Is fusion indicated for lumbar spinal disorders? *Spine* 1995;20:1385–1425.
9. Senegas J, Etchevers JP, Vital JM, Baulny D. Le recalibrage du canal lombaire, alternative è la laminectomie dans le traitement des sténoses du canal lombaire. *Rev Chir Orthop* 1988;74:15–22.
10. Senegas J. Le recalibrage du canal lombaire (Symposium canal lombaire étroit) SOFCOT. *Rev Chir Orthop* 1990;76[Suppl 1]:54–57.
11. Turner J, Ersek M, Herron L, Deyo R. Surgery for lumbar spinal stenosis. Attempted meta-analysis of the literature. *Spine* 1992;17:1–8.
12. Zdeblick TA. The treatment of degenerative lumbar disorders. An initial review of the literature. *Spine* 1995;20:1265–1375.

Lumbar Spinal Stenosis
edited by Robert Gunzburg and Marek Szpalski
Lippincott Williams & Wilkins, Philadelphia, © 2000.

35

Surgical Treatment of Severe Lateral and Foraminal Degenerative Lumbar Spinal Stenosis

The Benefits of Posterior Lumbar Interbody Fusion with Intervertebral Cages and Stabilization with Semirigid Posterior Fixation

Gilles Perrin

Department of Neurosurgery, Université C. Bernard Lyon I, 69373 Lyon, France

Lumbar degenerative nerve root compression may arise from a simple prolapsed disc or from vertebral bone lesions such as facet joint arthrotic deformation with lateral recess stenosis or degenerative spondylolisthesis (5). Nerve root compression also may be caused by foraminal stenosis due to combined discal collapse with arthrotic spurs and proliferative lesions. Sometimes nerve root decompression can be achieved only by restoration of the height of the intervertebral space and by a large opening of the lateral recesses and foramen. A large bone resection may be required. Decompression surgery for spinal stenosis due to degenerative arthrotic changes producing claudication is successful in patients. The main challenge in the surgical treatment of degenerative lumbar spinal stenosis is to achieve adequate decompression of the neural structures without inducing iatrogenic instability. According to the literature (7,11,13), the rate of further spinal instability ranges from 5% to 10%, and the risk of postoperative additional forward slip in degenerative spondylolisthesis is assessed between 10% and 18% of patients treated without fusion. Even if further horizontal dislocation did not lead to poorer clinical results (22), it is logical for surgical treatment not only to aim for the most efficient decompression of neurologic structures using adequate bone resection and restoration of intervertebral height by distractive interbody fusion, but also to prevent postoperative destabilization by using the same intervertebral fusion (8,9).

Unlike posterolateral intertransverse fusion, posterior lumbar interbody fusion (PLIF) is a biomechanically optimal fusion because the graft maintains the disc height (i.e., the lateral foraminal opening), protects the nerve roots, restores weight bearing to anterior structures, and immobilizes both horizontal and vertical instability. The cagelike implants (titanium or polyetherketone [PEEK] cages) meet the mechanical requirements for PLIF by serving both a mechanical function and a biologic bone growth function. The cages stretch the intervertebral space to its normal anatomic height and prevent postoperative collapse of the graft.

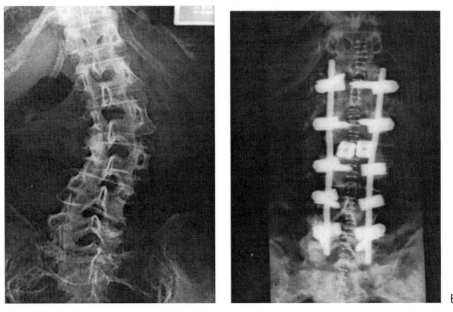

FIG. 1. Severe degenerative scoliosis with neurogenic claudication and right L3 radiculopathy **(A)**, treated by L2–3 posterior lumbar interbody fusion and L1–5 posterior fixation **(B)**.

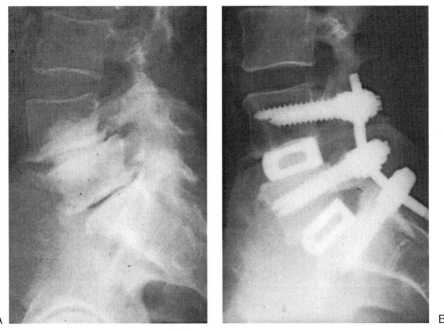

FIG. 2. Severe lumbar canalar and foraminal degenerative stenosis **(A)** treated by distractive interbody fusion with titanium cages as decompressive technique. Note restoration of intervertebral height and correction of slipping with the posterior fixation **(B)**.

TABLE 1. *Posterior lumbar interbody fusion performed on 1,000 patients from 1978 to September 1998*

	No. patients (%)
Isthmic lysis with spondylolisthesis	722 (72.2%)
Lateral and foraminal stenosis with collapsed disk	184 (18.4%)
Lumbar discoligamental instability	94 (9.4%)

The implant is packed with autologous bone graft with cancellous bone obtained from the laminectomy.

The purpose of posterior fixation is to (i) obtain temporary control of horizontal instability before achievement of the definitive bone fusion, (ii) enhance osteogenesis, and (iii) allow early mobilization without the need for a postoperative corset, to avoid external contention to prevent posterior muscle atrophy, loss of lordosis, and further destabilization at the adjacent level to the arthrodesis. Semirigid fixation significantly reduces the risk of screw fracture by absorption of stress on the interpedicular damper and improves bone fusion by maintaining constraints on the intervertebral implants.

Lumbar spine conditions that can be managed by fusion are degenerative spondylolisthesis, degenerative scoliosis with disc degeneration, facet joint arthrosis, severe foraminal stenosis and stretching of the compressed nerve root, iatrogenic segmental instability, and failed previous surgery (Figs. 1 and 2) (12).

From 1978 to September 1998, PLIF was performed on 1,000 patients with lumbosacral unstable lesions such as isthmic lysis with spondylolisthesis (722 patients) or discoligamentar instability (94 patients). PLIF also was performed for foraminal stenosis with collapsed disc in 184 patients (Table 1).

In the same period, 1,114 patients were operated on for radicular symptoms associated with degenerative lumbar stenosis. In 930 patients (83.5%) simple laminectomy without fusion was performed. Posterior lumbar interbody fusion was indicated for restoration of intervertebral height and for improving nerve root decompression in the foramen (Table 2).

RESULTS

Posterior lumbar interbody fusion formerly was performed using iliac crest graft with rigid posterior fixation. Collapse of the graft with loss of the restored intervertebral height was observed in 50% of cases. Some patients experienced breakage or dismantling of the rigid fixation system.

Since January 1994, 70 patients have been operated on using intervertebral titanium CH cages (55 patients) or carbon PEEK polymer CC cages (15 patients).

Posterior lumbar interbody fusion also was performed at one level in 53 patients, at two levels in 14 patients, and at three levels in 3 patients. Complementary interpedicular posterior fixation was performed using semirigid Isolock plates or rods (Figs. 3 and 4). No postoperative

TABLE 2. *Operation for degenerative lumbar stenosis performed on 1,114 patients from 1978 to September 1998*

	No. patients (%)
Simple laminectomy without fusion	930 (83.5%)
Decompression with posterior lumbar interbody fusion and posterior stabilization	184 (16.5%)

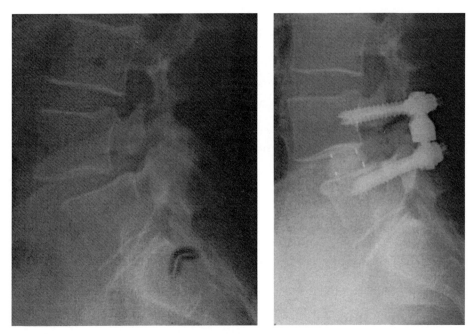

FIG. 3. L4−5 spondylolisthesis treated by posterior lumbar interbody fusion with CC radiolucent cages and monosegmental posterior fixation with Isolock semi-rigid plate.

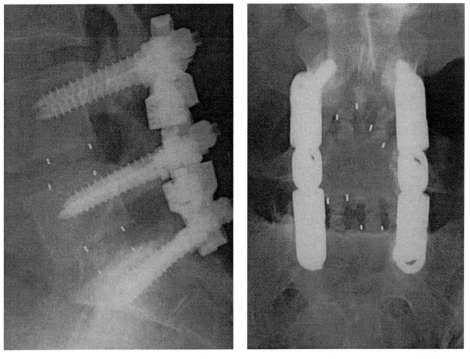

FIG. 4. Bisegmental arthrodesis using L4−5 and L5−S1 posterior lumbar interbody fusion and semirigid posterior fixation. Four-month postoperative radiologic control: note bone growth around the cages. The polymer structure of the cages with metallic wire fragments remain "black."

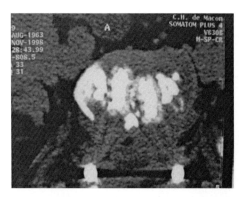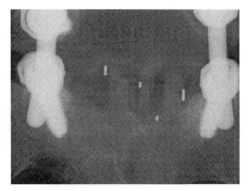

FIG. 5. Six-month postoperative computed tomographic scan and radiologic assessment of bone growth inside the CC cages and laterally to the implants.

corset or brace was necessary. Getting up and walking was allowed the day after the surgical procedure. The rehabilitation program started on the fifth postoperative day, with the aim to restore physiologic lumbar lordosis. The patient was ergonomically trained to prevent excessive flexion and axial rotation. In this series of 70 patients treated for degenerative lumbar stenosis using cages for PLIF and posterior fixation, no case of infection was observed. Transient postoperative radicular deficit was noted in two patients who recovered totally within 3 months. The first postoperative radiologic control performed after 3 months documented screw fracture or dismantling of the posterior fixation system. No fracture of the cage was observed. Intracorporeal penetration of the cages and loss of the restored intervertebral height occurred in two patients. No secondary anterior or posterior displacement of the intervertebral implants was noted. The two postoperative radicular deficits were not related to direct compression by the cages. No further surgical procedure was indicated in this series.

In 55 cases with long-term follow-up of more than 1.5 years, 54 patients (98.2%) demonstrated bone fusion. The bone growth in the group of patients operated on with the radiolucent CC polymer cages was evaluated as excellent within the cages and laterally to the implants.

If it was not possible to perform radiologic comparison of the bone growth inside the two different polymer or titanium cages due to the metallic density, the bone density and the osteogenesis alongside the lateral wall of the cages were significantly increased and enhanced on the front-view radiologic examination in the group of patients with polymer cages (Figs. 5 and 6).

TABLE 3. *Assessment of clinical outcome*

	Range of score
Importance of radicular pain	(1→5)
Consumption of analgesics	(1→5)
Evaluation of walking distance ability with treadmill test	(1→5)
Total of subscores = functional score	(3→15)

Post-/preoperative score = improvement of functional score	Clinical outcome
>50%	excellent
<50%	poor
0/−	bad

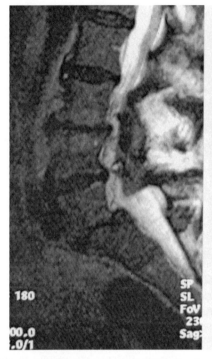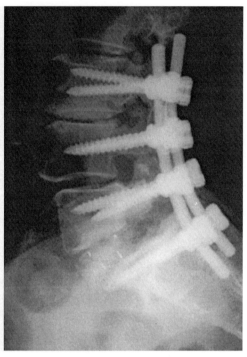

FIG. 6. L5–S1 isthmic spondylolisthesis with severe adjacent L3–5 degenerative stenosis. Large laminectomy L3–5 with foraminoplasty, L5–S1 interbody fusion with CC radiolucent cages, and L3–S1 posterior fixation using the TTL SYSTEM.

Clinical outcome assessed by the degree of radicular pain, consumption of analgesics, and evaluation of walking distance ability with the treadmill test was excellent in 44 patients (80%), with a mean 76% improvement of the functional score (Tables 3 and 4).

In this series, PLIF and posterior fixation were indicated in 16.5% of patients with radicular symptoms associated with degenerative lateral and foraminal lumbar stenosis.

Interbody fusion with cages and semirigid posterior fixation, avoidance of postoperative brace, early rehabilitation to achieve posterior remuscularization, and lordosis collectively meet all the requirements not only for pain relief but also for definitive stabilization without further iatrogenic spinal complication.

DISCUSSION

Some authors (3,6,24,25) advocate laminectomy without fusion, citing the comparable outcomes in the fusion and nonfusion operative groups of patients without preoperative insta-

TABLE 4. *Clinical outcome in 55 patients with follow-up for more than 1.5 years*

Outcome	No. patients (%)
Excellent	44 (81.5%)
Poor	8 (14.8%)
Bad	2 (3.7%)
Mean improvement of the functional score: 76%	

bility. Surgery for degenerative lumbar spinal stenosis can be successful in the majority of patients by wide laminectomy and medial facetectomy without the need for fusion or total facetectomy. However, early surgical failures (the mean rate of poor outcome is 20% in a large series of laminectomies) and late deteriorations due to iatrogenic instability (5% to 18%), restenosis (7%), or disc herniation at adjacent spinal levels (10%) are not nominal (15,23). Careful selection of patients for fusion must be performed using radiologic parameters (1,11,12,16,18). Radiologic factors predictive of greatest risk of postoperative destabilization are preoperative degenerative spondylolisthesis, abnormal motion on dynamic radiographs, and sagittally oriented facet joints demonstrated on computed tomographic scans. Patients who have these preoperative findings should be considered candidates for fusion. Stabilization also is peroperatively indicated in cases of total resection of the articular facets. The radiographic pseudarthrosis rate of posterolateral intertransverse grafting is high (12); PLIF is much more efficient. Interbody fusion should be considered not only if stability is threatened by overzealous or unavoidable sacrifice of supporting structures, but also as a distractive technique for restoration of intervertebral height and opening of the foramina to complete total nerve root decompression (6,14). In our series, only 16.5% of patients with severe lumbar spine stenosis required stabilization using PLIF with intervertebral cages and posterior interpedicular fixation. The intervertebral cages meet the requirements for definitive and efficient decompression by preventing the risk of graft collapse with subsequent loss of foraminal opening. Use of the radiolucent PEEK cage is well advisable to provide easy x-ray control of bone fusion. The material of the PEEK cage is able to improve fusion because its resilience is much closer to physiologic cortical bone elasticity than the too-rigid titanium alloys. The role of complementary posterior fixation is to (i) obtain temporary control of horizontal instability before achievement of the definitive bone fusion (2,4,10,17,19,21,26), (ii) enhance osteogenesis, and (iii) avoid external contention to prevent posterior muscle atrophy, loss of lordosis, and further destabilization at the adjacent level to the arthrodesis. The semirigid fixation system with interpedicular dampers meet the requirements for these purposes (20). The shock absorbers may prevent screw loosening or fixation breakage by absorbing most of the mechanical loads induced by early rehabilitation within the semirigid connecting element itself rather than letting them affect the bone-screw interface. Semirigid posterior fixation maintains physiologic sharing of the axial stress and anterior compression on the intervertebral implants with good mechanical conditions for early and enhanced fusion within and beside the cages.

REFERENCES

1. Airaksinen O, Herno A, Turunen V, Saari T, Suomlainen O. Surgical outcome of 438 patients treated surgically for lumbar spinal stenosis. *Spine* 1997;22:2278–2282.
2. Bridwell KH, Sedgewick TA, O'Brien MF. Role of fusion and instrumentation in the treatment of degenerative spondylolisthesis. *J Spinal Disord* 1993;6:461–472.
3. Brunon J, Chazal J, Chirossel JP, et al. When is spinal fusion warranted in degenerative lumbar spinal stenosis? *Rev Rhum Engl Ed* 1996;63:44–50.
4. Chang K, McAfee P. Degenerative spondylolisthesis and degenerative scoliosis treated with a combination segmental rod-plate and transpedicular screw instrumentation system: a preliminary report. *J Spinal Disord* 1989;1:247–256.
5. Cauchoix J, Benoist M, Chaissang V. Degenerative spondylolisthesis. *Clin Orthop* 1976;115:122–129.
6. Cloward RB. Spondylolisthesis: treatment by laminectomy and posterior interbody fusion. Review of 100 cases. *Clin Orthop* 1981;154:74–82.
7. Dall BE, Rowe DE. Degenerative spondylolisthesis. Its surgical management. *Spine* 1985;10:668–672.
8. Epstein NE. Primary fusion for the management of "unstable" degenerative spondylolisthesis. *Neuro-Orthopedics* 1998;23:45–52.
9. Feffer HL, Wiesel SW, Cuuckler JM, Rothman RH. Degenerative spondylolisthesis. To fuse or not to fuse? *Spine* 1985;10:287–289.

10. Fischgrund JS, Mackay M, Herkowitz HN, Brower R, Montgomery DM, Kurz LT. 1997 Volvo Award Winner in clinical studies: degenerative lumbar spondylolisthesis with spinal stenosis: a prospective randomized study comparing decompressive laminectomy and arthrodesis with and without spinal instrumentation. *Spine* 1997; 22:2807–2812.

11. Fox MW, Onofrio BM, Hanssen AD. Clinical outcomes and radiological instability following decompressive lumbar laminectomy for degenerative spinal stenosis: a comparison of patients undergoing concomitant arthrodesis versus decompression alone. *J Neurosurg* 1996;85:793–802.

12. Hanley EN Jr. The indications for lumbar spinal fusion with and without instrumentation. *Spine* 1995;20: 143S–153S.

13. Hopp E, Tsou PM. Postdecompression lumbar instability. *Clin Orthop* 1988;227:143–149.

14. Hutter CG. Spinal stenosis and posterior interbody fusion. *Clin Orthop* 1985;193:103–114.

15. Javid MJ, Hadar EJ. Long-term follow-up review of patients who underwent laminectomy for lumbar stenosis: a prospective study. *J Neurosurg* 1998;89:1–7.

16. Kotilainen E, Heinänen J, Gullichsen E, Koivunen T, Aro HT. Spondylodesis in the treatment of segmental instability of the lumbar spine with special reference to clinically verified instability. *Acta Neurochir (Wien)* 1997;139:629–635.

17. Lee TC. Transpedicular reduction and stabilization for postlaminectomy lumbar instability. *Acta Neurochir (Wien)* 1996;138:139–145.

18. Mardjetko SM, Connoly PJ, Shott S. Degenerative lumbar spondylolisthesis: a meta-analysis of the literature 1970–1993. *Spine* 1994;19:2256S–2265S.

19. Markwalder THM. Surgical management of neurogenic claudication in 100 patients with lumbar spinal stenosis due to degenerative spondylolisthesis. *Acta Neurochir (Wien)* 1993;120:136–142.

20. Perrin G. Usefulness of intervertebral titanium CH cages for PLIF and posterior fixation with semi-rigid Isolock plates. In: Szpalski M, Gunzburg R, Spengler DM, Nachemson A, eds. *Instrumented fusion of the degenerative lumbar spine: state of the art.* Philadelphia: Lippincott-Raven Publishers, 1996:271–279.

21. Rompe JD, Eysel P, Hopf CH, Heine J. Surgical management of central lumbar spinal stenosis. Results with decompressive laminectomy only and with concomitant instrumented fusion with the Cotrel-Dubousset instrumentation. *Neuro-Orthopedics* 1995;19:17–31.

22. Surin V, Hedelin E, Smith L. Degenerative lumbar spinal stenosis. Results of operative treatment. *Acta Orthop Scand* 1982;53:79–85.

23. Tuite GF, Doran SE, Stern JD, et al. Outcome after laminectomy for lumbar spinal stenosis. Part II: radiographic changes and clinical correlations. *J Neurosurg* 1994;81:707–715.

24. Turner JA, Ersek M, Herron L, Deyo R. Surgery for lumbar spinal stenosis. Attempted meta-analysis of the literature. *Spine* 1992;17:1–8.

25. Turner JA, Ersek M, Herron L, et al. Patient outcomes after lumbar spinal fusions. *JAMA* 1992;268:907–911.

26. Zdeblick T. A prospective, randomized study of lumbar fusion: preliminary report. *Spine* 1993;18:983–991.

Lumbar Spinal Stenosis
edited by Robert Gunzburg and Marek Szpalski
Lippincott Williams & Wilkins, Philadelphia, © 2000.

36

In Situ Noninstrumented Posterolateral Fusion versus Reduction and Anteroposterior Fusion with the SOCON Spinal System

Ralf H. Wittenberg, Roland E. Willburger, H. Knorth, and
*Reinhard Steffen

*Orthopaedic University Clinic, St. Josef Hospital, D-44791 Bochum, Germany; and
Department of Orthopaedics, Marienkrankenhaus, D-40489 Duesseldorf, Germany

Spondylolisthesis occurs in a variety of different entities and is classified into dysplastic, isthmic, degenerative, traumatic, and pathologic forms (18). Isthmic spondylolisthesis is seen in 5% to 6% of the population, with incidences for single segments of 82% L5–S1, 11.3% L4–L5, and 0.5% L3–4, and 2.2% for other segments (14).

According to current theory, a fatigue fracture through a congenitally weak pars interarticularis causes the entire vertebral body to slip (19). Although the exact origin of the initial lytic lesion of the pars still is unknown, a newer histologic study hypothesizes that uneven distribution of isthmic ossification of the pars interarticularis in the lower lumbar spine during fetal development makes the pars a target for fatigue fractures (15). Additionally, the fatigue fracture might fail to heal because of leakage of synovial fluid from upper or lower facet jonts into cavital defects of the pars articularis, thus creating a synovial pseudarthrosis (17).

Coexistence of disc degeneration is not of great relevance to the pathomechanism of isthmic spondylolisthesis, as indicated by the study of Sairyo et al. (16). In their study, anterior shearing force was applied to (immature calf) spines either with intact or dissected discs until displacement failure. The study revealed that load failures in both groups (973.8 vs. 986.4 N, respectively) did not appear at significantly different forces.

Generally, only a few patients with spondylolisthesis are symptomatic. The primary treatment is nonoperative and involves muscle reconditioning training, nonsteroidal antiinflammatory drugs, and corticosteroid injection. If these nonoperative treatment modalities fail, surgery is indicated. Surgical options range from single nerve root decompression to anteroposterior fusion techniques with reduction of the slip. Except for direct repair of the lyses with screws or hooks (10), all surgical techniques do not restore normal anatomy. Decompression and removal of facet joint tissue might even increase the instability (2).

The purpose of this chapter is to evaluate the clinical and radiological results after (i) noninstrumented, posterolateral *in situ* fusion and (ii) anteroposterior, instrumented stabilization and reduction.

METHODS

Patient Selection

Noninstrumented, posterolateral fusions with autologous iliac crest cancellous bone graft and an H-shaped tricortical iliac crest graft were performed for failed back surgery, lumbar instability without previous surgery, and spondylolisthesis. Twenty-two patients (mean age 50 years) with first- and second-degree spondylolisthesis are reported. There were 5 patients with spondylolisthesis L4–L5 and 17 with spondylolisthesis L5–S1. These 22 patients with tricortical bone graftings were matched with 20 spondylolisthesis patients who underwent posterior stabilization with the SOCON spinal system (Aesculap, Tutlingen, England). These 20 patients (mean age 45 years) were selected from another group of 72 patients who underwent anteroposterior, instrumented stabilization. Seven of these patients had listhesis at L4–5 and 13 at L5–S1.

Operative Techniques

In the posterolateral fusion group, the L4–S1 spinous processes and transverse processes are exposed in all patients. Careful decortication or the transverse processes is performed, the facet joints L5–S1 and L4–5 are destroyed, and the L5 spinous process is split and opened.

A tricortical graft from the upper ilium is harvested and a cancellous bone graft is removed from the ilium. The tricortical graft is wedged and inserted under tension between the L4 and S1 spinous processes, while the cancellous bone is used for posterolateral fusion L4–S1.

Patients are mobilized the day after surgery in a lumbar orthosis, which had to be worn 24 hours per day for an average of 4 months and a minimum of 3 months.

In instrumented, anteroposterior fusion, only the level involving either L5–S1 or L4–5 is exposed and the entry points for the pedicle screws are carefully prepared. Unlike posterolateral fusion, no exposure of the transverse processes or far lateral preparation is necessary. After cleaning the entry point of soft tissue, the cortex is removed with a nibbler and the probe is inserted under image intensifier control. The length of the screw path is measured and a screw of 6-mm major diameter was inserted to, or just through, the anterior cortex for best screw holding (21). After insertion of the pedicle screws, myelography is performed, and dural sac compression due to listhesis is documented. The spinal repositioning instrumentation is attached and the repositioning maneuver performed. First distraction to widen the foramen, then repositioning of the anterior slip is performed. After the repositioning maneuver is completed, the premounted clamps and rods are tightened, the spinal repositioning instrumentation is removed, and the clamp nuts are tightened with a momentum key.

A large tricortical bone graft is removed from the iliac crest and the wound is closed over three drains. The patient is turned around, and the disc is exposed from the anterior left-sided retroperitoneal approach. After excision of the disc, the upper and lower endplates are removed and the tricortical graft is shaped to fit into the intervertebral space. After insertion of the graft it can be secured additionally with a cancellous bone screw while a washer and a hemostatic is placed over the graft. The wound is closed, depending on the bleeding, with or without a drain. The patient is mobilized the day after surgery.

Although a brace is not needed for stabilization, it is given to some patients as a reminder and a motion restrictor.

Follow-up

Follow-up investigations were performed by an unbiased observer, who was not involved in any treatment of spine patients in our hospital. The minimum follow-up was 10 years in the posterolateral patients and 3 years in the anteroposterior instrumented patients.

After filling out the Oswestry questionnaire (6) and the visual analogue pain scale, which ranges from 0 = no pain to 10 = intractable pain, a thorough clinical examination was performed. Preoperative and postoperative roentgenograms, the latter not older than 6 months, were compared and evaluated.

RESULTS

Total surgery time was 4.5 hours for anteroposterior fusions and 3.4 hours for posterolateral fusion. Blood loss was higher in the patients with combined fusion than in patients with posterolateral fusion (average 1,120 ml vs. 870 ml).

In the posterolateral bone graft group, the anterior slip was not reduced. In the anteroposterior surgery group, the slip was completely reduced in 13 patients and reduced to more than 80% in 7. Myelography was performed in most of the instrumented fusions with reduction. Widening of the canal could be observed in all patients, and in some patients almost complete normalization could be seen (Fig. 1).

Only minor complications occurred in both groups. In the posterolateral group a hematoma at the graft harvesting site that needed no special therapy was seen in 3 patients (13.6%). In the anterior interbody fusion group venous lacerations that needed to be sutured during the anterior approach occurred in 2 patients (10%).

The pseudarthrosis rate was determined on anteroposterior, lateral, and flexion/extension x-ray films. There were two pseudarthroses in the posterolateral group and one in the anteroposterior group. In addition to the pseudarthroses, in 2 patients (10%) of the anteroposterior fusion group an anterior slippage was observed when the immediate postoperative and follow-up images were compared. Early in this series, four patients had loss of graft height due to insufficient removal of the endplates and subsequent partial graft deterioration. One graft was expulsed about 0.5 cm. One patient each in both groups required surgical revision.

Clinical follow-up showed a return-to-work rate to the same position of 88% in the posterolateral fusion group and 90% in the anteroposterior fusion group. Pain reduction was equal in both groups. More severe pain was seen in the anterior interbody fusion group, but the reduction of 5.3 points for the posterolateral fusion group and 5.6 points for the anterior interbody fusion group was not significantly different (Table 1).

The Oswestry score in the two groups was about the same before surgery; however, after anterior interbody fusion a significantly better functional outcome based on the Oswestry score was seen in the anteroposterior fusion group compared to the posterolateral fusion group (Table 2).

DISCUSSION

A limitation of the study is that it is not prospectively randomized to compare the two different surgical techniques; only a retrospective matched pair analysis is provided. Because of the relatively small number of patients in the two groups, only careful conclusions can be drawn from these results.

Nevertheless, it could be shown clearly that the fusion rate, especially of the noninstrumented fusion technique, is not as low as reported in the literature when instrumented and noninstrumented fusion techniques were compared (4,20). Comparison of the fusion rate of 95% in the instrumented fusion group and 91% in the noninstrumented fusion group cannot be used for discrimination between the two techniques. Both rates are very high compared to that reported in the literature, which shows a wide variety for noninstrumented fusion techniques (Table 3).

A study by Baski (2), who performed posterolateral fusion on 23 patients suffering from

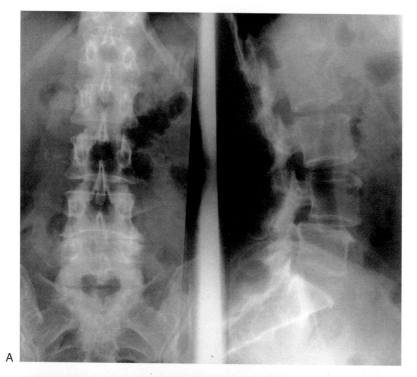

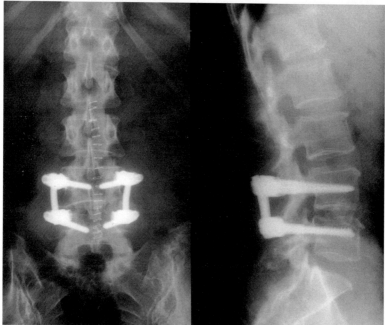

FIG. 1. A 50-year-old female patient with severe low back pain that did not improve after conservative treatment and leg pain with claudication. **A:** Preoperative image showing a decrease of disc height and anterior listhesis. **B:** Anteroposterior and lateral roentgenograms after complete reduction of the slip and increase of the disc height with posterior instrumentation (SOCON) and anterior tricortical bone graft. *(Figure continues.)*

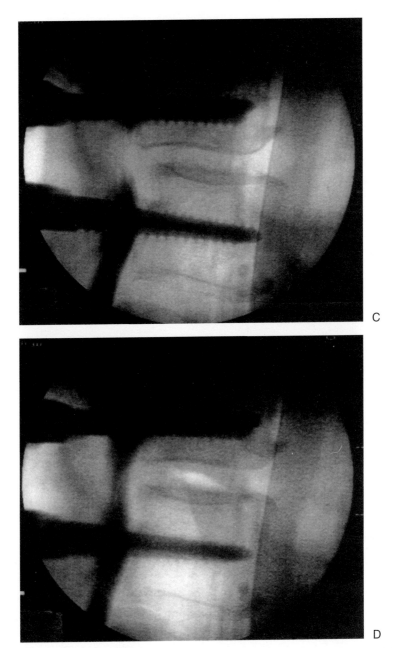

FIG. 1. *Continued.* **C:** Intraoperative myelography. Before reduction, compression of the dural sac is observed and demonstrated by filling defect. **D:** After complete reduction of the slip, myelography shows only little dural sac compression.

TABLE 1. *Preoperative and postoperative pain rating on a visual analogue scale from no to 10 intractable pain*

	Preoperative pain	Postoperative pain
Anteroposterior fusion	7.9	2.8
Noninstrumented posterolateral fusion	8.2	3.3

TABLE 2. *Oswestry score after surgery*

	No limitation	Little limitation	Moderate limitation	Severe limitation
Anteroposterior fusion	50%	25%	25%	0%
Noninstrumented posterolateral fusion	41%	32%	25%	0%

TABLE 3. *Results and complications after surgical therapy for isthmic spondylolisthesis using different fusion techniques*

Author (reference)	Study	Collective	n	Technique	Results	Complications
Carragee (3)	Prospective, randomized, clinical follow-up after 54 mo	Chronic low back patients with failed conservative treatment, isthmic spondylolistheses grade I/II	42	Posterolateral fusion	Satisfactory	Pseudarthroses
				Instrumented (n = 20)	90%	5%
				Uninstrumented (n = 22)	77.3%	13.6%
Jeanneret et al. (8)	Clinical follow-up	Isthmic spondylolistheses 25% to 81% (?)	20		Fusion 95%	Pseudarthroses 5%
				Anterior interbody fusion (n = 13)		
				L5/S1 posterior laminar screw fixation (n = 7)		
					Excellent and good results	Radicular pain
De Loubresse et al. (5)	Radiologic and clinical follow-up after 32 mo	Isthmic spondylolistheses grade I/II	48	Posterolateral fusion (n = 25)	88%	90%
				Posterolateral fusion and root release (n = 23)	65%	67.5%
Ricciardi et al. (13)	Radiologic and clinical follow-up after 30 mo	Symptomatic low-grade isthmic spondylolistheses	17	Instrumented (Luque pedicle screw plate) posterolateral arthrodesis	Fusion rate: 94.1% Satisfactory results 94.1% Return-to-work rate: 62%	
Poussa et al. (12)	Radiologic and clinical follow-up after 58 mo	Severe isthmic spondylolistheses slip >50%	22	Reduction (Magerl/Dick transpedicular screws) and posterior anterior fusion (n = 11)	Slip improvement (% points) 36.1	Improvement of sagittal rotation angle (°) 11
				Noninstrumented *in situ* fusion (n = 11)	7.7	2.8

lumbar spondylolisthesis, showed 48% excellent, 39% good, and 9% fair results. Only one patient showed a poor result. Other authors have not described their technique in detail. Careful surgical technique with thorough decortication and an autologous bone graft from the ilium might be responsible for a high percentage of fusions (9). This conclusion is supported by the data from the two large groups from which our patients were obtained. In those groups, the fusion rate was 86% in the posterolateral fusion group versus 97% for anteroposterior fusion group.

Complications were remarkably low in both groups and therefore cannot be used as a helpful discrimination between the two groups. When preoperative and postoperative pain was evaluated, there was no significant difference between the two groups. Compared to other studies, our data are in the upper range of pain reduction achieved. For subjective outcome it seems to be primarily important that a stable situation and not a perfect reduction be achieved. This was also shown by another study by O'Sullivan et al. (11), who evaluated the effects of stabilizing specific muscle training on 44 patients suffering from chronic back pain due to spondylolysis or spondylolisthesis, the exercise group showed a significant reduction of pain intensity.

The only significant difference between the two groups in our study occurred in the Oswestry functional score results, where the anteroposterior fusion group with reduction achieved a significantly better final outcome. More interesting, however, is what caused this difference. It can be attributed only partly to the age difference of 5 years. Possibly stabilization of one segment instead of two resulted in better lumbar spine motion, less stress on the other segments, and less muscle denervation during the surgery.

Neural damage must be considered as an important factor that partly affects or even determines the outcome after surgery. In this respect, the findings of Albrecht et al. (1) provided another twist to the story. They performed a study on 30 cadavers and found that in 46.7% of specimens the lumbosacral plexus was connected to pelvivertebral connective tissue through a special junction between the os sacrum and the nerve root of the fifth lumbar vertebra. In 20% of cases, sacral periostium provided additional neural fixation. *In vitro* repositioning of more than 20 mm (defining high-degree spondylolisthesis) caused an increase in perineural pressure greater than 30 mm Hg, resulting in nerve deformation.

Another reason for the discrepancies within the Oswestry score between the two groups might be that the contour of the spine with complete reduction is an important factor for load uptake and that good alignment and lumbar curvature result in more physiologic loading of the facet joints and discs in the upper lumbar spine.

CONCLUSION

Noninstrumented, posterior *in situ* fusion for isthmic spondylolisthesis results in a high fusion rate, pain reduction, and a good functional outcome. Posterior instrumentation, reduction, and anterior fusion of isthmic spondylolisthesis is also a safe and reliable method that has a slight tendency towards a better functional outcome.

REFERENCES

1. Albrecht S, Kleihues H, Gill C, Reinhardt A, Noack W. Repositioning injuries of nerve root L5 after surgical treatment of high degree spondylolistheses and spondyloptosis in vitro studies. *Z Orthop* 1998;136:182–192.
2. Baski DP. Sacrospinalis muscle-pedicle bone graft in posterolateral fusion for spondylolisthesis. *Int Orthop* 1998;22:234–240.
3. Carragee EJ. Single-level posterolateral arthrodesis, with or without posterior decompression, for the treatment of isthmic spondylolisthesis in adults. A prospective, randomized study. *J Bone Joint Surg* 1997;79:1175–1180.

4. Chang P, Seow KH, Tan SK. Comparison of the results of spinal fusion for spondylolisthesis in patients who are instrumented with patients who are not. *Singapore Med J* 1993;34:511–514.

5. De Loubresse CG, Bon T, Deburge A, Lassale B, Benoit M. Posterolateral fusion for radicular pain in isthmic spondylolisthesis. *Clin Orthop* 1996;323:194–201.

6. Fairbank JC, Couper J, Davies JB, O'Brien JP. The Oswestry low back pain questionnaire. *Physiotherapy* 1980; 66:271–273.

7. Hartwig E, Hoellen I, Kramer M, Wickstroem M, Kinzl L. Occupational disease 2108. Degeneration pattern in magnetic resonance tomography of the lumbar spine in patient with differential weight-bearing activity. *Unfallchirurg* 1997;100:888–894.

8. Jeanneret B, Miclau T, Kuster M, Neuer W, Magerl F. Posterior stabilization in L5-S1 isthmic spondylolisthesis with paralaminar screw fixation: anatomical and clinical results. *J Spinal Disord* 1996;9:223–233.

9. Kakiuchi M, Ono K. Defatted, gas-sterilised cortical bone allograft for posterior lumbar interbody vertebral fusion. *Int Orthop* 1998;22:69–76.

10. Morscher E, Dick W. Differentialindikation verschiedener operativer verfahren bei der spondylolisthesis. In: Matzen KA, ed. *Wirbelsäulenchirurgie spondylolisthesis*. Stuttgart: Thieme, 1990:34–44.

11. O'Sullivan PB, Phyty GD, Twomey LT, Allison GT. Evaluation of specific stabilizing exercise in the treatment of chronic low back pain with radiologic diagnosis of spondylolysis or spondylolisthesis. *Spine* 1997;22: 2959–2967.

12. Poussa M, Schlenzka D, Seitsalo S, Ylikoski M, Hurri H, Osterman K. Surgical treatment of severe isthmic spondylolisthesis in adolescents. Reduction or fusion in situ. *Spine* 1993;18:894–901.

13. Ricciardi JE, Pflueger PC, Isaza JE, Whitecloud TS 3rd. Transpedicular fixation for the treatment of isthmic spondylolisthesis in adults. *Spine* 1995;20:1917–1922.

14. Roche MB, Rowe GG. Incidence of separate neural arch and coincident bone variations. *Anat Rec* 1951;109: 233–252.

15. Sagi HC, Jarvis JG, Uhthoff HK. Histomorphic analysis of the development of the pars interarticularis and its association with isthmic spondylolysis. *Spine* 1998;23:1635–1639.

16. Sairyo K, Goel VK, Grobler LJ, Ikata T, Katoh S. The pathomechanism of isthmic lumbar spondylolisthesis. A biomechanical study in immature calf spines. *Spine* 1998;23:1442–1446.

17. Shipley JA, Beukes CA. The nature of spondylytic defect. Demonstration of a communicating synovial pseudarthrosis in the pars articularis. *J Bone Joint Surg* 1998;80:662–664.

18. Wiltse LL, Rothman LG. Inheritance and spondylolisthesis: classification, diagnosis, and natural history. *Semin Spine Surg* 1989;1:78–94.

19. Wiltse LL, Widell EH Jr, Jackson DW. Fatigue fracture: the basic lesion in isthmic spondylolisthesis. *J Bone Joint Surg Am* 1975;57:17–22.

20. Zdeblick TA. A prospective, randomized study of lumbar fusions. Preliminary results. *Spine* 1993;18:983–991.

21. Zindrick MR, Wiltse LL, Widell EH, et al. A biomechanical study of intrapedicular screw fixation in the lumbosacral spine. *Clin Orthop* 1986;203:99–112.

Lumbar Spinal Stenosis
edited by Robert Gunzburg and Marek Szpalski
Lippincott Williams & Wilkins, Philadelphia, © 2000.

37

Importance of Sagittal Adjustment in Lumbosacral Fusion

Radiologic and Functional Evaluation

J.-Y. Lazennec, S. Ramare, *N. Arafati, *C.G. Laudet, †M. Gorin,
‡B. Roger, S. Hansen, G. Saillant, §L. Maurs, and R. Trabelsi

*Service de Chirurgie Orthopédique and ‡Radiologie, Hôpital Pitie-Salpetriere, 75013
Paris; °Service d'Anatomie, Faculté Pitie-Salpetriere, 75013 Paris; †Clinique
Radiologique, 75009 Paris; and §Federation de Neurologie, Hôpital Pitie-Salpetriere,
75013 Paris, France*

Lumbosacral fusion with instrumentation has benefited from technical refinements provided by the development of better and more diverse internal fixation procedures (9–24,36,44,52,53) and of intersomatic grafting via either the posterior lumbar interbody fusion (PLIF) or anterior lumbar interbody fusion (ALIF) approach. Now, the main problem has shifted from obtaining vertebral fusion to achieving optimal spinal alignment (31,55,61).

Some authors, however, have reported harmful effects of flatback due to poorly aligned spinal fusion (6,10,35,38,40). Surgical correction of such flatback deformity has a complication rate of up to 60% (40), making prevention a top priority. "Normal" sagittal alignment is difficult to define, and the optimal degree of lordosis has not yet been determined (50–58). Although several studies have investigated normal lordosis in the standing, supine, or sitting position (2,4,21,22,35), the relationships between the components of the lumbopelvic complex remained unclear until the studies reported by Duval-Beaupere's group (34). Sagittal spinal alignment varies over time (3–5,18,22,28,59). Flatback syndrome generally is described as a manifestation of aging of the spine (43).

There are several reports in the literature of residual lumbosacral pain ascribed to the sacroiliac joints (11,19,23,26,32,57), sacrosciatic ligaments, and paraspinal muscles. In some cases, the pain was projected from the thoracolumbar junction (32,46). Few of these reports describe the pain as related to posture, and most place the blame primarily on changes in lumbar lordosis (12,13,49).

The objective of this study was to conduct a radiologic analysis of posture before and after lumbosacral fusion to evaluate the influence of spinal alignment during surgery on the occurrence and pattern of postsurgical pain, independently from the classic causes of failed back syndrome (graft nonunion, residual disc mobility, persistent nerve root compression, or technically faulty internal fixation). In addition to surgery-related changes in lumbar lordosis, we studied constitutional and functional pelvic parameters.

TABLE 1. *Indications and levels of lumbosacral fusion in 81 patients*

	n	Last mobile level	Last two mobile levels
Degenerative disk disease	44	16	8
Repeat surgery for disk herniation	12	6	6
Low-grade spondylolisthesis (grade I–II)	7	2	5
Revision of lumbar fusion	13	3	10
Revision of flexible instrumentation	1		1
Revision of ligamentoplasty	2		2
Grade III spondylolisthesis	2		2
Total	81	27	54

PATIENTS AND MATERIALS

The study included patients who underwent lumbosacral fusion and received follow-up at the Orthopedic Surgery Department of the Pitié Teaching Hospital between February 1991 and June 1997. Of the 103 cases identified by chart review, 10 were excluded because of psychopathology interfering with evaluation of surgical results, 7 because of inadequate radiologic documentation and possible persistent nerve root pain (n = 7), and 5 because of graft nonunion and unavailability of the patient for evaluation other than by telephone interview (n = 5). Therefore, 81 patients (49 men and 32 women, mean age 61 years, range 41 to 79) were studied. Mean follow-up was 2.8 years. Fifty-one patients had a history of low back surgery; among them, 47 had at least two prior surgical procedures on the low back.

The reason for the surgical procedure was degenerative disc disease in 44 patients, repeat surgery for disc herniation in 12, spondylolisthesis in 9, and a history of failed stabilization surgery in 16 (Table 1).

All 81 patients were positioned on the same type of operating table, with the hips flexed to 45 degrees and the knees to 90 degrees. A height-adjustable lumbar support was used to vary the degree of lordosis by changing the position of the iliac crests and the degree of flexion of the hips (Fig. 1).

We excluded patients who underwent ''suspended'' L4–5 fusion above a normal and/or mobile L5–S1 disc and those who had clinical neurologic abnormalities or other lesions of the lower limbs or spine. Nerve root pain was the dominant preoperative symptom in the 81 study patients. We also excluded patients with suspected or confirmed nonunion at last follow-up based on tomography or computed tomographic findings. None of the study patients had postoperative symptoms or residual nerve root impingement visible on imaging studies, which

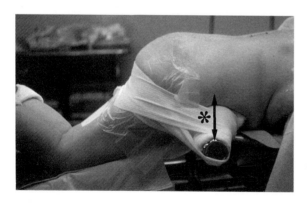

FIG. 1. Typical patient position on the operating table used in this series. The height-adjustable lumbar support (*) allows variations for the degree of lumbar lordosis as needed intraoperatively.

consisted of myelography in 13 cases, magnetic resonance imaging in 27, and computed tomography in 48.

None of the patients had evidence of significant psychopathology as assessed by a neuro-psychiatrist who was not involved in the study (54). Compensation, if any, was evaluated on a case-by-case basis.

Reference radiologic parameter values were obtained in 24 patients (12 men and 12 women, mean age 50 years) free of abnormalities of the spine, pelvis, and lower limbs.

METHODS

Clinical Study

The clinical study involved two phases:

1. A group of pain-free patients with a negative history for spinal surgery, spinal abnormali-ties, and pelvic abnormalities was studied to obtain reference data (nonfusion reference group, n = 24).
2. The 81 surgical patients in our series were studied (fusion group).

In the fusion group, patients with and without residual pain were studied separately (10). In the subgroup with residual pain, the pain was located in the lumbosacral area, with no typical nerve root radiation and no exacerbation with coughing or straining. The pain usually radiated to the groin area or buttock and to the posterolateral aspect of the thigh. The pain was analyzed based on whether it was described by the patients as present only or mainly when standing immobile or when sitting immobile, or as present in both positions (mixed).

Radiologic Study

Nonfusion Patients

Measurements were done on full-length lateral radiographs of the spine taken using large-size cassettes, with the patient standing or sitting with the arms folded across the chest (focal distance 2 m). In the standing position, the patients were asked to stand straight but relaxed, with the knees extended as fully as possible without causing discomfort. In the sitting position, the patients were positioned with the hips and knees in 90-degree flexion and the feet flat on the floor. Again, they were asked to sit straight but relaxed, with the arms folded across the chest.

The reference vertical line was the edge of the film corresponding to the edge of the cassette.

Fusion Patients

Lateral radiographs were taken of the entire thoracolumbar spine to allow analysis of the position of the femoral heads and sacrum, flexion contracture of the hips, position of the sacrum, and lumbar curvature.

Radiographs in the sitting position were taken preoperatively in 39 patients. In 49 patients, full-length lateral radiographs in the standing position taken before surgery that met the previously described criteria were available. In the remaining 32 patients, we only used long and large radiographs in a standing position, but without visualization of the upper femur.

At last follow-up after surgery, full-length lateral radiographs of the spine in the standing position were obtained in all patients.

Radiographic Parameters

Analysis of lumbopelvic parameters before surgery, during surgery, and at last follow-up after surgery was based on the criteria of Duval-Beaupere and colleagues (15,16) assessed on the standing radiographs. When the femoral heads were not exactly superimposed over each other, the middle of the segment connecting the femoral heads was used as the landmark. The sacral tilt (ST) angle in the standing position was defined as the angle formed by the line tangent to the upper edge of S1 (transecting the anterior and posterior angles of S1) and the horizontal plane (Fig. 2) (34). A smaller ST angle indicates a more vertical sacrum and a larger ST angle a more horizontal sacrum. On lateral radiographs, the sitting position is normally characterized by a decrease in lumbar lordosis and a shift of the sacrum toward a more vertical position, resulting in pelvic retroversion. During standing, in contrast, the sacrum moves to a more horizontal position, resulting in pelvic anteversion (Fig. 3).

We determined the ST angle at baseline (STbs) and at last follow-up (STfu).

Pelvic tilt (PT) is the angle formed by the vertical plane and the line connecting the center of the sacral plateau to the center of the axis of the hips. We determined PT at baseline (PTbs) and at last follow-up (PTfu). Pelvic tilt is larger in subjects with pelvic retroversion and a vertical sacrum. Conversely, a markedly horizontal sacrum is associated with a small or negative PT.

Another patient-related constitutional morphologic parameter was measured: the incidence angle (I) formed by the line perpendicular to the line tangent to the center of the sacral plateau

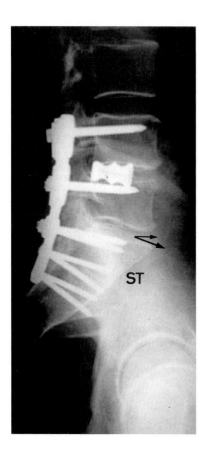

FIG. 2. Sacral tilt (ST) angle. In this case, fusion has been achieved in a very vertical position of the sacrum (ST angle = 19 degrees).

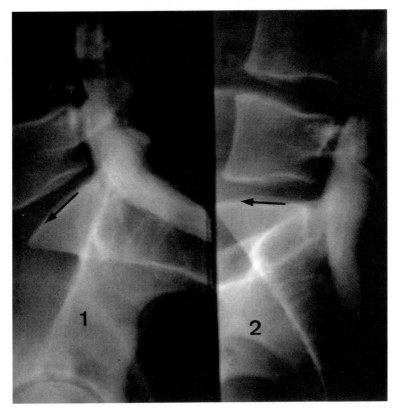

FIG. 3. Change in sacral tilt between the standing **(1)** and sitting **(2)** position. During sitting, the sacrum moves to a more vertical position, i.e, ST decreases.

and by the line connecting the center of the sacral plateau to the center of the axis of the hips (Figs. 4 and 5).

The angles that we determined are related by the formula $I = ST + PT$, which can be readily demonstrated geometrically. This formula shows that any change in ST is inevitably associated with a change in PT.

On the standing radiographs, the positions of T9, L1, L2, and L3 were calculated by measuring the angle formed by the vertical line drawn through the center of the femoral heads and the line connecting the center of the femoral heads to the center of the relevant vertebral body.

Overall lordosis was evaluated between the upper endplate of L1 and the upper endplate of S1. Segmental lordosis was assessed between L4 and S1 and between L5 and S1.

Data on S1 overhang were not analyzed because of substantial variability in results due to measurement difficulties (34). All measurements were done five times, during different measurement sessions, by each of three independent evaluators. Flexion contracture of the hip was evaluated only qualitatively, because reliable radiographic measurements were not available. The sacroiliac joints were evaluated radiologically before and after surgery.

Statistical Methods

Statistical analysis was done using the SAS package (SAS institute, Cary, NC). For comparisons of qualitative variables, either Pearson's Chi-square test or Fisher's exact test was used,

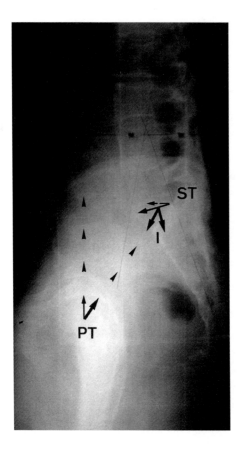

FIG. 4. Pelvic tilt (PT) angle and incidence angle I in a failed lumbosacral fusion (implant has been removed). Extreme pelvic retroversion with too important PT (30 degrees; normal 12 degrees). I = 46 degrees, with too low sacral tilt (ST) angle (16 degrees; normal 41 degrees). Note very low ST with relative hip flexum.

depending on sample size. Quantitative variables were compared either using Student's *t* test after verification that distribution of the variables was normal or using the nonparametric Kruskal-Wallis test if several groups were being compared. A multivariate logistic regression model was used to identify factors predicting postfusion pain, with the prefusion and postfusion radiologic parameters as the explanatory variables.

RESULTS

Clinical Results

Twenty-seven fusion patients were completely pain free and 54 experienced residual pain. Of these 54 patients, 30 reported pain only or primarily when standing immobile, 18 when sitting immobile, and 6 in both positions.

Accurate data on compensation were available for 61 patients. Of the 41 patients who received compensation, 21 had postfusion pain, whereas 19 of the patients who did not receive compensation were pain free after fusion, a statistically significant difference ($p = 0.001$).

Data allowing accurate evaluation of flexion contracture of the hip were available before fusion in 49 patients and after fusion in all 81 patients. Flexion contracture was present before fusion in 13 of 49 patients and after fusion in 23 of 81 patients. A significant association between flexion contracture of the hip and postfusion pain was found ($p = 0.015$).

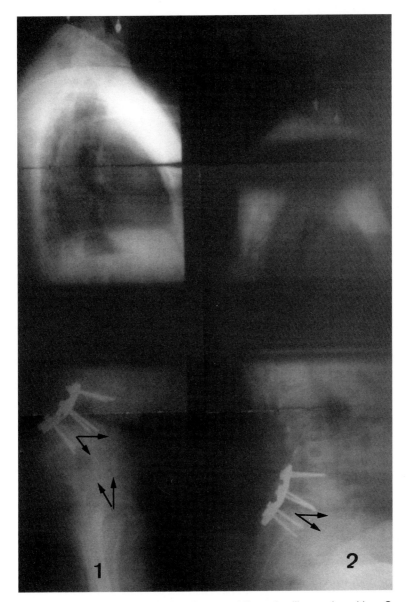

FIG. 5. Lumbosacral fusion with posterior plates and "standard" sacral position. Sacral tilt = 56 degrees in the standing position **(1)** and 35 degrees in the sitting position **(2)**. Pelvic tilt = 29 degrees.

Evaluation of Angles

The results of repeated angle measurements in the nonfusion reference group demonstrated satisfactory reproducibility: mean variability was 6 degrees for measurements obtained by placing a goniometer on the radiographs (none of the radiographs were digitized). Similar variability was noted in the fusion group, although ST measurement was more difficult because of vertebral endplate remodeling.

TABLE 2. *Angles in nonfusion patients (n–24)*

	Mean	Minimum	Maximum	Standard deviation
Sacral tilt	38.9	32	43	2.7
Pelvic tilt	17.9	5	35	7.4
Incidence angle	56.9	37	76	7.7
Overall sitting lordosis (L1–S1)			32 ± 12 degrees	
Overall standing lordosis (L1–S1)			46 ± 11 degrees	

Analysis of angles in the sitting position was unsuccessful because of difficulties in reading the films, despite the standardized acquisition protocol.

Evaluation of Nonfusion Patients

In our nonfusion reference group, ST was 39 degrees, PT was 18 degrees, and I was 57 ± 11 degrees (Table 2). Overall L1–S1 lordosis was 32 ± 12 degrees in the sitting position and 46 ± 11 degrees in the standing position.

Evaluation of Fusion Patients

Baseline values of ST, PF, and I on standing films in the fusion group showed no statistically significant differences with the nonfusion group. After surgery, in contrast, ST and PT in the fusion group showed significant differences versus the nonfusion group (Table 3).

Radiographic abnormalities of the sacroiliac joints (sclerosis, osteophytosis, or vacuum phenomenon) were seen before fusion in 11 patients and after fusion in 14 other patients; 18 of these 25 patients had postfusion pain.

Comparison of Fusion Patients with and without Postfusion Pain

Baseline Parameters

Baseline ST was 17.3 degrees overall, 12.4 degrees in the subgroup without postfusion pain, and 19.7 degrees in the subgroup with postfusion pain (Figs. 6 and 7, and Table 4). Corresponding values for PTbs were 41, 45.7, and 39.2 degrees. These data show that the subgroup with postfusion pain was characterized at baseline by a more vertical sacrum

TABLE 3. *Angles in fusion patients (n = 81)*

	Mean	Minimum	Maximum	Standard deviation
Sacral tilt at baseline	41.4	13	67	10.3
Sacral tilt at last follow-up	36.9	10	61	12
Pelvic tilt at baseline	17.3	−16	57	13
Pelvic tilt at last follow-up	22	−12	55	15
Incidence angle	58.6	39	77	9

	Preoperative	Postoperative
Overall sitting lordosis (L1–S1)	27 ± 7 degrees	25 ± 6 degrees
Overall standing lordosis (L1–S1)	40 ± 9 degrees	43 ± 10 degrees

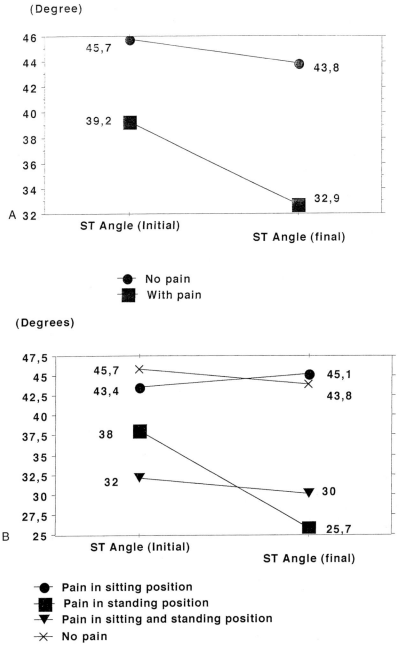

FIG. 6. Change in sacral tilt (ST) before and after fusion. Note the striking distribution of patients with postfusion pain, **A:** global analysis, **B:** detailed analysis according to pain type.

(degrees)

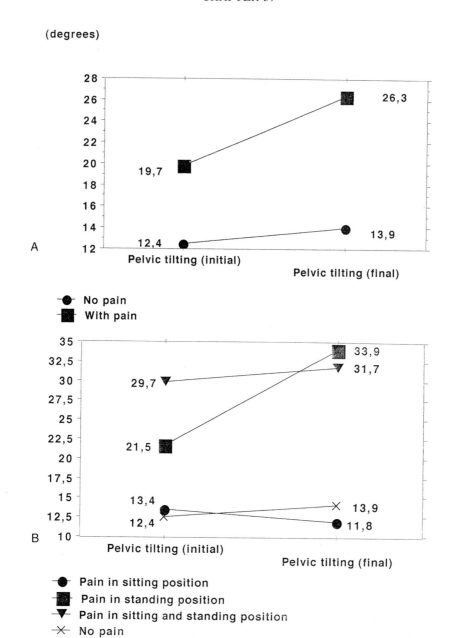

FIG. 7. Change in pelvic tilt (PT) before and after fusion. Note the striking distribution of patients with postfusion pain, **A:** global analysis, **B:** detailed analysis according to pain type.

TABLE 4. *Relationships between angles and pain*

	No pain	Pain while sitting	Pain while standing	Pain while sitting and standing	p Value by NP test
STbs	45.7	43.4	38	32	0.0033
STfu	43.8	45.2	25.8	30	<0.0001
PTbs	12.4	13.4	21.6	29.7	<0.0001
PTfu	13.9	11.7	33.9	31.6	<0.0001
ΔST	−1.9	+1.7	−12.3	−2	<0.0001
ΔPT	1.6	−1.6	12.3	2	<0.0001

PTbs, pelvic tilt at baseline; PTfu, pelvic tilt at follow-up; STbs, sacral tilt at baseline; STfu, sacral tilt at follow-up.

(smaller ST value) (p = 0.0062 by Student's t test) and by a greater degree of PT (p = 0.0160).

Parameters at Last Follow-up

Pelvic tilt at last follow-up was correlated with the presence of postfusion pain (p = 0.0003 by Student's t test). It was 22.2 degrees overall, 13.9 degrees in patients without postfusion pain, and 26.2 degrees in patients with postfusion pain. Thus, PT was almost twice the normal value in the patients with postfusion pain.

Sacral tilt at last follow-up in the standing position also was correlated with the presence of postfusion pain ($p < 0.0001$). It was 36.4 degrees overall, 43.8 degrees in the patients without postfusion pain, and 32.6 degrees in the patients with postfusion pain. Thus, the sacrum remained abnormally vertical in the subjects with postfusion pain.

No correlations were found between the presence of postfusion pain and the baseline or last follow-up values of I, the lordosis angles, or the positions of T9, L1, or L3.

Analysis of the Effect of Surgery-related Changes in Sacral Tilt and Pelvic Tilt on Presence of Postfusion Pain

The change in PT between baseline and last follow-up had a significant effect on the presence of postfusion pain (p = 0.0213 by Student's t test). The change in ST between baseline and last follow-up was significantly associated with the presence of postfusion pain (Nonparametric test, NP: p = 0.042). From baseline to last follow-up, ST decreased by 1.9 degrees in the pain-free patients versus 6.5 degrees in the patients with pain.

Analysis of Postural Pain Patterns

When postural pain patterns were analyzed, the patients were found to fall into two groups. Both at baseline and at last follow-up, patients who were either pain free or experienced pain only in the sitting position had roughly the same pattern of PT and ST as the nonfusion patients. Conversely, patients with pain in the standing position or in both the standing and sitting positions were characterized at baseline by a more vertical sacrum with a smaller degree of ST, according to the formula I = ST + PT.

Standardized radiologic evaluation in the sitting position proved disappointing. We were able to determine whether effective verticalization of the lumbopelvic complex was achieved, but could not take into account postural diversity in the sitting position across patients.

No correlations were found between the pattern of postfusion pain and values at baseline or last follow-up of I, the lordosis angles, or the positions of T9, L1, or L3.

Factors Predictive of Postfusion Pain

We evaluated the predictive value for postfusion pain of the following parameters: STbs, STfu, PTbs, PTfu, change in ST, and change in PT. The only factor significantly associated with postfusion pain was STfu ($p < 0.0001$).

DISCUSSION

Earlier studies established the importance of "normal" sagittal posture defined as alignment on the same vertical axis of the external auditory canals, the center of the bodies of C7 and L5, the centers of the femoral heads, and the center of the tibiotalar joint (36). However, there is no firm proof that sagittal imbalance is associated with spinal pain (44). Anterior displacement of the vertical weight-bearing axis carried down from the external auditory canal or the center of C7 may be associated with heavier loads through the lumbar spine (28,35). Sagittal alignment abnormalities may have harmful long-term effects, including degenerative disc disease at the level suprajacent to spinal fusion (14,62).

Fusion of a spinal level is generally thought to modify the mechanical behavior of the suprajacent and infrajacent intervertebral levels, exposing them to premature degenerative disc disease (6,7,33,34,41,42). It also has been suggested that mechanical alterations may occur at a distance from the fused level (21,26,45,60,61). However, there are no data in the literature regarding the influence of sagittal spinal alignment on the progression of these disturbances (54).

Instrumentation of the lumbosacral junction can result in flatback syndrome, characterized by loss of lumbar lordosis and sagittal imbalance with anterior displacement of the weight-bearing axis. However, some patients with treatment-related loss of lumbar lordosis remain free of symptoms, and there are few data in the literature on which postures are associated with pain (20,35). We found no influence on pain of postfusion lordosis angles or T9 position, which suggests that changes in the adjacent levels occurred to compensate for the fusion. None of our patients had preoperative loss of spinal motion, a feature that has been reported to be associated with postfusion pain in the hips, knees, and lower neck (27,31,32). Rather than the absolute degree of lordosis (35), the relevant parameters may be the "overall" and "useful" orientation of the lumbar segments in the sagittal plane. These parameters are directly governed by the position of the pelvis (14–16).

The description by Duval-Beaupere (15) of the pelvic incidence angle and its two components, PT and ST, provide a clear understanding of the relationship between the spine and pelvis. Pelvic tilt is the factor that ensures balance of the trunk around the femoral heads. Pelvic tilt varies with the incidence angle of each individual and is influenced by comorbid conditions and surgery-related alignment changes.

Our study also focused on "morphologic angles" inherent in the structure of each individual (incidence angle I) and on "postural angles" amenable to modification (PT and ST). We elected to use those angles, because this method provides better information on postural status than the junctional couple described by Vidal and Marnay (39–57), which neither separates the contributions of sacral position and pelvic position nor takes into account constitutional anatomic variations.

"Narrow" incidence angles theoretically could result in limited compensation possibilities and in pain, because they leave little room for angle changes to occur. "Wide" incidence angles should allow to achieve better alignment.

None of our nonfusion or fusion patients had incidence angles below the usual range (the situation theoretically associated with limited compensation possibilities). All the subjects included in our study had normal or wide incidence angle values.

For our measurements, we used "full-length" radiographs in the standing position taken with the arms folded on the chest. Other investigators used radiographs taken with the arms extended on arm rests placed in front of the chest (48). We found in a walking platform study that this arm position was associated with substantial changes in the center of gravity.

Our overall study population (nonfusion patients and fusion patients with and without pain after surgery) was homogeneous regarding our study parameters. At baseline, no significant differences were found among these groups regarding I, PT, or ST. These values were consistent with those reported by Duval-Beaupere and Robain (15) and Mangione and Senegas (38).

The numeric data abstracted from each medical record confirmed that $I = ST + PT$. I represents the angle of "sacroiliac joint opening" and is a morphologic parameter characteristic of each individual. It is independent of the position of the pelvis and does not vary in a given individual beyond the age when walking is learned. In our study, the incidence angle I was not significantly associated with the presence of postfusion pain.

Pelvic tilt and ST at baseline both were associated with the presence of postfusion pain, most notably in the sacroiliac area. Sacroiliac joint dysfunction too often is overlooked due to insufficient postural analysis (47,56). Nevertheless, the influence of gluteus maximus muscle, sacrotuberous ligament, and hamstring muscles has been proved in sacrum nutation and spine-pelvis relationship.

A striking finding from our study is that patients who later were found to have postfusion pain were characterized at baseline by a more vertical sacrum (i.e., a smaller ST) and by greater PT than the nonfusion patients or the fusion patients who were free of pain at last follow-up. This result suggests that a subset of patients may be at high risk for poor functional results of lumbosacral fusion. Similarly, our analysis of PT and ST at baseline showed that patients with a more vertical sacrum and greater PT were more likely to have postfusion pain. Furthermore, in the patients whose sacrum was more vertical at baseline than in the nonfusion group, the surgical procedure was associated with further sacral verticalization, which may have resulted in additional postfusion pain.

Anterior spinal imbalance due to poor spinal alignment displaces the center of gravity forward. This should normally be compensated for by extension of the hip with an increase in PT (27).

Mangione and Senegas (38) reported that patients with degenerative lumbar kyphosis had pelvic retroversion with a normal incidence angle, indicating that the morphotype initially was normal. Loss of lordosis was associated with anterior displacement of the center of gravity and progressive sagittal imbalance characterized by an increase in PT and a decrease in ST, i.e., verticalization of the sacrum. These changes were partly compensated for at the hips, which moved to a hyperextended position, to the extent permitted by the frequent presence of hip osteoarthritis.

If hip extension is limited by osteoarthritis, retroversion of the pelvis around the center of rotation of the hips becomes extreme, and compensation for the imbalance occurs at the knees. Therefore, caution needed in patients in whom the presurgical evaluation discloses flexion contracture of the hips or abnormalities of the knees. The usefulness of full-length radiographs of the lower limbs in the standing position cannot be overemphasized.

We found that evaluation of the femoropelvic angle as advocated by Mangione and Senegas

(38) was difficult on available radiographic documents because of the curvature of the femur and of difficulties in interpreting findings near the edges of the films. In our study, flexion contracture of the hips, which often was asymmetric, could be evaluated only in a qualitative manner, which probably reduced the significance of this parameter.

Our analysis of postural postfusion pain patterns demonstrated a significant difference between patients who had pain in the standing position and those who had pain only in the sitting position. The patients with postfusion pain while standing had a more vertical sacrum after the fusion procedure. In the patients with pain only while sitting, none of the study parameters showed significant differences versus nonfusion patients. There are no data in the literature on the interpretation of postural pain patterns (17,30,35,59). Studies of large lateral radiographs in the sitting position probably would provide interesting information, although preliminary work would be needed to define a reference sitting position and to evaluate individual variations.

CONCLUSION

Lumbosacral fusion by no means focuses only on neurologic objectives or segmental mechanical factors. Achieving a strong fusion is not the only goal. Appropriate position of the fused vertebras also is of paramount importance to minimize muscle work during posture maintenance. Caution is necessary in patients in whom the presurgical evaluation discloses flexion contracture of the hips or abnormalities of the knees.

The main risk is fixing or causing excessive retroversion with a vertical sacrum, which leads to a sagittal alignment that replicates the sitting position. This situation often is accompanied by loss of lumbar lordosis and adversely affected stiff or degenerative hips.

Sagittal alignment should be done with the goal of minimizing muscle work during posture maintenance (16).

The main merit of our study is that it emphasizes the difficulty of achieving optimal sacral alignment under the lumbar column during lumbosacral fusion. Alignment is obtained by adjusting the position of the patient (1,8,32,40,49,51,53) and the internal fixation material. The main risk is fixing or causing excessive retroversion of a vertical sacrum, a situation that often is accompanied by loss of lumbar lordosis—as occurs during aging of the spine—and that leads to sagittal alignment replicating the sitting position. This results in pain in the standing position because of undue stress on the sacroiliac joints and on the hips. Increased extension of the hips occurs to reduce loads through the adjacent spinal levels and to protect the lumbopelvic complex, most notably the sacroiliac joints.

Lumbosacral morphotype and therefore the incidence angle vary across individuals. It is preferable to move the sacrum to a more horizontal position, i.e., to increase standing ST and to decrease PT (especially in patients with preoperative abnormalities in these parameters). However, we cannot make any recommendations for avoiding the theoretical risk of predominant pain in the sitting position in patients with a markedly horizontal sacrum or with normal parameters before surgery.

REFERENCES

1. Aaro S. The effect of Harrington instrumentation on the sagittal configuration and mobility of the spine in scoliosis. *Spine* 1983;8:570–575.
2. Adams MA, Hutton WC. The effect of posture on the lumbar spine. *J Bone Joint Surg Br* 1985;67:625–629.
3. Bernhardt M, Bridwell KH. Segmental analysis of the sagittal plane alignment of the normal thoracic and lumbar spines and thoracolumbar junction. *Spine* 1989;14:717–721.
4. Bogduk N. The anatomical basis for spinal pain syndromes. *J Manipulative Physiol Ther* 1995;18:603–605.

5. Bradford DS. Failed back syndrome secondary to previous spondylolisthesis surgery. *Chir Organi Mov* 1994; 79:109–110.

6. Brodsky .E. Post-laminectomy and post-fusion stenosis of the lumbar spine. *Clin Orthop* 1976;115:130–139.

7. Brodsky AE, Hendricks RL, Khalil MA, Darden BV, Brotzman TT. Segmental (''floating'') lumbar spine fusions. *Spine* 1989;14:447–450.

8. Callahan RA, Brown MD. Positioning techniques in spinal surgery. *Clin Orthop* 1981;154:22–26.

9. Cauchoix J, David T. Lumbar arthrodesis: results after more than 10 years. *Rev Chir Orthop* 1985;71:263–268.

10. Daum WJ. The sacroiliac joint: an underappreciated pain generator. *Am J Orthop* 1995;24:475–478.

11. Deburge A, Vaquin G, Lassale B, Benoist M. Sciatica caused by lateral stenosis of the spinal canal. *Rev Chir Orthop* 1989;75:90–97.

12. Drummond DS, Breed AL, Narechania R. Relationship of spine deformity and pelvic obliquity on sitting pressure distributions and decubitus ulceration. *J Pediatr Orthop* 1985;5:396–402.

13. Drummond DS, Narechania R, Rosenthal AN, Breed AL, Lange TA, Drummond DK. A study of pressure distributions during balanced and unbalanced sitting. *J Bone Joint Surg Am* 1972;54:492–510.

14. During J, Goudfrooij H, Keessen W, Beeker TW, Crowe A. Toward standards for posture. Postural characteristics of the lower back system in normal and pathologic conditions. *Spine* 1985;10:83–87.

15. Duval-Beaupere G, Robain G. Visualization on full spine radiographs of the anatomical connections of the centres of the segmental body mass supported by each vertebra and measured in vivo. *Int Orthop* 1987;11: 261–269.

16. Duval-Beaupere G, Schmidt C, Cosson P. A barycentremetric study of the sagittal shape of spine and pelvis: the conditions required for an economic standing position. *Ann Biomed Eng* 1992;20:451–462.

17. Farfan HF, Huberdau RM, Dubow HI. Lumbar intervertebral disc degeneration. *J Bone Joint Surg Am* 1972,54: 492–510.

18. Fernand R, Fox DE. Evaluation of lumbar lordosis. A prospective and retrospective study. *Spine* 1985;10: 799–803.

19. Fortin JD, Aprill CN, Ponthieux B, Pier J. Sacroiliac joint: pain referral maps upon applying a new injection/arthrography technique. Part II: Clinical evaluation. *Spine* 1994;19:1483–1489.

20. Froning EC, Frohman B. Motion of the lumbosacral spine after laminectomy and spine fusion. Correlation of motion with the result. *J Bone Joint Surg Am* 1968;50:897–918.

21. Frymoyer JW, Hanley EN Jr, Howe J, Kuhlmann D, Matteri RE. A comparison of radiographic findings in fusion and nonfusion patients ten or more years following lumbar disc surgery. *Spine* 1979;4:435–440.

22. Frymoyer JW, Howe J, Kuhlmann D. The long-term effects of spinal fusion on the sacroiliac joints and ilium. *Clin Orthop* 1978;134:196–201.

23. Gelb DE, Lenke LG, Bridwell KH, Blanke K, McEnery KW. An analysis of sagittal spinal alignment in 100 asymptomatic middle and older aged volunteers. *Spine* 1995;20:1351–1358.

24. Gerard Y, Schernberg F, Thirion Y. Results of postero-lateral grafts in the lumbosacral vertebrae. *Acta Orthop Belg* 1981;47:636–642.

25. Goutallier D, Vigroux JP, Sterkers Y. Results of intersomatic arthrodeses in essential lumbalgia. *Rev Rhum Mal Osteoartic* 1990;57:91–97.

26. Ha KY, Schendel MJ, Lewis JL, Ogilvie JW. Effect of immobilization and configuration on lumbar adjacent-segment biomechanics. *J Spinal Disord* 1993;6:99–105.

27. Hasday CA, Passof TL, Perry J. Gait abnormalities arising from iatrogenic loss of lumbar lordosis secondary to Harrington instrumentation in lumbar fractures. *Spine* 1983;8:501–511.

28. Jackson RP, McManus AC. Radiographic analysis of sagittal plane alignment and balance in standing volunteers and patients with low back pain matched for age, sex, and size. A prospective controlled clinical study. *Spine* 1994;19:1611–1618.

29. Junghans H. Der lumbosakralwinkel. *Dtsch Z Chir* 1929;213–332.

30. Keegan JJ. Alteration of the lumbar curve related to posture and seating. *J Bone Joint Surg Am* 1988;19: 383–393.

31. Lagrone MO. Loss of lumbar lordosis. A complication of spinal fusion for scoliosis. *Orthop Clin North Am* 1988;19:383–393.

32. Lagrone MO, Bradford DS, Moe JH, Lonstein JE, Winter RB, Ogilvie JW. Treatment of symptomatic flatback after spinal fusion. *J Bone Joint Surg Am* 1988;70:569–580.

33. Lee CK, Langrana NA. Lumbosacral spinal fusion. A biomechanical study. *Spine* 1984;9:574–581.

34. Legaye J, Duval-Beaupere G, Hecquet J, Marty C. Pelvic incidence: a fundamental pelvic parameter for three dimensional regulation of spinal sagittal curves. *Eur Spine J* 1998;7:99–103.

35. Lord MJ, Small JM, Dinsay JM, Watkins RG. Lumbar lordosis. Effects of sitting and standing. *Spine* 1997; 22:2571–2574.

36. Maigne JY, Aivaliklis A, Pfefer F. Results of sacroiliac joint double block and value of sacroiliac pain provocation tests in 54 patients with low back pain. *Spine* 1996;21:1889–1892.

37. Maigne R. Low back pain of thoracolumbar origin. *Arch Phys Med Rehabil* 1980;61:389–395.

38. Mangione P, Senegas J. Sagittal balance of the spine. *Rev Chir Orthop Reparatrice Appar Mot* 1997;83:22–32.

39. Marnay TH. Equilibre du rachis et du bassin. Cahiers d'enseignement de la SOFCOT. Conférences d'enseignement. 281–313. Expansion scientifique française, Paris, 1988.

40. Peterson MD, Nelson LM, McManus AC, Jackson RP. The effect of operative position on lumbar lordosis. A radiographic study of patients under anesthesia in the prone and 90–90 positions. *Spine* 1995;20:1419–1424.
41. Rahm MD, Hall BB. Adjacent-segment degeneration after lumbar fusion with instrumentation: a retrospective study. *J Spinal Disord* 1996;9:392–400.
42. Rolander SD. Motion of the lumbar spine with special reference to the stabilizing effect of posterior fusion. An experimental study on autopsy specimens. *Acta Orthop Scand* 1966;90[Suppl]:1–144.
43. Roy-Camille R. L'instabilité rachidienne. *Rachis* 1994;6:107–112.
44. Roy-Camille R, Benazet JP, Desauge JP, Kuntz F. Lumbosacral fusion with pedicular screw plating instrumentation. A 10-year follow-up. *Acta Orthop Scand Suppl* 1993;251:100–1004.
45. Saillant G, Rolland E, Benazet JP, Roy-Camille R. Destabilization after surgical treatment of narrow lumbar canal: when should arthrodesis be performed? *Chirurgie* 1996;121:597–600.
46. Schlegel JD, Smith JA, Schleusener RL. Lumbar motion segment pathology adjacent to thoracolumbar, lumbar, and lumbosacral fusions. *Spine* 1996;21:970–981.
47. Schwarzer AC, Aprill CN, Bogduk N. The sacroiliac joint in chronic low back pain. *Spine* 1995;20:31–37.
48. Shaffer WO, Spratt KF, Weinstein J, Lehmann TR, Goel VK. The consistency and accuracy of roentgenograms for measuring sagittal translation in the lumbar vertebral segment. *Spine* 1990;15:741–750.
49. Smith RM, Emans JB. Sitting balance in spinal deformity. *Spine* 1992;17:1103–1109.
50. Stagnara P, De Mauroy JC, Dran G, et al. Reciprocal angulation of vertebral bodies in a sagittal plane: approach to references for the evaluation of kyphosis and lordosis. *Spine* 1982;7:335–342.
51. Sypert GW. Low back pain disorders: lumbar fusion? *Clin Neurosurg* 1986;33:457–483.
52. Tan SB, Kozak JA, Dickson JH, Nalty TJ. Effect of operative position on sagittal alignment of the lumbar spine. *Spine* 1994;19:314–318.
53. Temple HT, Kruse RW, van Dam BE. Lumbar and lumbosacral fusion using Steffee instrumentation. *Spine* 1994;19:537–541.
54. Turner RS, Leiding WC. Correlation of the MMPI with lumbosacral spine fusion results. Prospective study. *Spine* 1985;10:932–936.
55. Van Horn JR, Bohnen LM. The development of discopathy in lumbar discs adjacent to a lumbar anterior interbody spondylodesis. A retrospective matched-pair study with a postoperative follow-up of 16 years. *Acta Orthop Belg* 1992;58:280–286.
56. Van Wingerden JP, Vleeming A, Snijders CJ, Stoekart R. A functional anatomical approach to spine pelvis mechanism: interaction between the biceps femoris muscle and the sacrotuberous ligament. *Eur Spine J* 1993; 2:140–144.
57. Vidal J, Marnay T. Sagittal deviations of the spine, and trial of classification as a function of the pelvic balance. *Rev Chir Orthop Reparatrice Appar Mot* 1984;70[Suppl 2]:124–126.
58. Voutsinas SA, MacEwen GD. Sagittal profiles of the spine. *Clin Orthop* 1986;210:235–242.
59. Waisbrod H, Krainick JU, Gerbershagen HU. Sacroiliac joint arthrodesis for chronic lower back pain. *Arch Orthop Trauma Surg* 1987;106:238–240.
60. Williams MM, Hawley JA, McKenzie RA, van Wijmen PM. A comparison of the effects of two sitting postures on back and referred pain. *Spine* 1991;16:1185–1191.
61. Wood KB, Schendel MJ, Pashman RS, et al. In vivo analysis of canine intervertebral and facet motion. *Spine* 1992;17:1180–1186.
62. Yoganandan N, Pintar F, Maiman DJ, et al. Kinematics of the lumbar spine following pedicle screw plate fixation. *Spine* 1993;18:504–512.

Lumbar Spinal Stenosis
edited by Robert Gunzburg and Marek Szpalski
Lippincott Williams & Wilkins, Philadelphia, © 2000.

38

Concept and Clinical Aspects of Computer-Assisted Spine Surgery

Heiko Visarius

Medivision, CH-4436 Oberdorf, Switzerland

Spinal fixation relying on transpedicular screws was introduced by Roy-Camille et al. (12,13) in 1963 and recently was the focus of increased attention (4,6–8,16,18). It is widely accepted that pedicle screw systems provide reliable spinal fixation. However, even with advanced surgical techniques, several potential problems and possible complications still are involved in the process of screw insertion (2,3,19).

To successfully insert a pedicle screw, the accurate screw axis must be identified. Mathematically, this axis is completely defined by the three-dimensional location of two different points along its length. Clinically, this definition involves identification of an entry point and correct spatial orientation, i.e., angles in the sagittal and transverse planes. In addition, the depth of insertion must be controlled (5). Any major deviation causes perforation of the pedicular or vertebral cortex and may result in neurologic or vascular damage.

High failure rates in screw location have been reported with intraoperative pedicle cortex perforations ranging from 5.5% up to 39.9% (3,4,11,16). Even with screws inserted *in vitro,* failure rates up to 21% have been documented (18).

Various techniques have been proposed to safely insert pedicle screws. Identification of the entry point commonly is based on anatomic landmarks. Information for the proper angulation of the screw axis may be gained from morphometric data or preoperative planar and tomographic images as well as intraoperative planar images.

Most of the reported improvements are associated with the use of image intensifiers that may increase operation time as well as radiation exposure to patient and staff. Furthermore, none of the existing techniques provides accurate skeletal registration, i.e., a direct and accessible transformation between the "virtual world" of the image and the "real world" in the operation room. They all rely on the three-dimensional perception of the surgeon.

In light of these problems with anchoring posterior instrumentation systems, insertion of pedicle and sacral screws was chosen as the first clinical application of our system for computer-assisted orthopedic surgery. Following an accuracy study and *in vitro* evaluation of the proposed system (9,10), clinical introduction of this technique began 1994. Today, the first studies describing the encouraging clinical results achieved with the introduction of computer-assisted orthopedic surgery are available (14,15).

CONCEPT

A first complete description of principles and devices for stereotaxis was reported in 1906 in the classic paper by Clarke and Horsley (1). With the availability to the medical community

TABLE 1. *Components of the generalized stereotactic concept*

Component	Example[a]
Navigational objects	Pointer
	Pedicle awl or probe
	Pneumatic drill
	Dynamic reference bases
	Calibrated C-arm or ultrasound probe
Surgical objects	Vertebra
	Bone fragments
	Implant components
Virtual objects	Computed tomography
	Magnetic resonance imaging
	Calibrated C-arm or ultrasound probe
Other objects	Virtual keyboard
	Bending device
	Screw Head localizer
	Calibration unit

[a] Examples are given for application in spine surgery.

of computed tomography, applications of computer-assisted surgery became practical. It stimulated pioneering research and clinical applications in the area of frame-based tumor stereotaxis using different types of stereotactic apparatus for navigation. Certain advancements were made with the use of articulated arms and medical robots. However, inherent to these navigators is the limitation that only one object at a time can be controlled and guided and the need for a rigid connection of the navigator to the surgical object. These disadvantages can be avoided by using modern marker-based optoelectronic motion analysis systems for navigation.

It is assumed that all surgical components involved can be treated mechanically as rigid bodies. Usually this is done by associating a separate local coordinate system with each rigid body. By attaching a sufficient number of markers to each component, their motion (three translations and three rotations) can be computed from the location of these markers as recorded by the optoelectronic camera. Basic components of such a surgical system are (a) one surgical object, e.g., the vertebra, (b) the associated virtual object, e.g., its tomographic image, and (c) at least one surgical tool. However, this concept can be generalized, incorporating various navigational, surgical, and virtual objects as summarized in Table 1. Furthermore, other objects can be considered, which may provide an advanced man-machine interface. Note that some components can be categorized as either a navigational object or a virtual object depending on their specific use. This is exemplified by an acoustic probe, which may be used either to generate contours of bones for the matching procedure (navigational object) or to create a data set for image reconstruction (virtual object).

COMPONENTS

Hardware

The SurgiGATE system (Medivision, Oberdorf, CH) used consists of an optoelectronic camera that can precisely (0.1 mm) locate light-emitting diodes in a large field of view (cube with 1.5-m side length). These diodes send out an infrared signal and are mounted on standard instruments for spine surgery (Stratec Medical, Medivision, Oberdorf, Switzerland), e.g., the Synthes USS pedicle awl and probe. Further tools include a calibration unit for on-the-fly calibration of surgical instruments, a dynamic reference base to compensate for patient motion

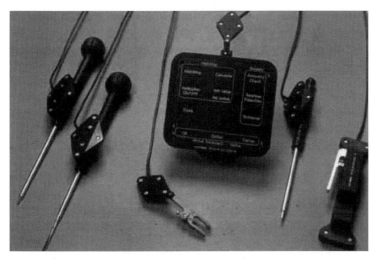

FIG. 1. Standard tool set used for computer-assisted spine surgery includes the USS pedicle awl, USS pedicle probe, dynamic reference base, and virtual keyboard, space pointer, and calibration unit.

during the surgical procedure, and a virtual keyboard, which, in combination with a foot switch, allows the surgeon to control the system directly without the need for an on-site system engineer (17). The standard tool set for spine surgery is shown in Fig. 1. All tools have a cable attached, which is plugged into a distributor box. The plug further contains a chip for self-identification of all instruments.

The electronics for the camera, workstation computer, and monitor for use by the surgeon are stored on a movable cart (Fig. 2).

Software

The SurgiGATE software installed on the workstation provides modules for image data acquisition from various scanners, preoperative diagnosis, planning, and simulation, tool check and calibration, skeletal registration (matching) based on paired points as well as surface, and two different modules for intraoperative support. The software is structured clearly, with only six main buttons that guide the surgeon through the procedure. Inherent hierarchies help to control the program flow, e.g., the matching modules cannot be accessed until a patient is loaded and tools are calibrated. The use of the specific modules is integrated into the next section.

SURGICAL PROCEDURE

Preoperative Planning

Tomographic scans of all vertebrae to be operated on are obtained from the associated radiologic department by hospital network, tape, or magnetooptical disc. The acquisition module reads image and header data and displays the patient. Using the mouse, the surgeon can select any view of the image data including nonorthogonal cuts through the image volume. A three-dimensional model of the patient can be created in a semiautomatic fashion within minutes.

Within the image, four to six anatomic landmarks are selected via mouse click, labeled,

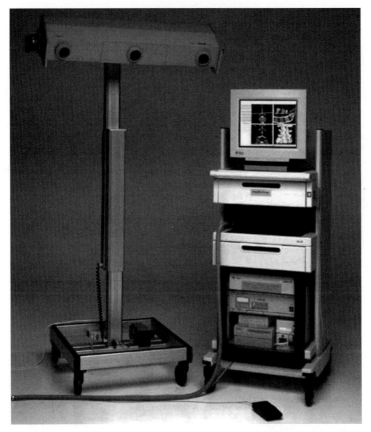

FIG. 2. Components of a system used for computer-assisted surgery. The computer cart contains the electronic components. From here, connections are made to the camera and to the navigation instruments.

and stored for intraoperative use during the matching procedure. Optionally, the surgeon can plan the procedure by defining an optimal axis for the pedicle screw (trajectory) by selection of an entry and target point in the image, respectively. The chosen path can be displayed, thus simulating the surgery, and, if desired, optimized further.

System Setup

The computer cart and the camera cart are positioned in the operating room during normal preparation of room. Conceptually, cart and camera positions are arbitrary, but they should be chosen to ensure good vision of the screen for the surgeon and of the situs/tools for the camera. A possible setup is shown in Fig. 3. During the standard posterior surgical exposure of the dorsal vertebral elements, the assistant can prepare the navigation instruments. The plugs are dropped and connected to the distributor box, and the instruments are checked and calibrated by insertion into the calibration unit. This procedure should not take longer than 5 minutes total and does not delay the operation, as it can be performed simultaneously with the surgical exposure.

The dynamic reference base (DRB) is mounted to a suitable anchor point, usually the

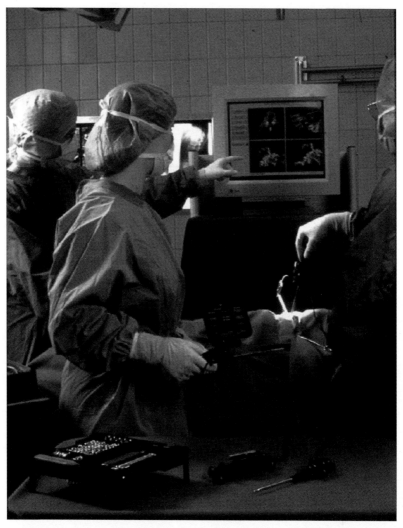

FIG. 3. Arrangement of computer-assisted surgery components in the operating room. The pedicle probe or drill is in the surgeon's hand. A marker carrier with light-emitting diode markers is attached to the standard USS tool (Stratec Medical). The dynamic reference base can be seen on the patient's anatomy. The tool position is shown in the image.

spinous process, by the surgeon. Attaching the dyamic reference base to the patient compensates for any patient and/or camera motion during the procedure, because all instruments are tracked in the local, patient-fixed dynamic reference base coordinate system.

Skeletal Registration (Matching)

In the next step, the patient's anatomy must be registered with the medical image. For spine surgery, a paired-point technique is used to find the transformation between the real world of the patient and the virtual world of the image. The preoperatively stored anatomic landmarks (typically, the facet joints and the spinous process are used) are shown on the screen one by one and subsequently located and digitized on the patient. Schlenzka et al.

(14) reported an average time of 3.48 minutes for this procedure. Alternatively, a set of 12 to 15 surface points digitized anywhere on the bone can be used (surface matching). After determination of the transformation, the overall accuracy of the system is checked. To do so, an instrument is located somewhere on the bony surface (e.g., the spinous process), and the surgeon confirms that the system indicates the exact same position on the screen. The system now is ready for use. Using the virtual keyboard, the surgeon can select a module for intraoperative guidance as described in the following.

Real-time Trajectory

The real-time trajectory module (Fig. 4) provides the surgeon with a transverse and a sagittal cut through the tomographic volume at the location indicated by the tip of the tool. Further, seven image slices perpendicular to the current tool orientation are computed in different depths and indicate the future path of the tool. It could be described as the ''what would happen if I drill in this direction'' view. The surgeon can see the position of the pedicle screw in the bone before any tissue is penetrated.

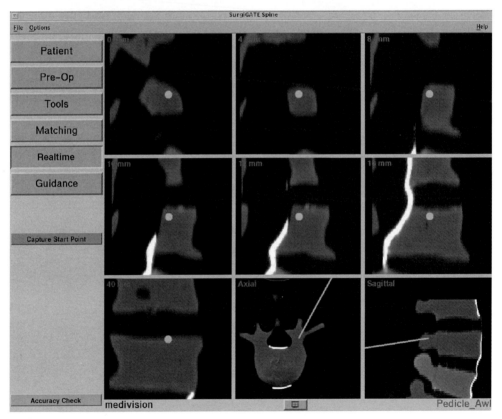

FIG. 4. Real-time trajectory. Seven image slices perpendicular to the axial orientation of the tool are computed and displayed in real time. The first slice is directly at the tip of the tool, slices 2 through 7 are at 4, 8, 10, 12, 18, and 40 mm, respectively. The eighth and ninth image show cuts defined by a plane through the tool axis (quasiaxial and quasisagittal). The *circles* in slice 1 through 7 simulate a 6-mm pedicle screw positioned in line with the tool's axis. In slice 8 and 9 the tool is displayed as a *line*.

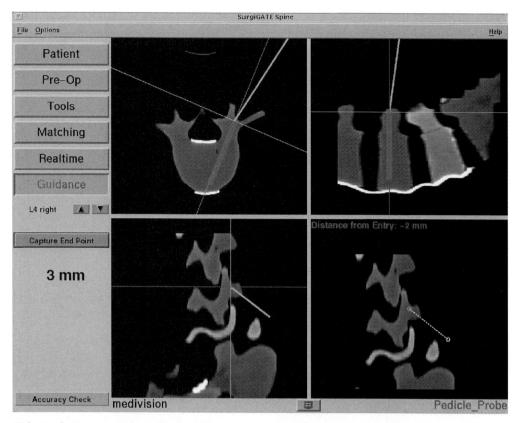

FIG. 5. Guidance module. This module allows for precise guidance toward a preoperatively defined target. The target position is indicated by the *thick line*; the current tool position is indicated by the *thin line*. The window on the lower right indicates deviation of the tip as well as orientation of the instrument with respect to the planning.

Pedicle Navigator (Guidance)

If preoperative planning for a pedicle screw location was stored, it can be recalled intraoperatively and compared with the current tool position (Fig. 5). The guidance window (lower right) also indicates the deviation of the tip and the orientation of the tool relative to the optimal path. The insertion depth is indicated on the upper left of that window.

CLINICAL EXPERIENCE

The system described has been in clinical use at several medical centers since June 1994. To date, two scientific studies have been reported (14,15). In both of these studies, the misplacement rate for pedicle screws was found to be drastically reduced as compared to standard values without computer assistance reported in the literature.

Schlenzka et al. (14) served as a trial clinic for the preversion of the SurgiGATE system and performed a controlled study of 151 screws in 25 patients. Compared to a 9.4% miss rate without surgical navigation, the miss rate of screws inserted with support from the system was 2.5% overall and 1.2% for the last 13 cases performed with the new technique.

Schwarzenbach et al. (15) analyzed the first 150 screws inserted using the SurgiGATE system by postoperative computed tomographic imaging. Despite these being the introductory cases of a novel technology, only three screws (2.0%) injured the pedicle cortex and no screw was located outside of so-called ''safe zone'' as defined by Gertzbein et al. (3).

DISCUSSION AND CONCLUSION

The combination of surgical action and medical image information has led to a substantial improvement in precision and accuracy for a difficult surgical procedure where enormous variability in pedicular anatomy diameter as well as angulation aggravates precise placement of implant components based only on conventional aids.

Because the preoperative image is used and cuts of interest are calculated in real time, there is no intraoperative radiation induced by use of image intensifiers. Further, the surgeon is provided with true cuts through a three-dimensional volume rather than two-dimensional projections. Improving from a two-dimensional printout (film) to a three-dimensional data set gives surgeons the opportunity to select any angle for inspection of patient anatomy and preoperative planning and simulation of surgical procedures.

Intraoperatively, this system can be controlled directly using advanced man-machine interfaces such as the virtual keyboard without the need for an operator on site. The surgeon is provided with knowledge of the current tool position relative to the individual anatomic situation at any time during the operation.

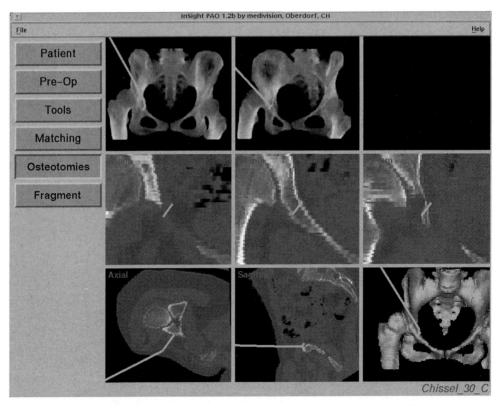

FIG. 6. Pelvic osteotomy module. This module allows for guidance in cases of pelvic osteotomies. All current procedures (Ganz, Tönnies, Wagner) can be supported.

Development of support for orthopedic procedures will continue. Encouraged by the clinical results of the spine module, further applications already are being developed or in clinical trial. This includes intraoperative visualization of acetabular osteotomies (Fig. 6), minimally invasive procedures for spine surgery, and applications in the field of traumatology.

REFERENCES

1. Clarke RH, Horsley V. On a method for investigating the deep ganglia and tracts of the central nervous system (cerebellum). *Br Med J* 1906;2:1799–1800.
2. Esses SI, Sachs BL, Dreyzin V. Complications associated with the technique of pedicle screw fixation. *Spine* 1993;18:2231–2239.
3. Gertzbein SD, Robbins SE. Accuracy of pedicular screw placement in vivo. *Spine* 1990;15:11–14.
4. Jerosch J, Malms J, Castro M, Wagner R, Wiesner L. Accuracy of pedicle screws in dorsal lumbar spinal fusion (in German). *Z Orthop* 1993;130:479–483.
5. Krag MH. Depth of insertion of transpedicular vertebral screws into human vertebrae: effect upon screw-vertebra interface strength. *J Spinal Disord* 1989;4:287–294.
6. Krag MH. Biomechanics of thoracolumbar spinal fixation. *Spine* 1991;16:84–99.
7. Magerl F. Stabilization of the lower thoracic and lumbar spine with external skeletal fixation. *Clin Orthop* 1984; 189:125–141.
8. Moran JM, Berg WS, Berry JL, Geiger JM, Steffee AD. Transpedicular screw fixation. *J Orthop Res* 1993;7: 107–114.
9. Nolte LP, Zamorano LJ, Jiang Z, Wang Q, Langlotz F, Berlemann U. Image-guided insertion of transpedicular screws—a laboratory setup. *Spine* 1995;20:497–500.
10. Nolte LP, Zamorano L, Visarius H, et al. Clinical evaluation of a system for precision enhancement in spine surgery. *Clin Biomech* 1995;10:293–303.
11. Roy-Camille R. Experience with Roy-Camille fixation for the thoraco-lumbar and lumbar spine. Acute spinal injuries: current management techniques. University of Massachusetts Continuing Medical Education Course, Sturbridge, Massachusetts, 1987.
12. Roy-Camille R, Saillant G, Mazel C. Internal fixation of the lumbar spine with pedicle screw plating. *Clin Orthop* 1986;203:7–17.
13. Roy-Camille R, Saillant G, Berteaux D, Marie-Anne S, Mamoudy P. Vertebral osteosynthesis using metal plates. Its different uses. *Chirurgie* 1979;105:579–603.
14. Schlenzka D, Laine T. Computer assisted pedicle screw insertion—first clinical experience. In: Nolte LP, Ganz R, eds. *CAOS—computer assisted orthopaedic surgery.* Bern: Hogrefe & Huber, 1999, 99–103.
15. Schwarzenbach O, Berlemann U, Jost B, et al. Accuracy of computer assisted pedicle screw placement—an in vivo CT analysis. *Spine* 1996;22:452–458.
16. Steinmann JC, Herkowitz HN, El-Kommos H, Wesolowski P. Spinal pedicle fixation: confirmation of an image-based technique for screw placement. *Spine* 1993;18:1856–1861.
17. Visarius H, Gong J, Scheer C, Nolte LP. Man-machine interfaces in computer assisted surgery. In: Nolte LP, Ganz R, eds. *CAOS—computer assisted orthopaedic surgery.* Bern: Hogrefe & Huber, 1999, 228–232.
18. Weinstein JN, Spratt KF, Spengler D, Brick C, Reid S. Spinal pedicle fixation: reliability and validity of roentgenogram-based assessment and surgical factors on successful screw placement. *Spine* 1989;14:1012–1018.
19. Weinstein JN, Rydevik BL, Rauschning W. Anatomic and technical considerations of pedicle screw fixation. *Clin Orthop* 1992;284:34–46.

SECTION VII

Economic and Ethical Considerations in the Management of Spinal Stenosis

Lumbar Spinal Stenosis
edited by Robert Gunzburg and Marek Szpalski
Lippincott Williams & Wilkins, Philadelphia, © 2000.

39

Economic Evaluation in Health Care

Christian Melot

Intensive Care Department, Erasme University Hospital, and Free University of Brussels, 1070 Brussels, Belgium

The myth of unlimited resources for health care belongs in the past. In nations that provide universal health care at public expense, budget limits have been exceeded and some draconian measures have been enacted. As a consequence, budget constraints increasingly determine the provision of health care services. One of the promises of economic evaluation is that it can demonstrate how to maximize the health care benefits attainable with a specific budget.

HEALTH CARE EXPENDITURES: THE DANAIDES' JAR THAT NEEDS ECONOMIC EVALUATION

Economic evaluation, sometimes referred to as efficiency evaluation, aims to ask the following questions. Is this health procedure, service, or program worth doing compared with other things we could do with these same resources? Are we satisfied that the health care resources, required to make the procedure, service, or program available to those who could benefit from it, should be spent this way rather than some other way?

It is important to note that although economic evaluation provides important information to decision makers, it addresses only one dimension of health care program decisions. Economic evaluation is most useful and appropriate when preceded by three other types of evaluation, each of which addresses a different question: (i) *Can it work?* Does the health procedure, service, or program do more good than harm to people who fully comply with the associated recommendations or treatments? This type of evaluation is concerned with efficacy. (ii) *Does it work?* Does the procedure, service, or program do more good than harm to those people to whom it is offered? This form of health care evaluation, which considers both the efficacy of a service and its acceptance by those to whom it is offered, is the evaluation of effectiveness or usefulness. (iii) *Is it reaching those who need it?* Is the procedure, service, or program accessible to all people who could benefit from it? Evaluation of this type is concerned with availability (4).

However, economic evaluation has been criticized for setting health care priorities in a way that violates people's values. For example, many people value equity in the distribution of health care resources, yet equity is not accounted for in economic analyses (15). As a result, the medical profession is being forced to reconcile its role as advocate for the individual patient with its role for rational deployment of the resources available (16).

WHAT DOES ECONOMIC EVALUATION MEAN?

Two features characterize economic analysis, regardless of the activities to which it is applied. First, it deals with both the inputs and the outputs, sometimes called costs and

COSTS   CONSEQUENCES

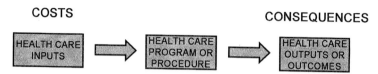

FIG. 1. Economic evaluation of a health care program or procedure defines the costs (health care inputs) and consequences (health care outputs or outcomes) related to the program or procedure.

consequences, of activities (Fig. 1). It is the linkage of costs and consequences that allows us to reach our decision. Second, economic analysis concerns itself with choices. Resource scarcity, and our consequent inability to produce all desired outputs, necessitates that choices must, and will, be made in all areas of human activity. These two characteristics of economic analysis lead us to define economic evaluation as the comparative analysis of alternative courses of action in terms of both their costs and consequences. Therefore, the basic tasks of any economic evaluation are to identify, measure, value, and compare the costs and consequences of the alternatives being considered. Figure 2 illustrates that an economic evaluation usually is formulated in terms of a choice between competing alternatives A and B. The general rule when assessing treatments A and B is that the difference in costs is compared with the difference in consequences, in an incremental analysis.

These two characteristics of economic analysis can be used to distinguish and label several evaluation situations commonly encountered in the health care evaluation literature. The answers to two questions—(i) is the comparison of two or more alternatives and (ii) are both the costs (inputs) and outcomes or consequences (outputs) of the alternatives examined—define six possible methods for evaluation (Table 1) (4).

When no comparison between alternatives is made (i.e., a single service or program is being evaluated), there is no true evaluation because evaluation requires comparison, but only a description of the service or program. When only consequences are examined the evaluation is labeled an outcome description. When only costs are examined it is called a cost description. The literature on cost of illness, or burden of illness, falls into this category

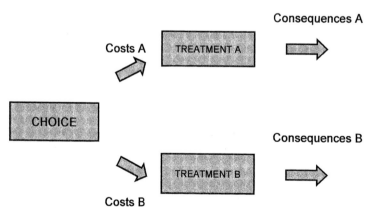

FIG. 2. A full economic evaluation is formulated in terms of a choice between competing alternatives. Here we consider the choice between two treatments, A and B. The difference in costs will be compared with the difference in consequences or outcomes. (Adapted from ref. 4.)

TABLE 1. *Partial and full economic evaluations*

	Outcomes only	Costs only	Both costs and outcomes
	Partial economic evaluation		Partial economic evaluation
No comparison	Outcome description	Cost description	Cost-outcome description
	Partial economic evaluation		Full economic evaluation
Comparison	Efficacy or effectiveness evaluation	Cost analysis	Cost-minimization analysis Cost-effectiveness analysis Cost-utility analysis Cost-benefit analysis

Adapted from ref. 4.

(3). These studies describe the cost of disease to society, but they are not full economic evaluations because alternatives are not compared. When both outcomes and costs of a single service or program are described without any comparison with an alternative, the study is a cost-outcome description (10).

When outcomes are compared in two or more alternative programs or services, the term efficacy or effectiveness evaluation is used. This is the case of most of the randomized clinical trials. When the costs of the alternatives are only examined, the study is called cost analyses (7,14).

The previous economic evaluations or descriptions, often labeled partial economic evaluations, will not allow us to answer efficiency questions. For this we need studies labeled full economic evaluation as cost-minimization, cost-effectiveness, cost-utility, or cost-benefit analyses. The outcomes or consequences are defined differently for each type of analysis, whereas costs are uniformly defined in terms of monetary expenditure (Table 2).

Cost-minimization analysis focuses on the differences in total costs associated with the study treatments. In this type of analysis, the treatments to be compared are considered to be equally efficacious based on previous research, and thus only treatment costs are compared. The objective of cost-minimization analysis is to identify the most efficient treatment method.

Cost-effectiveness analysis is perhaps the most widely used economic methodology. Consequences are expressed in terms of nonmonetary units; thus, this type of analysis can only be used to compare interventions that produce similar outcomes (5,13). Cost-effectiveness analysis also may compare resource use associated with different therapies (1). The objective of this type of analysis is to determine the least costly method of achieving a given outcome.

Cost-utility analysis is a variation of cost-effectiveness analysis that considers patient preferences for the effects of the therapy (8). The patient preferences usually are measured in quality-adjusted life-years using either the standard gamble or the time-tradeoff methods (9); however, both are time consuming and complex methods. Recently, alternative methods based

TABLE 2. *Measurement of outcomes or consequences in full economic evaluations*

Type of study	Measurement/valuation of consequences
Cost-minimization analysis	None
Cost-effectiveness analysis	Health effects in natural units (e.g., life-years gained, blood pressure reduction, disability-days saved)
Cost-utility analysis	Patient preference measured in quality-adjusted life-year
Cost-benefit analysis	Monetary units estimated by willingness-to-pay, wage-risk, human capital approach

Adapted from ref. 4.

on prescored multiattribute health status classification systems such as quality of well-being (QWB), health utilities index (HUI), and EuroQol (EQ-5D) have been used (4).

Cost-benefit analysis defines both benefits and costs in monetary terms. Benefits typically are defined as costs avoided by the use of the intervention. Such costs may include hospitalization, days of disability, or lost productivity due to premature death. The objective is to determine if the cost saving realized outweighs the costs incurred from the therapy. Because therapeutic benefits are translated into monetary units, this type of analysis is ideal for comparing the value of treatments that have different therapeutic outcomes (1). Cost-benefit analysis is advanced as the gold standard among the economic approaches because it forces decision makers to explicitly value both the cost and health consequences of alternative health care program. However, its usefulness is limited by the reluctance of many to accept the assignment of a monetary value to patient health outcomes.

WHAT ARE THE RELEVANT COSTS IN THE ECONOMIC EVALUATION?

Most economists would define a cost as the consumption of a resource that otherwise could have been for another purpose. Because the resource has been used, the opportunity to use it for another purpose is lost. Therefore, its value in the next best use, which is no longer possible, is called its opportunity cost. Strictly speaking, economic evaluation should seek to value all inputs in terms of their opportunity costs. For more practical purposes, however, it is usual to use market prices unless there is evidence to suggest that they diverge from opportunity costs.

The precise nature of the costs (C) to be considered are shown in Fig. 3. The resources consumed by the program are considered to be in three sectors. In each case their quantities

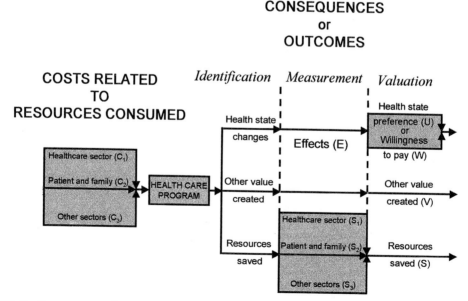

FIG. 3. Components of economic evaluation in health care. See text for explanation. (Adapted from ref. 4.)

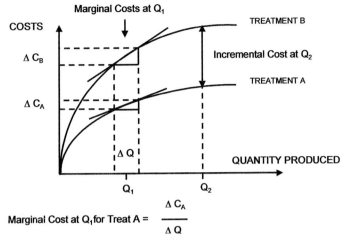

FIG. 4. Difference between marginal costs and incremental costs, which often are used interchangeably in the literature. See text for explanation. (Adapted from ref. 4.)

(q) would be measured and total cost calculated by multiplying the quantities by the relevant prices (p):

$$C = q \times p.$$

The health sector resources (C_1) consist of items such as drugs, equipment, hospitalization, and physician visits. It is important to note that these include not only the costs of providing the initial program (e.g., a heart transplant) but also all the continuing care costs (e.g. immunosuppressive drugs, treatment of infections).

The patient and family resources (C_2) consist of out-of-pocket expenses incurred when traveling to hospital, various copayments, and expenditure in the home (e.g., adapting a room to accommodate a home dialysis machine). However, one of the most important patient and family resources consumed in treatment is time. This could be time of family members in providing informal nursing support at home. The time could either be from leisure activities or work time, which would affect its valuation.

The other sectors resources (C_3) used are likely to depend on the nature of health care program being evaluated. For example, some programs, such as those for the elderly or mentally ill, consume resources from other public agencies (e.g., homemaker services, nursing home care). Moreover, many health care programs rely on resource inputs from the voluntary sector.

In making these determinations of cost, it is important to separate costs that are fixed (and would not be reduced in the short term by a change in the number of services provided, such as the overhead of building maintenance) from costs that are variable (those that vary with the volume of services provided). The terms marginal and incremental costs often are used interchangeably. However, strictly speaking, the marginal cost relates to the cost of producing one extra unit of output. The term incremental cost is used to refer to the difference in cost between the two treatments being compared in the evaluation (Fig. 4).

WHAT ARE THE RELEVANT OUTCOMES OR CONSEQUENCES IN THE ECONOMIC EVALUATION?

Turning to the outcomes or consequences, it can be seen that these consist of three main categories (Fig. 3).

TABLE 3. *Possible formulations of economic evaluation*

Cost-minimization analysis	Health care resources only: $C_1 - S_1$ All resources: $(C_1 + C_2 + C_3) - (S_1 + S_2 + S_3)$	Costs minus Savings
Cost-effectiveness analysis (efficiency)	Health care resources only: $(C_1 - S_1)/E$ All resources: $\{(C_1 + C_2 + C_3) - (S_1 + S_2 + S_3)\}/E$	Costs minus Savings divided by the Effects measured in natural units
Cost-utility analysis	Health care resources only: $(C_1 - S_1)/U$ All resources: $\{(C_1 + C_2 + C_3) - (S_1 + S_2 + S_3)\}/U$	Costs minus Savings divided by health state preferences (Utility)
Cost-benefit analysis	Health care resources: $W - C_1$ All resources: $(W + V + S_1 + S_2 + S_3) - (C_1 + C_2 + C_3)$	Valuation minus Costs

E and U represent changes in effectiveness or health status compared to an alternative.
Adapted from ref. 4.

First, the patients health state usually will be improved. This can be measured in terms of effects (E) (e.g., life-years gained or disability-days reduced) in a cost-effectiveness analysis, but also valued, in terms of either health state preferences (U) in a cost-utility analysis or willingness to pay (W) in a cost-benefit analysis.

Second, other value (V) can be created by health state. This could include the value of information or reassurance about one's health. Some authors argued that patients obtain utility or value from the process of receiving care, independent of the outcome (2). Although a separate component of the value of health care programs, V usually is incorporated in the measurement of U or W.

Third, resources can be saved by health care programs (5). Risk reduction (e.g., lowering serum cholesterol) will lead to cost savings (12). The health effects resulting from health care program also may improve the patient's social functioning and ability to work (6). These savings (S_1 to S_3) mirror the costs (C_1 to C_3) and are measured and valued in a similar way. These savings (S_1 to S_3) are the costs (C_1 to C_3) not spent on the alternative program. All the measurements of consequences are comparative to an alternative.

Moreover, there are a number of possible formulations of economic evaluation depending on the perspective adopted by the analysts (health care resources only or all resources) depending on the point of view taken (society, payer, provider, or patient) and the evaluation methods they use (Table 3).

ASSIGNING MONEY VALUES TO HEALTH OUTCOMES: A DIFFICULT TASK

The major disadvantage of cost-benefit analysis is the requirement that human life and quality of life must be valued in monetary units. Many decision makers find this difficult or unethical or do not trust analyses that depend on such valuations (17). There are three general approaches to the monetary valuation of health outcomes: (i) human capital, (ii) wage-risk approach, and (iii) willingness to pay (contingent valuation) (4).

Human Capital Approach

The utilization of a health care program can be viewed as an investment in a person's human capital. In measuring the payback on this investment, the value of the healthy time produced can be quantified in terms of the person's renewed or increased production in the market place. Hence, the human capital method places monetary weights on healthy time using market wage rates and the value of the program is assessed in terms of the present value of future earnings. We can distinguish between two uses of the human capital concept: (i) as the sole basis for valuing all aspects of health improvements, and (ii) as a method of valuing part of the benefits of health care interventions, using earnings data as a means of valuing productivity changes only. In addition to some of the practical measurement problems of using the human capital approach, it came under attack in the 1970s by economists who argued that this production-based method for valuing health improvements was not consistent with the theoretical foundation of cost-benefit analysis from welfare economics. The proposition (and judgment) is that social welfare should comprise individuals welfare and that individuals should be considered the best source of information on their own welfare.

Wage-risk Approach

A number of wage-risk studies have been reported, in which the goal was to examine the relationship between particular health risks associated with a hazardous job and wage rates that individuals require to accept the job. This approach is consistent with the welfare economics framework, because it is based on individual preferences regarding the value of increased (or decreased) health risk, such as injury at work, as a tradeoff against increased (or decreased) income. The wage-risk approach is based on actual consumer choices involving health versus money, rather than hypothetical scenarios and preference statements. It is why such studies are labeled as revealed preference studies.

Willingness-to-pay Approach

The willingness-to-pay approach uses survey methods to present respondents with hypothetical scenarios about the program or problem under evaluation. These studies are labeled as stated preference or contingent valuation studies. Respondents are required to think about the contingency of an actual market existing for a program or health benefit and to reveal the maximum they would be willing to pay for such a program or benefit. Briefly, the maximum willingness to pay is evaluated using a questionnaire (Fig. 5). The willingness-to-pay question is introduced by the following statement: "Since the treatment uses a lot health care resources, it is possible that in the future government will withdraw funding and patients will have to pay all, or a large proportion of treatment costs. For this question assume that this will be the case. Remember that any money you spend for treatment costs will not be available for you to spend on other things" (11).

Why are we interested in the maximum willingness to pay? Consider a simple consumer decision to buy a commodity. A measure of how much she values the commodity is the maximum that she would be willing to pay. The difference between this value and the price she has to pay in the market is known as consumer surplus. This consumer surplus may be improvements in health status, whereas others may be attributed to the value associated with the process of care itself (2). It is the aggregation of this consumer surplus—which can be large or small, positive or negative—across individuals that forms the basis of the cost-benefit calculus. In recent years there has been a rapid growth in the number of willingness-to-pay studies reported in the health care literature (4).

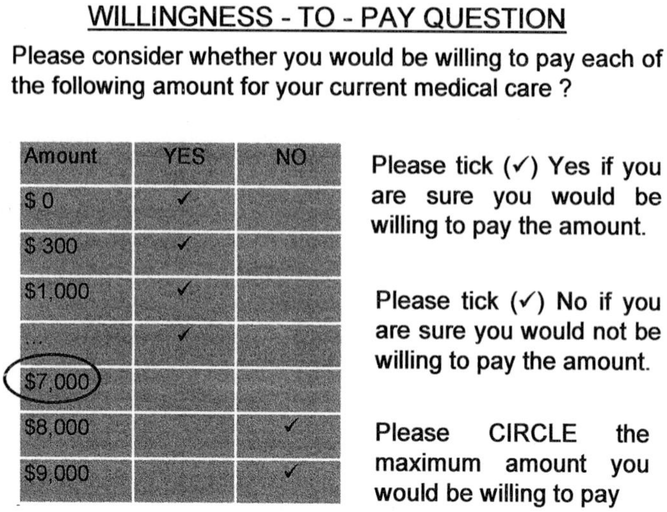

WILLINGNESS - TO - PAY QUESTION

Please consider whether you would be willing to pay each of
the following amount for your current medical care ?

Amount	YES	NO
$ 0	✓	
$ 300	✓	
$1,000	✓	
...	✓	
$7,000		
$8,000		✓
$9,000		✓

Please tick (✓) Yes if you are sure you would be willing to pay the amount.

Please tick (✓) No if you are sure you would not be willing to pay the amount.

Please CIRCLE the maximum amount you would be willing to pay

FIG. 5. The willingness-to-pay question presented to the patient in a survey to evaluate the maximum willingness to pay. (Adapted from ref. 11.)

CONCLUSION

All would agree that physicians should refrain from providing services that offer no additional healthy outcomes for substantial increases in cost. The difficulty arises when there are too few resources to allow all patients to receive all care that does have a chance to improve health. Thus, tradeoffs must be made among services. This approach is in conflict with the concept of equity developed in the medical ethics. The health care economic evaluation techniques reviewed in this chapter are tools for comparing options in medical practice. These may help clinicians to achieve the societal goal of achieving the greatest benefit for the most people, thus maximizing the utility of medical care for the resources used. The principles and methods of health care economic evaluation allow physicians to be more critical users of newly available information about the costs and effects of clinical practice. Clinicians who can critically assess data on costs and effectiveness will more likely be able to retain their roles as their patients' advocates while being responsible participants in hospitals, insurance plan, health maintenance organizations, and society at large.

REFERENCES

1. Conrad DA, Deyo RA. Economic decision analysis in the diagnosis and treatment of low back pain. A methodologic primer. *Spine* 1994;19:2101s–2106s.
2. Donaldson C, Shackley P. Does "process utility" exist? A case study of willingness to pay for laparoscopic cholecystectomy. *Soc Sci Med* 1997;44:699–707.
3. Drummond MF. Cost of illness studies: a major headache? *PharmacoEconomics* 1992;2:1–4.
4. Drummond MF, O'Brien BJ, Stoddart GL, Torrance GW, eds. *Methods for the economic evaluation of health care programmes,* 2nd ed. Oxford, UK: Oxford University Press, 1997.
5. Javid MJ. Chemonucleolysis versus laminectomy. A cohort comparison of effectiveness and charges. *Spine* 1995;20:2016–2022.
6. Koopmanschap MA, Rutten FFH. Indirect costs. The consequence of production loss or increased costs of production. *Med Care* 1996;34[Suppl]:DS59–DS68.
7. Lowson KV, Drummond MF, Bishop JM. Costing new services: long-term domiciliary oxygen therapy. *Lancet* 1981;ii:1146–1149.
8. Malter AD, Weinstein J. Cost-effectiveness of lumbar discectomy for the treatment of herniated intervertebral disc. *Spine* 1996;21:1048–1055.

9. Mélot C. Principles of cost-benefit analysis. In: Szpalski M, Gunzburg R, Pope MH, eds. *Lumbar segmental instability*. Philadelphia: Lippincott Williams & Wilkins, 1999:259–273.
10. Reynell PC, Reynell MC. The cost-benefit analysis of a coronary care unit. *Br Heart J* 1972;34:897–900.
11. Ryan M. Using willingness to pay to assess the benefits of assisted reproductive techniques. *Health Economics* 1996;5:543–558.
12. Shalowitz M, Heaton AH. Cost-effectiveness of risk reduction: the managed care perspective. *Am J Med* 1996; 101[Suppl 4A]:71s–75s.
13. Skargren EI, Carlsson PG, Öberg BE. One year follow-up comparison of the costs and effectiveness of chiropractic and physiotherapy as primary management for back pain. *Spine* 1998;23:1875–1884.
14. Stevenson RC, McCabe CJ, Findlay AM. An economic evaluation of a clinical trial to compare automated percutaneous lumbar discectomy with microdiscectomy in the treatment of contained lumbar disk herniation. *Spine* 1995;20:739–742.
15. Ubel PA, DeKay ML, Baron J, Asch DA. Cost-effectiveness analysis in a setting of budget constraints. Is it equitable. *N Engl J Med* 1996;334:1174–1177.
16. Weinstein MC. Spine update. Editorial comment. *Spine* 1996;21:651–652.
17. Weinstein MC, Fineberg HV, eds. *Clinical decision analysis*. Philadelphia: WB Saunders, 1980:240.

Lumbar Spinal Stenosis
edited by Robert Gunzburg and Marek Szpalski
Lippincott Williams & Wilkins, Philadelphia, © 2000.

40

Scientific Evidence on the Management of Lumbar Spinal Stenosis

Gordon Waddell and *J.N.A. Gibson

*Department of Orthopaedic Surgery, Gladsgow Nuffield Hospital, Gladsgow G12 OPJ, United Kingdom; and *Department of Orthopaedic Surgery, The University of Edinburgh, and Princess Margaret Rose Orthopaedic Hospital, Edinburgh EH10 7ED United Kingdom*

Lumbar spinal stenosis has been defined as any type of narrowing of the spinal canal, nerve root canal(s), or tunnel(s) of the intervertebral foramina (9).

It was only after Verbiest (14) set out the definitive clinical and pathologic findings of the rare condition of developmental spinal stenosis and gave the first description of its surgical treatment that the condition began to be recognized clinically. There is now increasing recognition that spinal stenosis due to degenerative lumbar spondylosis is a cause of low back and leg pain, particularly in older patients. Spinal stenosis is now the most common and fastest growing reason for spinal surgery in adults older than 65 years of age (3). Yet despite the large number of surgical procedures being performed, there is still uncertainty about the diagnostic criteria and natural history of spinal stenosis, the indications for surgery and choice of surgical procedures, and the clinical or patient characteristics associated with a favorable outcome.

Degenerative lumbar spondylosis (degenerate disc disease) is, to at least some extent, a normal, age-related finding in most adults. Associated symptoms are variable and have a relatively low correlation with the severity of anatomic or radiologic changes. Only a small proportion of patients undergo surgery. Surgical treatment may consist of either decompression of nerve root(s) or the cauda equina, with the goal of relieving nerve root pain or neurogenic claudication, and/or fusion with the goal of relieving discogenic and facet pain. In general terms, spinal or root canal stenosis is treated by decompression, whereas severe disc degeneration, malalignment, and instability (either pathologic or surgically induced) are treated by fusion. However, decompression and fusion often are combined. Decisions about surgery usually are based not only on the nature of the localized pathology and associated symptoms and disability, but also allow for other factors such as the patient's occupation, athletic or recreational activity, and economic pressures. The choice of procedure also may be influenced by the surgeon's beliefs about the role of surgery in these spinal disorders, and the surgical instrumentation and skills available. Different procedures are reported to give a wide range of good, fair, and poor results. All have specific complications, the most important of which are spinal instability and progressive slip following decompression and pseudarthrosis following fusion.

REVIEW OF THE SCIENTIFIC EVIDENCE ON TREATMENT
OF SPINAL STENOSIS

We have not been able to locate any good scientific evidence or randomized controlled trials (RCTs) on the effectiveness of any form of conservative treatment for lumbar stenosis.

Cochrane Review

The Cochrane Review of surgical treatments for degenerative lumbar spondylosis and the associated pathologies and clinical syndromes of back pain, instability, spinal stenosis and degenerative spondylolisthesis was accepted in November 1998 and went on-line in January 1999 (5). At present it contains 14 RCTs on various surgical treatments of lumbar spinal spondylosis, including five RCTs dealing with surgery for spinal stenosis. This is a very heterogeneous group of trials with a number of methodologic weaknesses. The trials:

- are few in number and generally small in size
- are poorly randomized
- compare heterogeneous pathologies
- provide outcome assessments that often are not blinded
- commonly consider technical surgical outcomes only.

All of the trials identified in this review compared two or more surgical techniques. There are no published RCTs on the efficacy of any form of surgery for degenerative lumbar spondylosis compared with natural history, placebo, or any form of conservative treatment. There is little information on patient-centered outcomes such as relief of pain, disability, and return to work.

One trial considered techniques of decompression for spinal stenosis by comparing laminectomy with multiple laminotomy (10). This study had several confounding factors. Nine of the 35 patients scheduled for laminotomy actually had a laminectomy for technical reasons, and several patients in each group also had an intertransverse arthrodesis for degenerative spondylolisthesis. This trial did not demonstrate any difference in clinical outcomes or spondylolisthesis progression between the two treatment methods.

Three trials considered whether some form of posterolateral fusion, with or without instrumentation, was a useful adjunct to decompression alone (1,6,7). They provided data on a total of 139 patients with 99% follow-up at 2 to 3 years. Comparison of the three trials showed no difference in outcomes between a fusion of any type or a laminectomy (odds ratio 1.15, 95% confidence interval 0.46 to 2.91) as rated by the surgeon 18 to 24 months after the procedure. Grob et al. (6) considered fusion with and without instrumentation in patients with degenerative spinal stenosis with no evidence of instability. They showed no difference in clinical outcomes or relief of pain, provided the posterior elements were preserved at operation. The other two trials considered the role of adjunct fusion in spinal stenosis associated with single- or two-level degenerative spondylolisthesis. Herkowitz and Kurz (7) studied noninstrumented fusion and showed that fusion produced significantly less self-reported back pain and leg pain and significantly better surgeon's ratings of outcome. Bridwell et al. (1) studied both instrumented and noninstrumented fusion. They showed that patients who had a successful fusion had less spondylolisthesis progression and better patient's rating of improvement. However, these results were only statistically significant in the group with an instrumented fusion, whereas noninstrumented fusion produced no such benefit.

Carragee (2) compared the results of fusion alone, or fusion plus laminectomy and decompression, for patients with an isthmic L5–S1 spondylolisthesis. The trial was confounded by the fact that nonsmokers had fusion by bone grafting alone, whereas smokers had their fusion supplemented by instrumentation. In neither group did the addition of decompression to the arthrodesis appear to improve the clinical outcomes.

These five RCTs permit very limited conclusions (from the Cochrane review):

- There is *limited evidence* that adjunct fusion to supplement decompression for degenerative spondylolisthesis produces less progressive slip and better clinical outcomes than decompression alone.
- There is *limited evidence* that fusion alone may be as effective as combined decompression and fusion for patients with grade I or II isthmic spondylolisthesis and no significant neurology.

Other Systematic Reviews

There are three published meta-analyses: two on the surgical treatment of lumbar spinal stenosis (9,13) and one on the surgical treatment of degenerative lumbar spondylolisthesis (8).

An attempted meta-analysis of largely retrospective case series by Turner et al. (13) suggested that 64% of patients treated surgically for lumbar spinal stenosis had good or excellent outcomes, but that varied widely from 26% to 100%. Deyo et al. (4) and Ciol et al. (3) analyzed a very large Medicare cohort and found that mortality within 1 year increased from less than 0.8% in those aged less than 75 years to 2.3% in those aged more than 80 years. The complication rate was double in the older age group. Eleven percent of all patients had repeat back surgery within 6 years.

Niggemeyer et al. (9) undertook a more recent meta-analysis of 1,668 patients who had primary surgery for lumbar spinal stenosis in 30 studies published between 1975 and 1995. They compared the results of decompression alone, decompression plus fusion without instrumentation, and decompression plus instrumented fusion. They excluded patients with degenerative spondylolisthesis. Overall, there was no difference between the techniques, and only subgroup analysis showed any statistically significant findings. These authors suggested that if the clinical history was less than 8 years, decompression alone might give the best results and fewest complications, particularly in elderly, unfit patients. For patients with a clinical history of more than 15 years, decompression combined with instrumented fusion seemed to give better results. They could not identify any other preoperative features that predicted success or failure.

Mardjetko et al. (8) reviewed degenerative spondylolisthesis, including 3 reports of nonoperative management/natural history, 11 of decompression alone, 6 of decompression plus fusion without instrumentation, and 4 of decompression plus instrumented fusion. Their meta-analysis suggested that decompression without fusion gave 69% satisfactory outcomes, although many reports described progressive vertebral slip following surgery. Addition of fusion to the decompression appeared to give 90% satisfactory outcomes and 86% solid fusion. Addition of instrumentation appeared to improve the fusion rate but did not further improve clinical outcomes.

All three of these meta-analyses were based mainly on uncontrolled, retrospective, case series that reported widely varying results, and they do not permit any firm conclusions. They suggest that decompression alone is the safest procedure and may give better results for patients with spinal stenosis, for those with less than 8-year clinical history, and in elderly unfit patients. They also suggest that decompression combined with instrumented fusion may have some place in patients with degenerative spondylolisthesis or in those with a history of more than 15 years, but it has a higher complication rate.

There is no evidence as to whether surgical management for lumbar spinal stenosis is effective in returning patients to work [see reviews by Taylor (12) and Scheer et al. (11)].

DISCUSSION

There is a serious lack of scientific evidence on the efficacy of conservative or surgical treatment of lumbar spinal stenosis. The Cochrane Review does not include any RCTs on the efficacy of surgery compared with natural history, placebo, or any form of conservative treatment. This is of particular concern given the magnitude of the clinical problem and the numbers and costs of surgical procedures being performed.

The few and diverse RCTs on decompression for lumbar spinal stenosis permit very limited conclusions. There is no clear evidence about the most effective technique of decompression for spinal stenosis. There is limited evidence that adjunct fusion to supplement decompression for degenerative spondylolisthesis produces less progressive slip and better clinical outcomes than decompression alone. There also is limited evidence that fusion alone may be as effective as fusion combined with decompression for patients with grade I or II isthmic spondylolisthesis and no significant neurology. There is no clear scientific evidence on different techniques of fusion, and, at present, the available scientific evidence from RCTs does not support the routine clinical use of instrumented fusion for degenerative lumbar spondylosis (5).

There is an urgent need for scientific evidence on the clinical efficacy and cost effectiveness of surgical decompression and/or fusion for specific pathologic and clinical syndromes associated with degenerative lumbar spondylosis if we are to justify the resources and risks of lumbar stenosis surgery. This will require high-quality RCTs that compare these surgical treatments with natural history, placebo, or conservative treatment. In view of the generally poor quality of many of these trials of spinal surgery, surgeons should seek expert methodologic advice when planning trials.

The authors will be pleased to receive information about any other RCTs of the surgical management of lumbar spinal stenosis to add to the Cochrane Review (5).

CONCLUSION

At present:

There is *no acceptable scientific evidence* on the effectiveness of any form of conservative or surgical management for lumbar spinal stenosis compared with natural history or placebo.

There is *no evidence* on whether any form of conservative or surgical management for lumbar spinal stenosis is effective in returning patients to work.

There is *no evidence* on the cost effectiveness of any form of conservative or surgical management for lumbar spinal stenosis.

There is *limited evidence* on the relative efficacy of different surgical techniques for particular pathologies.

REFERENCES

1. Bridwell KH, Sedgewick TA, O'Brien MF, Lenke LG, Baldus C. The role of fusion and instrumentation in the treatment of degenerative spondylolisthesis with spinal stenosis. *J Spinal Disord* 1993;6:461–72.
2. Caragee EJ. Single-level posterolateral arthrodesis, with or without posterior decompression, for the treatment of isthmic spondylolisthesis in adults. A prospective, randomised study. *J Bone Joint Surg* 1997;79A:1175–1180.
3. Ciol MA, Deyo RA, Howell E, Krief S. An assessment of surgery for spinal stenosis: time trends, geographic variations, complications and re-operations. *J Am Geriatr Soc* 1996;44:285–290.

4. Deyo RA, Cherkin D, Loeser JD. Morbidity and mortality in association with operations on the lumbar spine: the influence of age, diagnosis, and procedure. *J Bone Joint Surg Am* 1992;74:536–543.

5. Gibson JNA, Waddell G, Grant IC. The surgical management of degenerative lumbar spondylosis (Cochrane Review). In: *The Cochrane Library Issue 1 1999.* Oxford: Update Software, 1999.

6. Grob D, Humke T, Dvorak J. Degenerative lumbar spinal stenosis. Decompression with and without arthrodesis. *J Bone Joint Surg* 1995;77A:1036–1-41.

7. Herkowitz HN, Kurz LT. Degenerative lumbar spondylolisthesis with spinal stenosis. A prospective study comparing decompression with decompression and intertransverse process arthrodesis. *J Bone Joint Surg* 1991;73A:802–808.

8. Mardjetko SM, Connolly PJ, Shott S. Degenerative lumbar spondylolisthesis: a meta-analysis of literature 1970–93. *Spine* 1994;19:2256S–2265S.

9. Niggemeyer O, Strauss JM, Schulitz KP. Comparison of surgical procedures for degenerative lumbar spinal stenosis: a meta-analysis of the literature from 1975 to 1995. *Eur Spine J* 1997;6:423–429.

10. Postacchini F, Cinotti G, Perugia D, Gumina S. The surgical treatment of central lumbar stenosis. Multiple laminotomy compared with total laminectomy. *J Bone Joint Surg* 1993;75B:386–392.

11. Scheer SJ, Radack KL, O'Brien DR. Randomized controlled trials in industrial low back pain relating to return to work. Part 2. Discogenic low back pain. *Arch Phys Med Rehabil* 1996;77:1189–1197.

12. Taylor ME. Return to work following back surgery: a review. *Am J Ind Med* 1989;16;79–88.

13. Turner JA, Ersek M, Herron L, Deyo R. Surgery for lumbar spinal stenosis. Attempted meta-analysis of the literature. *Spine* 1992;17:1–8.

14. Verbiest H. A radicular syndrome from developmental narrowing of the lumbar vertebral canal. *J Bone Joint Surg* 1954;36B:230–237.

Lumbar Spinal Stenosis
edited by Robert Gunzburg and Marek Szpalski
Lippincott Williams & Wilkins, Philadelphia, © 2000.

41

Surgery for Lumbar Spinal Stenosis

Surgical Rates, Fitness for Work, and Costs

Marc Du Bois and Peter Donceel

*Department of Occupational and Insurance Medicine, School of Public Health,
Department of Medical Direction, Katholieke Universiteit Leuven, 3000 Leuven, Belgium*

Based on autopsy findings and on clinical practice, the frequency of lumbar spinal stenosis is rather low, estimated to be 5% and 2%, respectively (11). Nevertheless, lumbar spinal stenosis deserves attention because it is a major cause of low back and lower extremity discomfort resulting in disability in older adults (4). It is a condition that imposes an important social and economic burden on society. It underscores the need for treatment modalities, whether conservative or invasive, to improve the effectiveness of care at an acceptable cost. Because conservative therapy for this condition seldom results in sustained improvement, many patients must consider surgery, which includes decompressive laminectomy with or without concomitant arthrodesis. In the United States, more than 30,000 surgical procedures for degenerative spinal stenosis are performed annually, at a direct medical cost of approximately $1 billion (8). To our knowledge, no such figures about the Belgian population are available.

Reported success rates for lumbar spinal stenosis vary from 57% to 85% (5,8,10,14). These varying estimates of success rates may result partly from methodologic differences. In most studies, the criteria used to evaluate the outcome are not standardized, and assessment of results is made by the operating surgical team, which results in possible observer bias.

Patients with poor outcomes from primary surgery represent a specific medical challenge to physicians and an economic concern, because they often experience long-term sequelae and rarely achieve complete pain relief by any combination of therapeutic measures. It is assumed that patients who failed to benefit adequately from primary lumbar disc surgery tend to become very costly patients, as they usually receive a complex array of medical therapies, expensive diagnostic measures, repeat surgery, and a work incapacity benefit or allowance.

The goals of this study were fourfold:

1. To describe the trends in surgical rates for lumbar spinal stenosis in Belgium
2. To describe the 2-year outcome of surgery for lumbar spinal stenosis in terms of return to work
3. To identify the factors that are related to return to work in patients operated on for lumbar spinal stenosis
4. To delineate the costs related to surgery for lumbar spinal stenosis.

METHODS

The present investigation was based on patient record files from the largest Belgian Sickness Fund. It covers approximately 45% of the population in Belgium, where sickness insurance is legally mandated. All 866 claims files of the Christian Sickness Fund that were related to a surgical intervention for lumbar spinal stenosis performed in 1994 were reviewed. Details about diagnosis or clinical or radiologic signs were not available in this administrative database. Patient records were followed for 2 years after surgical intervention. The database is based on the Belgian fee list for surgical interventions ("procedure code"). The Belgian procedure code is a numerically encoded system that refers to the official description of a surgical intervention with regard to the financial reimbursement as defined in the Belgian sickness and invalidity legislation. The surgeon must register every performed intervention for lumbar disc herniation according to this procedure code.

The surgical interventions correspond with the following nomenclature descriptions:

- Laminectomy without opening the dura mater
- Laminectomy with concomitant arthrodesis
- Flavectomy and ligamentectomy
- Resection of the posterior lamina
- Lumbar laminarthrectomy for congenital or acquired cauda equina syndrome.

Trends in Surgery Rates

We obtained data on lumbar spinal stenosis interventions performed from 1994 to 1997 from Christian Sickness Fund claims files (Fig. 1). Surgery rates were calculated by dividing the number of treated patients by the year-specific total sickness fund enrollees for 1994 to 1997. Rates were not adjusted for age and sex. Additional data on the number of providers enabled us to investigate the association between surgical rate and density of surgeons.

Fitness for Work

Patients were evaluated by medical advisers of the sickness fund. Individual medical evaluations took place regularly from about 1 month after surgical intervention until patients were judged fit for resuming work according to the legal criteria in the sickness and invalidity insurance. In the first 6 months of work incapacity, the medical adviser evaluates fitness for work with regard to the patient's last job. After an incapacity period of 6 months, the criterion is extended to all occupations the patient may have access to, according to his or her professional career and education. The return-to-work rate after surgery for lumbar spinal stenosis

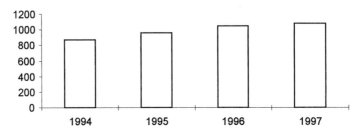

FIG. 1. Annual number of surgeries for lumbar spinal stenosis in the Christian Sickness Fund population.

TABLE 1. *Worker's compensation population characteristics (N = 225)*

Variable	No. (%)/median
Gender	
Male	158 (70.2)
Female	67 (29.8)
Professional status	
Self-employed	15 (6.7)
Salaried	210 (93.3)
Job category	
Blue collar worker	162 (72.0)
White collar worker	48 (21.3)
Period of work incapacity before intervention (d)	95
Age (yr)	46
Instrumented surgery	50 (22.2)

was determined from claim files of patients belonging to the working population who were operated on in 1994. There were 67 women and 158 men in the study. The available preoperative features were obtained through a review of the individual files of the claimants. The retrieved information is shown in Table 1. Patients who returned to work within 1 year were classified as good outcomes.

Analysis of Costs

In Belgium, health care and sickness benefits are insured by a social security system that is financed by contributions from both employees and employers. For health care insurance, tariff agreements are made among health care providers, government, and sickness funds. In this system, each medical act or intervention is valued at a fixed price. A daily lump sum is provided for hospitals to finance medical equipment, nursing, lodging, and administration. Patients who belong to the working population also are compensated during the recovery period until they are fit for work. They receive a daily compensation in accordance with their previous salary level. The expenditures for medical procedures, work incapacity compensation, hospital nursing, lodging, and administration add up to the social insurance costs.

The cost-assessment phase of the study determined the social insurance cost for a follow-up of 2 years postoperatively. In view of the retrospective design of the present study, we were not able to rule out medical care costs unrelated to lumbar spinal stenosis intervention.

Patient's claims files were broken down into the following cost items: visits to a practitioner (general and specialist), corset/bracing, diagnostic procedures such as plain x-ray films, myelography, computed tomography, magnetic resonance imaging, the cost of a neurostimulator, physiotherapy, kinesitherapy, rehabilitation, and instrumentation. Hospital costs were not traced separately. For the working population, daily sickness fund payments compensating for work time lost after 1 month of work incapacity were calculated. No information about compensation payments during the first month of sick leave was available (to be paid by the employer in the Belgian social security system). All costs are expressed in 1997 dollars.

Statistics

Analyses were performed with the SPSS statistical package. Chi-square test was used to identify the factors crucial for ability to work postoperatively. Logistic regression was used to identify factors independently associated with the return-to-work status 1 year after intervention. $p < 0.05$ was considered significant. The variables tested were duration of work incapacity before the operation, gender, age, strenuousness of occupation (light, moderately light, heavy, or moderately heavy), and professional status (salaried or self-employed). Kruskal-Wallis one-way analysis of variance was used to analyze costs. Kaplan-Meier curves and trend figures were drawn using SPSS and Excel 5.0 for Windows.

RESULTS

Trends in Surgery Rates

Current rates of lumbar spinal stenosis surgery were obtained from the Christian Sickness Fund claims files. These data are used primarily for reimbursement purposes. These administrative data may be subject to erroneous and biased coding.

There were 3,959 cases of lumbar spinal stenosis surgery performed on Christian Sickness Fund enrollees from 1994 to 1997. The 1994 annual rate of lumbar spinal stenosis surgery was 19.3 per 100,000 enrollees. There was an overall upward trend in total lumbar spinal stenosis surgery in the Christian Sickness Fund population over the 4-year period from 1994 to 1997, with an increase of 24%. This trend reflects the internationally rising surgical rate in the treatment of disorders of the lumbar spine. In the same period, the number of orthopedists and neurosurgeons in Belgium increased approximately 15%.

Fitness for Work

There were 225 patients (67 women and 158 men; mean age 46 years) in working population who had an intervention for lumbar spinal stenosis in 1994 (Fig. 2). After operation, 111 (49.3%) patients returned to work within 1 year after the operation. Comparison of the features among the bad and good outcome groups showed that there was no significantly statistical difference in work capacity between blue collar and white collar workers. The professional category had no effect on postoperative work capacity.

Period of work incapacity before surgical intervention affected the postoperative work capacity: 75% who were out of work less than 1 month at the time of operation were able to return to work after 1 year. For patients who were out of work for more than 6 months

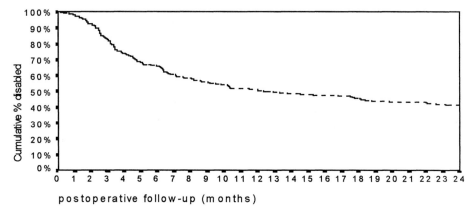

FIG. 2. Work incapacity after surgery for lumbar spinal stenosis in the workers compensation population (n = 225).

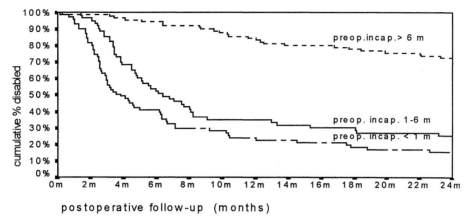

FIG. 3. Impact of work incapacity period on return-to-work rates before surgery for lumbar spinal stenosis.

because of medical reasons, only 16.5% were able to work 12 months after operation (Fig. 3).

Age was significantly associated with return to work. Sixty percent of the patients who were younger than 40 years resumed work in comparison with 40% of the patients in the older age category (Fig. 4).

Significantly more patients who were not able to resume work within 1 year after surgery had instrumented lumbar spinal stenosis surgery ($p < 0.01$).

In the regression analysis, the duration of work incapacity before the operation was significantly ($p < 0.001$) associated with a return to work within 1 year after operation. This variable explained substantially the variance in return to work (partial correlation coefficient = 0.23).

Analysis of Costs

The administrative database also provides information on costs (Table 2). Charges for 866 lumbar spinal stenosis patients totaled $10 million 2 years after operation.

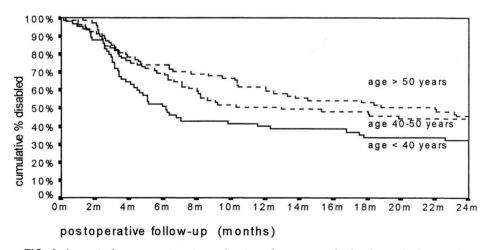

FIG. 4. Impact of age on return to work rates after surgery for lumbar spinal stenosis.

TABLE 2. *Frequency and average number of expenditures after surgery for lumbar spinal stenosis and median costs per case over the 2-year follow-up period*

	Frequency per 866 cases (%)	Average number (mean ± SD)	Median cost per case
General practioner office visits	94.5%	28.1 ± 40.5	$267
Specialist office visits	93.7%	10.18 ± 8.8	$79
Orthosis	11.7%	1.1 ± 0.2	$343
Computed tomography/nuclear magnetic resonance	43.7%	1.8 ± 1.3	$116
Myelography	11.7%	1.9 ± 0.7	$105
Plain radiographs	55.3%	2.8 ± 2.7	$114
Physiotherapy sessions	34.2%	24.2 ± 51.8	$100
Kinesitherapy sessions	74.0%	11.8 ± 33.9	$352
Neurostimulator	0.01%	—	$6512
Rehabilitation center	4.6%	—	$531
Instrumentation	14.4%	—	$3574

Including hospitalization, the costs of the procedure itself, and the mean cost per case of diagnostic procedures and follow-up visits by physicians and physiotherapists, the costs of primary lumbar spinal stenosis surgery were found to be approximately $12,000 over a 2-year period after intervention. The average cost per procedure and number of procedures are listed in Table 1. Instrumentation was used in 14.4% of patients, in 11.7% of cases an orthosis was prescribed, and 4.6% were referred to a specific rehabilitation center. The median number of office visits during the follow-up period was 21 for general practitioner consultations versus 8 for specialist office visits ($p < 0.001$). Additionally, patients had more kinesitherapy sessions than physiotherapy sessions ($p < 0.001$). During follow-up, more plain radiographs were performed than computed tomographic scans and myelography ($p < 0.001$).

Patients who experience a good outcome entail fewer costs than patients who were incapacitated to resume work. The savings associated with good outcomes comes primarily from fewer (i) worker compensation payments, (ii) consultations and kinesitherapy sessions, and (iii) plain radiographs after surgery.

DISCUSSION

This study had the unavoidable shortcomings of all retrospective studies. Therefore, it was impossible to provide information concerning preoperative symptoms, coexisting diseases, prior back surgery, duration of symptoms, myelographic findings, and complications such as scar formation, scoliosis, and instability (11). Any information about the indications for surgery and the intraoperative measurement of the midsagittal diameter of the spinal canal also was lacking. Nevertheless, the minor variables that were included were sufficiently reliable.

Trends in Surgery Rates

The rising trend in surgical rates in Belgium reflects the internationally rising surgical rate in the treatment of disorders of the lumbar spine (12,15). It goes along with the increasing use of computed tomography and magnetic resonance imaging leading to more patients with radiologically defined lumbar spinal stenosis. Additionally, the growing rates of lumbar spinal stenosis are not surprising in view of the aging population. The growing number of orthopedists and neurosurgeons in Belgium also may be a factor influencing the surgical rates.

Fitness for Work

Because loss of work due to illness or early retirement as a result of back pain is the most important consequence to society, the patient's return to work is the most relevant and objective outcome measure of the effectiveness of medical care (16). During the follow-up period, no changes were noticed in conditions under which sickness pensions are granted. There also were no other major changes in the labor market that may have affected the patient's work capacity. We found that 50% of all operated patients were still unable to resume work after 1 year postoperatively. There are few studies in the literature about the postoperative work capacity of operated lumbar spinal surgery patients (6,13). The corresponding variations in return-to-work rates from different studies probably are due to patient selection, different back diagnoses, mean age of patients, job-related factors, labor market issues, and different invalid pension laws.

Herno et al. (6) found that clinical findings did not predict work capability. Because of the lack of information on clinical examination in the database of the sickness fund, we could not investigate the evidence for this conclusion (3).

We found that the period of work incapacity before the intervention was the strongest factor related to the professional outcome. This finding was in agreement with that of Alaranta et al. (1), who showed that after several months of sick leave only 30% of low back pain patients return to work and after 1 year the proportion is as low as 10% (2,6). Because conservative therapy seldom results in substantial pain or disability relief, it is assumed that the best result can be achieved if lumbar spinal surgery patients are operated on as soon as possible.

Older age had an obvious negative impact on the patient's ability to return to work after operation. This finding also was observed by Alaranta et al. (1) and Nykvist et al. (13). Nonetheless, the effect of age in the univariate analysis did not sustain in the logistic regression procedure. This effect obviously is due to the significant positive correlation between period of preoperative work incapacity and age.

The strenuousness of occupation had no effect on postoperative work capacity, which had been observed in other studies. However, this finding does not imply that patients are expected to return to heavy work, for it was shown by many authors that patients returned to light or sedentary work (6).

Furthermore, it was demonstrated that instrumented lumbar spinal surgery was associated with a bad outcome. Because instrumented surgery adds to the cost of lumbar spinal surgery interventions, this finding needs to be confirmed in prospective settings.

Analysis of Costs

The general conclusion that can be drawn from the cost-assessment phase is that benefits of work incapacity become more important in the ongoing recovery period after surgery to the extent that they obviously outweigh health care expenditures within 2 years postoperatively. Therefore, physicians must be oriented toward the patient's early professional rehabilitation, e.g., either gradual or partial resumption in former or other work activities. This policy can be obtained best in a multidisciplinary way, where surgeon, general practitioner, occupational physician, and medical adviser collaborate in the rehabilitation process.

A striking conclusion in the cost analysis was the dramatic variation in use of radiology and follow-up physician visits (7,9). This finding elicits questions about quality and uniformity of health care. Nevertheless, these questions must be addressed correctly within the retrospective analysis of an administrative database where no information about indications for surgery and preoperative health status were available. Confirmation in prospective studies is scientifically necessary (3).

ACKNOWLEDGMENT

This investigation was funded by grant 3.0272.95 from the Research Program of the Fund for Scientific Research-Flanders, Belgium (F.W.O).

REFERENCES

1. Alaranta H, Hurme M, Knuts LR. Invalidity pension after lumbar disc operation. *Ann Chir Gynaecol* 1984;73: 78–82.
2. Andersson GB, Svensson HO, Oden A. The intensity of work recovery in low back pain. *Spine* 1983;8:880–884.
3. Deyo RA, Taylor VM, Diehr P, et al. Analysis of automated administrative and survey databases to study patterns and outcomes of care. *Spine* 1994;19[18 Suppl]:2083S–2091S.
4. Fritz JM, Delitto A, Welch WC, Erhard RE. Lumbar spinal stenosis: a review of current concepts in evaluation, management, and outcome measurements. *Arch Phys Med Rehabil* 1998;79:700–708.
5. Hall S, Bartleson JD, Onofrio BM, Baker HL Jr, Okazaki H, O'Duffy JD. Lumbar spinal stenosis. Clinical features, diagnostic procedures, and results of surgical treatment in 68 patients. *Ann Intern Med* 1985;103: 271–275.
6. Herno A, Airaksinen O, Saari T, Svomalainen O. Pre- and postoperative factors associated with return to work following surgery for lumbar spinal stenosis. *Am J Ind Med* 1996;30:473–478.
7. Katz JN, Lipson SJ, Lew RA, et al. Lumbar laminectomy alone or with instrumented or noninstrumented arthrodesis in degenerative lumbar spinal stenosis. Patient selection, costs, and surgical outcomes. *Spine* 1997; 22:1123-1131.
8. Katz JN, Lipson SJ, Chang LC, Levine SA, Fossel AH, Liang MH. Seven- to 10-year outcome of decompressive surgery for degenerative lumbar spinal stenosis. *Spine* 1996;21:92–98.
9. Katz JN. Lumbar spinal fusion. Surgical rates, costs, and complications. *Spine* 1995;20[24 Suppl]:78S–83S.
10. Katz JN, Lipson SJ, Larson MG, McInnes JM, Fossel AH, Liang MH. The outcome of decompressive laminectomy for degenerative lumbar stenosis. *J Bone Joint Surg Am* 1991;73:809–816.
11. Lange M, Hamburger C, Waidhauser E, Beck OJ. Surgical treatment and results in patients suffering from lumbar spinal stenoses. *Neurosurg Rev* 1993;16:27–33.
12. Nilasena DS, Vaughn RJ, Mori M, Lyon JL. Surgical trends in the treatment of diseases of the lumbar spine in Utah's Medicare population, 1984 to 1990. *Med Care* 1995;33:585–597.
13. Nykvist F, Knuts LR, Alaranta H, et al. Clinical, social, and psychological factors and outcome in a 5-year follow-up study of 276 patients hospitalized because of suspected lumbar disc herniation. *Int Disabil Stud* 1990; 12:107–112.
14. Sanderson PL, Wood PL. Surgery for lumbar spinal stenosis in old people [see comments]. *J Bone Joint Surg Br* 1993;75:393–397.
15. Taylor VM, Deyo RA, Cherkin DC, Kreuter W. Low back pain hospitalization. Recent United States trends and regional variations. *Spine* 1994;19:1207–1212.
16. Waddell G. Evaluation of results in lumbar spine surgery. Clinical outcome measures—assessment of severity. *Acta Orthop Scand Suppl* 1993;251:134–137.

Lumbar Spinal Stenosis
edited by Robert Gunzburg and Marek Szpalski
Lippincott Williams & Wilkins, Philadelphia, © 2000.

42

Cost of Surgical Decompression across Europe

Per Wessberg and *Björn Rydevik

*Department of Orthopaedic Surgery and *Orthopaedics, Sahlgrenska University Hospital, Göteborg University, Göteborg SE-41345, Sweden*

With gradually increasing financial constraints on the health care system, the importance of the economic aspects of various treatment modalities has become more apparent. Such considerations include both the actual costs as well as the consequences for the patients in terms of improvement in quality of life and increased ability to function in daily activities. Within the European Union (EU) it is likely that various conditions, such as health care systems, for people in different nations gradually will become more uniform. Health care market economic systems have gradually developed in some countries (8). It is not unlikely that we might see EU regulations regarding health care systems in the future, which possibly might lead to a common health care market in the EU. However, currently there seem to be major variations in the rate of back surgery among various countries. A comparative study found that the rate of back surgery in the United States (US) was at least 40% higher than in any other country and was more than five times the rate of back surgery in England and Scotland (2). Several authors in the US have noted a marked increase over time in the rate of surgery for spinal stenosis and of fusions for these conditions (3,5,7,11). A study of the use of back surgery in the Utah Medicare population found that the increase in back surgery rates was dependent on the use of surgery for the treatment of spinal stenosis and not to an increase in the number of surgeons performing back surgery (11).

Comparisons regarding costs of surgical decompression among various countries have inherent difficulties. The most accurate way to estimate such costs is to determine the costs per case and the rate of surgery. Moreover, comparisons over time should be made to establish if there is an ongoing increase in the rate of surgery. When analyzing these problems, one may divide the questions into the following components:

1. Rate of the particular type of surgery in various countries
2. Cost of the surgical procedure
3. Cost/effectiveness of the procedure.

It should be noted that this implies an ideal situation with full access to this kind of information. In reality, little information of this kind is available from published sources. The following text provides a review and discussion of some data from the author's own institution and some published and publicly available information. Based on such data, the costs for spinal stenosis surgery are estimated for other countries.

INCIDENCE OF LUMBAR SPINAL STENOSIS AND RATE OF SURGICAL DECOMPRESSION

In a survey conducted in Sweden, Johnsson (4) investigated the annual incidence of lumbar spinal stenosis in two cities in Sweden. He reported that the annual incidence between 1982 and 1991 was between 45 and 59 new cases per million inhabitants in the two communities studied. Johnsson also reported that there were few severe neurologic symptoms. It should be noted that this study is limited to the incidence of patients consulting orthopedic departments and may not reflect the true incidence of lumbar spinal stenosis in the population.

In the material evaluated in the retrospective study by Johnsson (4), surgical decompression for lumbar spinal stenosis was found to be 30 to 40 operations per million inhabitants per year. This frequency of operating treatment is about 50% higher than that found by Verbiest (13), which may be an indication of the increasing rate of decompression surgery over the last 10 to 20 years. One may suspect that there will be an increased need for surgical treatment of lumbar spinal stenosis during the next decade in developed countries due to an aging population. This fact will most likely result in more cases of lumbar spinal stenosis. Moreover, elderly people are relatively healthy and probably will have an increased demand on ability to move around, thus provoking neurogenic claudication (10).

COST OF SURGERY

In our institution, the costs for surgical treatment of lumbar spinal stenosis in 1997 and 1998 are reported by the fiscal office of the department. Cost for treatment can be derived according to specified diagnoses (ICD codes) and specified surgical procedures coded according to *Classification of Surgical Procedures* (Swedish version, 1997, the Nordic Medical Statistics Committee]. The costs reported are built up from a fixed part and a variable part. The fixed part represents the cost per day care in the whole hospital, i.e., capital costs for buildings and inventory, and costs for personnel and basic medications. The variable part represents direct patient-related costs for certain investigations, the surgical procedure (per time), postoperative care (per time), implants when used, and certain medications. Decompression alone (M 48.0 and ABC 5) was found to cost SEK 33,700 or EUR 3,800 (exchange rate of late January 1999 1 EUR = 8.95 SEK), decompression and posterolateral noninstrumented fusion (M 48.0, ABC 5, and NAG 6) SEK 53,000 or EUR 5,900, and decompression including instrumented fusion (M48.0, ABC 5, and NAG 7) SEK 83,000 or EUR 9,300). The mean cost for spinal stenosis surgery was SEK 56,900 or EUR 6,400.

Tables 1 and 2 show calculated values of the number of lumbar surgeries performed per

TABLE 1. *Calculated values of the total number of lumbar surgeries performed in 1998*

	Back surgery rate ratio to US	Lumbar surgery rate (per million)	Population 1998 (million)	Total no. of lumbar surgeries in 1998
United States	1	1,103	270.3	298,100
The Netherlands	0.73	805	15.7	12,600
Denmark	0.64	706	5.3	3,700
Finland	0.56	618	5.1	3,200
Norway	0.49	540	4.4	2,400
Austria	0.44	485	8.1	3,900
Sweden	0.33	364	8.9	3,200
England	0.19	210	48.1	10,100
Scotland	0.13	143	5.7	800

Rate ratio to the United States (US) are values published by Cherkin et al. (2). The US rate is calculated by dividing 279,000 lumbar surgeries per annum (1990) with the US population that year (253 million).

TABLE 2. *Total number of lumbar spinal stenosis surgeries calculated as 30% of the total number of lumbar surgeries from Table 1*

	Total no. of LSS surgeries in 1998	1998 Cost (million EUR)
United States	89,400	572.2
The Netherlands	3,800	24.3
Denmark	1,100	7.0
Finland	900	5.8
Norway	700	4.5
Austria	1,100	7.0
Sweden	1,000	6.4
England	3,000	19.2
Scotland	200	1.3

Cost calculated using the mean cost for lumbar spinal stenosis (LSS) surgery at Sahlgrenska University Hospital, Göteborg, Sweden, 1997–1998 (EUR 6,400, exchange rate 1 EUR = 8.95 SEK).

annum in certain European countries, the number of lumbar surgeries for spinal stenosis (estimated to be 30% of the total number of lumbar surgeries), and the subsequent cost using the mean cost for spinal stenosis surgery at the authors' institution as the norm. The rates of lumbar surgeries are calculated from the ratios to the US rate reported by Cherkin et al. (2) multiplied by the 1990 US rate. This calculation was performed by dividing the total number of low back operations in the US 1990 (279,000) (5) by the US population for that year (253 million). The rates then were multiplied by the US population for 1998 to obtain an appreciation of the total number of lumbar surgeries for this year.

COST-EFFECTIVENESS CONSIDERATIONS

The reason for studying costs of different therapeutic procedures is usually to make comparisons among them. When doing so, it is imperative to consider not only the costs but also the gains achieved by the treatments, and to study the relationship of costs and gains. Different techniques applicable in different situations are available (9). If the therapeutic procedures have a similar outcome, a simple comparison of costs can be made (cost-minimization analysis). If the effects of the procedures can be appreciated by a common outcome measure (e.g., survival), the cost can be put in relation to this measure (e.g., costs per life-year gained). This method of calculation is the cost-effectiveness technique. If the different therapies cannot be appreciated by a common outcome measure, the effects of treatment can be evaluated according to its *use* to the patient. Utility, i.e., the improved quality of life that the patient has experienced as a result of the treatment, is used as effect measure (cost-utility analysis) (Fig. 1). If monetary effects are considered (usually future costs saved), a cost-benefit analysis can be made.

Lumbar spinal stenosis mainly affects persons over the age of retirement; therefore, cost-benefit analysis probably will prove less beneficiary for the treatment of lumbar spinal stenosis because, in most countries, society provides for the patient and successful treatment will not give the patient the ability to provide for himself or herself (for age reasons alone). However, costs for extra care, hospitalization, walking aids, etc., could be considered. The cost-effectiveness technique could not be used because lumbar spinal stenosis probably does not affect life expectancy, and comparisons to other treatments, such as hip replacement surgery and coronary artery bypass surgery, precludes the use of a common outcome measure. The most appropriate way to compare the effects of lumbar spinal stenosis treatment is probably by cost-utility analysis.

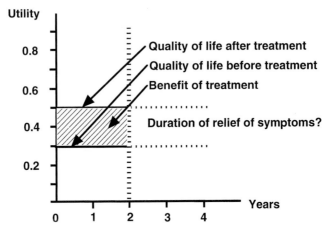

FIG. 1. Possible levels of quality of life before and after treatment for lumbar spinal stenosis.

To our knowledge, studies demonstrating utilities before and after lumbar spinal stenosis surgery have not reported. This makes cost-utility assessments impossible. Outcomes have been studied, and success rates of 64% in a meta-analysis by Turner et al. (12) and 62% in a retrospective large study by Airaksinen (1) were reported. However, as pointed out by Katz (6), the success rate is difficult to judge solely by looking at outcomes such as pain and functional abilities. A better way would be to incorporate preoperative data and patient expectations. This is probably true for results after many other types of back surgery as well.

Even though, to date, the cost-effectiveness of lumbar spinal stenosis surgery cannot be assessed properly, some reflections can be made. The procedures used for surgical treatment are relatively inexpensive. In the cost analysis of Sahlgrenska University Hospital in Sweden 1997 to 1998, the costs range from EUR 3,800 for a simple decompressive laminectomy to EUR 6,400 for decompression and instrumented fusion. The mean treatment cost was EUR 6,400. Even with a moderate improvement of half of what can be seen after hip replacement surgery (where utility improvement can be 0.4 utility) and with the effects maintained for 2 years, the cost per quality-adjusted life-year (QUALY) would be in the range of 9,430 to 23,190 EUR/QUALY. Looking at these estimated figures in view of various published QUALY league tables, one can assume that the cost effectiveness of lumbar spinal stenosis surgery probably is good. An even greater utility gain and a longer duration of symptom relief would lower the cost/QUALY ratio even further.

In conclusion, even though we cannot provide any hard data and our extrapolating calculations involve some obvious weaknesses, the level of estimated costs indicates that lumbar spinal stenosis, relative to other conditions, is not a very expensive condition to treat surgically and the cost-utility relationship probably is favorable.

REFERENCES

1. Airaksinen O, Herno A, Turunen V, Saari T, Suomlainen O. Surgical outcome of 438 patients treated surgically for lumbar spinal stenosis. *Spine* 1997;22:2278–2282.
2. Cherkin DC, Deyo RA, Loeser JD, Bush T, Waddell G. An international comparison of back surgery rates. *Spine* 1994;19:1201–1206.
3. Ciol MA, Deyo RA, Howell E, Kreif S. An assessment of surgery for spinal stenosis: time trends, geographic variations, complications, and reoperations. *J Am Geriatr Soc* 1996;44:285–290.
4. Johnsson KE. Lumbar spinal stenosis. A retrospective study of 163 cases in southern Sweden. *Acta Orthop Scand* 1995;66:403–405.

5. Katz JN. Lumbar spinal fusion. Surgical rates, costs, and complications. *Spine* 1995;20:78S–83S.

6. Katz JN. Point of view. *Spine* 1997;22:2282.

7. Katz JN, Lipson SJ, Lew RA, et al. Lumbar laminectomy alone or with instrumented or noninstrumented arthrodesis in degenerative lumbar spinal stenosis. Patient selection, costs, and surgical outcomes. *Spine* 1997;15:22:1123–1131.

8. Maynard A. Developing the health care market. *Econ J* 1991;101:1277–1286.

9. Melot CA. Principles of cost-benefit analysis. In: Szpalski M, Gunzburg R, Pope MH, eds. *Lumbar segmental instability*. Philadelphia: Lippincott Williams & Wilkins, 1999:259–273.

10. Nachemson AL. Spinal disorders. Overall impact on society and the need for orthopedic resources. *Acta Orthop Scand Suppl* 1991;241:17–22.

11. Nilasena DS, Vaughn RJ, Mori M, Lyon JL. Surgical trends in the treatment of diseases of the lumbar spine in Utah's Medicare population, 1984 to 1990. *Med Care* 1995;33:585–597.

12. Turner JA, Ersek M, Herron L, Deyo R. Surgery for lumbar spinal stenosis. Attempted meta-analysis of the literature. *Spine* 1992;17:1–8.

13. Verbiest H. Stenosis of the lumbar vertebral canal and sciatica. *Neurosurg Rev* 1980:3:75–89.

Lumbar Spinal Stenosis
edited by Robert Gunzburg and Marek Szpalski
Lippincott Williams & Wilkins, Philadelphia, © 2000.

43

Role of the Generalist versus the Specialist

"Doing the Right Things Right"

James N. Weinstein

Department of Community and Family Medicine, Center for Evaluative Clinical Sciences, Dartmouth Medical School, Hanover, New Hampshire 07055 and The Dartmouth-Hitchcock Medical Center, Lebanon, New Hampshire 03756

There continues to be a great deal of debate, in the ever-changing health care system, about the role of the specialist versus the generalist. Should gatekeepers determine when patients receive care and from whom?

As the supply of health care providers grows, there is increasing competition between the generalist and the specialist. In this supply-induced demand health care system, there has been an attempt to control access to specialists as a means to decrease health care costs. Although the idea is not new, it has spurred a series of studies by interested parties. Those advocates of the gatekeeper model believe that patients can get most of their needs met by the generalist, whereas the specialist argues that he or she is more cost effective in the long run. As the United States health care system approaches the trillion dollar level, many people are interested in how they can play a part and in some cases obtain a piece of the action. Thus, motivation to change comes in many flavors and with many conflicting interests.

"Where should we be headed?" is a different question than "Where are we headed?" In this chapter I will address the limited information available regarding the generalist versus the specialist but ask that we not delimit ourselves to this seemingly self-serving question. At the end I will suggest that we look beyond the specialist versus generalist question and begin a dialogue about "what is right" and how we as a profession and as nations can begin to take a higher ground and "do the right thing right."

The issues regarding generalist versus specialist often are framed in the genre of cost effectiveness. Cost effectiveness is not, and must not be, the only criterion by which a health care system or a patient is asked to choose between the generalist who has the "holistic" approach and the specialist who has a great deal of "expert" knowledge but who in some cases is not cost effective. Let us review what has been written and then play the role of devil's advocate.

Results have suggested that specialists may have better outcomes. This is particularly true for patients who have acute myocardial infarction, strokes, asthma, acute monoarthritis, and rheumatoid arthritis. However, this does not appear to be true for the treatment of hypertension, diabetes, and acute low back pain, where there is little difference in outcomes between generalist and specialist (1). Regarding cost, there generally is no contest: specialists usually are more expensive. Their processes of care may be different, i.e, use of medication(s), procedures (surgery and angioplasty as done by a specialist), and assessment of outcomes (e.g., using generic instruments for the generalist vs. the specialist's use of disease-specific measures).

In reviewing the limited literature in this area, one is struck by the paucity of good comparative studies. Thus, there are problems with trying to understand the treatments of generalists versus specialists. Many of the studies are observational studies when it comes to the generalist, and many are interventional studies when it comes to the specialist. Each is problematic in its selection bias of patients and techniques.

As an example, in the area of acute low back pain, one can reach mixed conclusions. There are many types of providers with this near-epidemic problem, with no consistent differences across providers. However, there is more satisfaction with chiropractic care even though, in some cases, it is more expensive (1,7). Another argument against the specialist is access. The issue of direct access to the specialist is an important one when considering surgery. Today some systems are trying to determine the feasibility and acceptability of direct access to surgery for general practitioners and their patients. If this is to work, there must be accuracy of general practitioners' diagnoses within a range of specified surgical conditions, and one needs to determine whether direct access to surgery could be carried out without attracting inappropriate referrals of patients needing more extensive preoperative investigation or management (6). Is the surgeon just a mechanic who then would rely on the generalist to determine surgical candidacy and simply fill their schedule with generalist referrals? I suggest not. Not if the patient wants to discuss with his or her surgeon the specifics of the case or the specific risk and/or benefits of such a surgery. I still maintain that the surgeon should see and make an independent evaluation of the patient contemplating a surgical intervention. The patient must understand from that surgeon the potential risk and/or benefits of the specific surgical intervention. Not only must the risks of the surgery be considered, but also the risks associated with general anesthesia. The generalist may not be able to relate these risks to the patient. The American Society of Anesthesiologists classification of physical status becomes important in referring patients from the generalist to the specialist in that one needs to be aware of the comorbid conditions:

Grade 1: Normally healthy patient
Grade 2: Mild systemic disease, with no functional limitations
Grade 3: Severe systemic disease, with definite functional limitations
Grade 4: Severe systemic disease that is a consistent threat to life
Grade 5: Moribund patient not expected to survive for 24 hours or without an operation.

Obviously, these comorbidities play a significant role in the risk of anesthesia and point to the necessity of having a specialist involved in determining a patient's candidacy for surgical intervention. When we think of direct access to surgery, we need to think about the operations that are performed most commonly, which include operations for inguinal hernias, skin lesions or lumps, vasectomies, cholecystectomies, varicose veins, epididymal cysts, and nutritional supplementation. Most of these are outpatient procedures (except for cholecystectomies, which usually are done on an inpatient basis; also some hernias). Some of these conditions might lend themselves to direct referral, but spine surgery does not.

The issue of specialist versus generalist is one that is yet to be resolved. Based on the literature, it remains undecided which provider one should see for acute back pain. There is a lack of effectiveness and efficacy studies; therefore, there are only random reflections of what currently exists. Scientific evaluation of various medical interventions generally have not been translated into clinical practice, yet there are clearly areas where specialty care seems to be better, such as with acute myocardial infarction.

To address the predominant concerns of clinicians, one should use research designs that begin to address whether generalists or specialists are more appropriate in a given situation. The dilemma in designing such studies often means traveling from the high ground of research-based theory to what some call the lowlands of "clinical reality." There is some limited information, yet patients' expectations are not yet satisfied, and patients are not involved in any meaningful way in understanding the differences between seeing a generalist versus a specialist for various medical problems.

What are possible solutions? We should put into context the available information so it is clinically applicable when patients are trying to decide about complicated issues, such as relative risk, probabilities, and odds ratios, to understand the difference between what the generalist offers versus what the specialist offers. We need to communicate more effectively what things are clear and what things are *not* so as to empower patients to make decisions. Between the specialist and the generalist there are many issues a health plan or patient might consider before diagnostic and/or therapeutic decisions are made. For example, if I undergo magnetic resonance imaging and my disc is found to be bulging, then I may be facing an unnecessary surgical decision because perhaps I should not have had the test in the first place.

Some have suggested that consensus or evidence-based clinical guidelines may be the right approach. I remain concerned about the relevant aspects of guidelines. In one's daily practice, guidelines generally provoke a negative reaction and often are not compatible with current practice. More work is necessary to understand how to implement guidelines into clinical practice. However, despite these controversies there is information that suggests that evidence-based recommendations are better followed in practice than those that are not based on scientific evidence. Precise definitions of recommended performance to improve the use of guidelines and testing the feasibility and acceptance of clinical guidelines in a target group remain important steps for effective implementation.

People who work in the development and implementation of guidelines need to understand the attributes of effective guidelines. Guidelines that are hard to implement will not be used no matter how good they are. It takes a significant effort to write guidelines and even more effort to implement them. There remains a disparity in proven medical management and implementation of the obvious. A clear example is that of patients who had an acute myocardial infarction. Despite clinical evidence that aspirin and beta blockers improve survival, there is a lack of compliance in nearly 50% of the cases, with tremendous variation in compliance depending on where one lives (2–5).

In summary, the issues of specialists versus generalists has not been well studied, and much more work is needed. The preceding information is based on the author's review of the literature and his own personal perspective. Without more information and evidence, one cannot completely decide on the best approach for a given diagnosis. However, when good information is available, it appears that specialists, although they are more costly, seem to come to diagnostic certainty sooner and, in some cases, have better outcomes.

So where are we headed and, more importantly, where should we be headed? As stated earlier, "doing the right thing right" is a good place to start. Market forces should not drive the utilization of resources. When there is disparity in care based on the availability of resources rather than on the basis of evidence, we see tremendous variability and this variability is costly. If, as is the case in the United States, geography can partly determine resource utilization and supply is a factor, we have much work ahead. The issues here go beyond the generalist versus specialist debate to the basic issues of our hippocratic principles. Following purely the evidence of what works and what does not may sound simple, but in fact is the core of our need for health care reform. Further, if as intended, we shared medical information in a format in which our patients' values and utilities were part of the health care decision process and we provided equity across the system, there would be more than enough for all. We must find rationality in our health care system, and we must do this by making patients active partners now and in the future. The issue of the generalist and the specialist is a symptom of a diseased health care system, and it is time to diagnose this illness and start on a treatment course that deals with the real questions before us. These issues can be best summarized as my colleague and mentor Dr. Wennberg has put forth in the *Darmouth Atlas of Health Care*: supply-induced demand, workforce, hospital beds, inequity in the reimbursement system, and lack of patient involvement in health care decisions. When we have the courage to address these issues we will see where the real problems in health care lie and we can begin to feel better that we are, in fact, able to make a difference and are ''doing the right things right.''

REFERENCES

1. Carey T, Garrett J, Jackman A, McLaughlin C, Fryer J, Smucker D. The outcomes and costs of care for acute low back pain among patients seen by primary care practitioners, chiropractors, and orthopaedic surgeons. *N Engl J Med* 1995;333:913–917.
2. *Effective healthcare: implementing clinical practice guidelines: can guidelines be used to improve clinical practice?* Leeds: Nuffield Institute for Health, University of Leeds; College of Health Economics and NHS Center for Reviews and Dissemination, University of New York; Research Unit, Royal College of Physicians; 1994.
3. Grimshaw J, Russell I. Effect of clinical guidelines on medical practice: a systematic review of rigorous evaluations. *Lancet* 1993;342:1317–1322.
4. Grol R, Dalhuijsen J, Thomas S, Veld C, Rutten G, Mokkink H. Attributes of clinical guidelines that influence use of guidelines in general practice: observational study. *Br Med J* 1998;317:858–861.
5. O'Connor GT, Quinton HB, Traven ND, et al. Geographic variation in the treatment of acute myocardial infarction: the Cooperative Cardiovascular Project. *JAMA* 1999;281:627–633.
6. Smith F, Gwynn B. Direct access surgery. *Ann R Coll Surg Engl* 1995;77:94–96.
7. Solomon D, Bates D, Panush R, Katz J. Costs, outcomes and patient satisfaction by provider type for patients with rheumatic and musculoskeletal conditions: a critical review of the literature and proposed methodologic standards. *Ann Intern Med* 1997;127:52–60.

Subject Index

Page numbers followed by *f* refer to figures; page numbers followed by *t* refer to tables.